Current Techniques in

NEUROSURGERY

Michael Salcman

The George Washington University
School of Medicine
Washington, D.C.

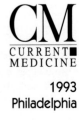

CURRENT■
MEDICINE

1993
Philadelphia

Current Medicine
20 North Third Street
Philadelphia, PA 19106

ISBN: 1-878132-01-6
ISSN: 1068-4093

Developmental editor: Maureen McNally
Art director: Paul Fennessy
Illustration director: Larry Ward
Typesetting director: Bill Donnelly
Production manager: David Myers
Managing editor: Diana Merritt

Printed in Singapore
Produced by Imago
5 4 3 2 1

*For my children
Joshua and Dara*

Preface

The publishers and I welcome you to this first edition of *Current Techniques in Neurosurgery*. We believe that it represents a new concept in the field of neurosurgical publications, one that is based on the success of similar volumes in the Current Medicine series. Each edition of *Current Techniques in Neurosurgery* will represent a unique combination of fully illustrated authoritative reviews of the most exciting topics in contemporary neurosurgery and up-to-date annotated bibliographies of the leading articles in the field. In addition, each author will give a personal perspective on the topic and describe his or her own methods for tackling the subject.

Among the many outstanding contributions this year are several on brain tumor surgery and biology. Even the surgery of skull base meningiomas, a subject conventionally thought to be a purely technical exercise, is shown by Wright and Sekhar to be based on scientific principles. No doubt the future practice of neurosurgery will be strongly affected by new developments in the molecular biology of brain tumors, many of which are so clearly explained by Kim and Harsh. Although the use of radiosurgery in the treatment of malignant brain tumors, metastases, and chordomas is in its infancy, Kondziolka and Lunsford provide an authoritative review of its application to such benign tumors as acoustic schwannoma and meningioma. New developments in magnetic resonance angiography, as described by Zimmerman and Naidich, are just as likely to affect surgical planning for tumors as they are the surgery of vascular disease. The implications of three-dimensional reconstruction of the cerebral gyri and surface vasculature are truly far-reaching. Similarly, the use of positron emission tomography in the selection of patients for epilepsy surgery, as described by Wyler, represents yet another major modification of clinical practice based on advances in neuroimaging.

In the area of cerebrovascular disorders, Weber and Mayberg remind us of the importance of randomized clinical trials, not just in the evaluation of a surgical procedure or medical treatment but also in the study of the natural history of a disease. The combination of such knowledge and technical advances in the operating room, intensive care unit, and imaging suite has resulted in attempts to surgically treat the poor-grade aneurysm patient. Le Roux and Winn provide us with their management protocols as well as new information on the usefulness of infusion computed tomography scanning. In addition to providing a beautifully illustrated exposition of their surgical techniques, Shin and Al-Mefty carefully describe the patient selection process employed prior to cavernous sinus surgery.

Friedman and Bova are no less scholarly in their discussion of radiosurgery for arteriovenous malformations while Guterman and colleagues provide us with the latest overview on the intravascular treatment of aneurysms and arteriovenous malformations.

Central to the treatment of all neurologic emergencies is a careful evaluation of the patient with a depressed level of consciousness and proper understanding of neuronal resuscitation. Marshall and colleagues highlight the latest findings from the Traumatic Coma Data Bank like a series of news bulletins, presenting new classifications of head injury and intensity of therapy based in part on criteria derived from imaging. Henson and colleagues provide us with a comprehensive review of the latest developments in the pharmacology of cerebral protection, a topic of great importance in both head injury and cerebrovascular disease.

In the areas of spine and peripheral nerve surgery, this edition incudes three contributions of immediate interest. Sonntag and Dickman provide a careful analysis of the data available on the various techniques and instrumentation systems currently being used for cervical spine fusion. The key points in each method are beautifully illustrated and carefully described. Maroon and colleagues review their considerable experience in automated percutaneous lumbar diskectomy, and Millesi brings us up to date on the latest biochemical and mechanical considerations involved in the treatment of peripheral nerve injuries.

Several themes are common to virtually all the subjects covered in this initial volume. The first is the considerable dependence of contemporary neurosurgery on the development of modern neuroimaging. The second is the emergence of a new and more sophisticated body of biologic knowledge as the basis for further improvements in the care of our patients. The third is the growing recognition that there is no substitute for careful and scientifically organized clinical observation. These three methodologic principles have allowed us the luxury of more properly selecting patients increasingly complex and better-targeted procedures. I expect these trends to continue, and I anticipate that every succeeding volume of *Current Techniques in Neurosurgery* will contain fresh insights and improved procedures of direct benefit to our patients.

Michael Salcman, MD
The George Washington University
School of Medicine, Washington, DC

Contributor list

ARVIND AHUJA, MD
Clinical Instructor of Neurosurgery
School of Medicine and Biomedical Sciences
State University of New York
Buffalo, New York

OSSAMA AL-MEFTY, MD, FACS
Loyola University Medical School
Professor, Division of Neurological Surgery
Maywood, Illinois

FRANK J. BOVA, PhD
Departments of Neurosurgery and
  Radiation Oncology
College of Medicine
University of Florida
Gainesville, Florida

SHARON BOWERS MARSHALL, RN
University of California, San Diego
Division of Neurosurgery
San Diego, California

RANDALL M. CHESNUT, MD
University of California, San Diego
Division of Neurosurgery
San Francisco, California

CURTIS A. DICKMAN, MD
Associated Chief, Spine Section
Director, Spinal Research
Division of Neurological Surgery
Barrow Neurological Institute
Phoenix, Arizona

WILLIAM A. FRIEDMAN, MD
Edward Shedd Wells Professor of Stereotactic
  Radiosurgery
Departments of Neurosurgery and Radiation Oncology
College of Medicine
University of Florida
Gainesville, Florida

JENNIFER B. GREEN, MD
University of Virginia
Health Sciences Center
Department of Neurosurgery
Charlottesville, Virginia

LEE R. GUTERMAN, PhD, MD
Clinical Instructor of Neurosurgery
School of Medicine and Biomedical Sciences
State University of New York at Buffalo
Buffalo, New York

GRIFFITH R. HARSH, IV, MD
Department of Neurological Surgery
Massachusetts General Hospital
Harvard Medical School
Boston, Massachusetts

SCOTT L. HENSON, MD
University of Virginia
Health Sciences Center
Department of Neurosurgery
Charlottesville, Virginia

LEO N. HOPKINS, MD
Professor and Chairman of Neurosurgery
Professor of Radiology
School of Medicine and Biomedical Sciences
State University of New York at Buffalo
Buffalo, New York

NEAL F. KASSELL, MD
University of Virginia
Health Sciences Center
Department of Neurosurgery
Charlottesville, Virginia

DONG H. KIM, MD
Department of Neurological Surgery
School of Medicine
University of California, San Francisco
San Francisco, California

MELVILLE R. KLAUBER, MD
University of California, San Diego
Division of Neurosurgery
San Francisco, California

DOUGLAS KONDZIOLKA, MD, MSc, FRCS(C)
Assistant Professor of Neurological Surgery
Specialized Neurological Center
Presbyterian University Hospital
University of Pittsburgh Medical Center
Pittsburgh, Pennsylvania

KEVIN S. LEE, MD
University of Virginia
Health Sciences Center
Department of Neurosurgery
Charlottesville, Virginia

PETER D. LE ROUX, MD
Department of Neurological Surgery
University of Washington
School of Medicine
Seattle, Washington

L. DADE LUNSFORD, MD
Director
Specialized Neurological Center
Presbyterian University Hospital
University of Pittsburgh Medical Center
Pittsburgh, Pennsylvania

JOSEPH C. MAROON, MD
Professor of Neurological Surgery
Medical College of Pennsylvania
Chairman, Neurosurgery Department
Allegheny General Hospital
Pittsburgh, Pennsylvania

LAWRENCE F. MARSHALL, MD
University of California, San Diego
Division of Neurosurgery
San Francisco, California

MARC R. MAYBERG, MD
Associate Professor
Department of Neurological Surgery
University of Washington School of Medicine
Seattle, Washington

HANNO MILLESI, MD
Professor of Plastic Surgery
Head, Department of Plastic and
  Reconstructive Surgery
First Surgical Clinic
University of Vienna Medical School
Director, Ludwig-Boltzmann Institute for
  Plastic and Reconstructive Surgery
Vienna, Austria

THOMAS P. NAIDICH, MD
Department of Radiology
Baptist Hospital
Miami, Florida

GARY ONIK, MD
Associate Professor of Neurosurgery
Medical College of Neurosurgery
Head, Department of Cryomedicine
Allegheny General Hospital
Pittsburgh, Pennsylvania

LALIGAM N. SEKHAR, MD, FACS
Associate Professor of Neurological Surgery
Center for Cranial Base Surgery
University of Pittsburgh Medical Center
Pittsburgh, Pennsylvania

KYU MAN SHIN, MD
Division of Neurological Surgery
Loyola University Medical Center
Maywood, Illinois

VOLKER K. H. SONNTAG, MD
Vice Chairman, Division of Neurological Surgery
Chairman, BNI Spine Section
Clinical Professor of Surgery
Barrow Neurological Institute
Phoenix, Arizona

DANKO VIDOVICH, MD
Senior Research Associate
Neurosurgery Department
Allegheny General Hospital
Pittsburgh, Pennsylvania

JED P. WEBER, MD
Department of Neurological Surgery
University of Washington School of Medicine
Seattle, Washington

H. RICHARD WINN, MD
Professor and Chairman
University of Washington School of Medicine
Department of Neurological Surgery
Seattle, Washington

DONALD C. WRIGHT, MD
Associate Professor
Department of Neurological Surgery
Center for Cranial Base Surgery
University of Pittsburgh Medical Center
Pittsburgh, Pennsylvania

ALLEN R. WYLER, MD
Swedish Medical Center
Seattle, Washington

ROBERT A. ZIMMERMAN, MD
Department of Radiology
The Children's Hospital of Philadelphia
Philadelphia, Pennsylvania

Contents

Chapter 1

Advances in Brain Tumor Biology: The Genetics of Astrocytoma

Dong H. Kim
Griffith R. Harsh, IV

An explosion of knowledge over the past 10 years has yielded profound insights into the nature of cancer. Tumors arise from genetic alterations that lead to uncontrolled cellular proliferation [1]. The elucidation of the basic genetic defects that result in tumors provides the best chance for developing effective therapies. Understanding the molecular changes resulting from these genetic defects will provide new opportunities for therapeutic intervention. This chapter reviews the current understanding of the oncogenesis of astrocytomas, the most common type of primary brain tumor.

Alterations in two types of genes contribute to tumorigenesis: oncogenes and tumor suppressor genes. Inappropriate expression of oncogenes can foster tumor development by stimulating cell proliferation. These changes in oncogene expression can arise from genetic alterations such as carcinogen-induced mutation or viral transformation. Such alterations may be manifested oncogenically even though they affect only one of two alleles [1,2]. In contrast, tumor suppressor genes—genes that normally inhibit cell proliferation—become tumorigenic as a result of inactivation, either through mutations or through chromosomal loss. For the loss of tumor suppressor genes to be oncogenic, both copies must be affected [3,4].

The discovery of oncogenes resulted from early observations that genes inserted into cells by retroviruses (*eg*, Rous sarcoma virus) can cause tumors. These viral genes, named *oncogenes*, were found to be highly homologous or identical to normal cellular genes named *protooncogenes* [1]. The hypothesis that defects in protooncogenes produce cancers that are not caused by viral infection has proved true, and over 30 protooncogenes that are involved in a wide variety of tumors have been identified.

The concept of a tumor suppressor gene evolved from the study of retinoblastoma, a rare childhood tumor of the eye. Twenty years ago, Knudson [5] postulated that this tumor developed following two successive lesions in the cell genome. Cytogenetic observation of an interstitial deletion at chromosome 13q14 in cells from these tumors led to the discovery of the retinoblastoma gene. A tumor forms when both copies of this gene are inactivated. The retinoblas-toma gene encodes a nuclear phosphoprotein with an ability to bind DNA, suggesting that the protein plays a role in transcriptional regulation. This protein alternates between a hyperphosphorylated and an unphosphorylated state, depending on the phase of the cell cycle, and it is thought to play an important role in the regulation of this cycle [4].

Oncogenesis in most cases requires numerous chromosomal abnormalities that involve a combination of oncogenes and tumor suppressor genes. Identification of the genetic basis for a particular type of tumor has thus proved difficult. Perhaps the best understood is colorectal carcinoma. Carcinogenesis in the colon involves a progression of steps, from adenomatous polyps with varying dysplasia to noninvasive and then invasive carcinomas. This sequence is analogous to the progression of astrocytoma from low-grade glioma to anaplastic astrocytoma to glioblastoma multiforme (Figure 1.1).

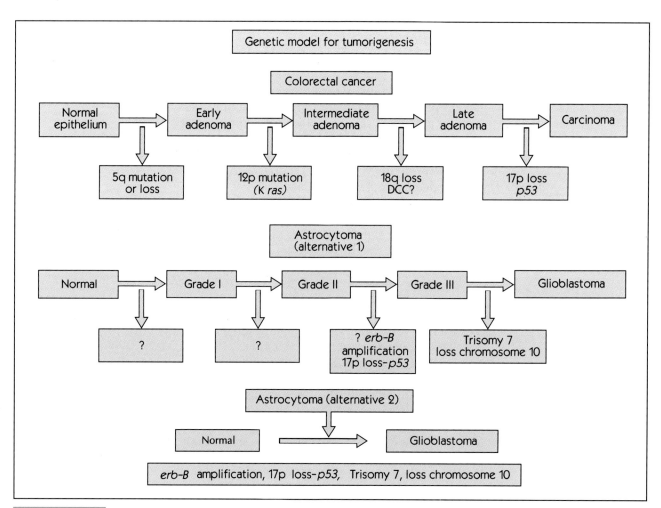

A model for tumorigenesis. The well-characterized progression depicts colorectal cancer. Two models for glioblastoma formation are presented, the first showing a progression from lower grade tumor, the second showing glioblastoma arising from normal brain. (*From* Fearon and Vogelstein [14]; with permission.)

Approximately 50% of colorectal carcinomas and adenomas greater than 1 cm in size carry the mutated, activated allele of the *ras* oncogene [6–8]. In contrast, fewer than 10% of adenomas less than 1 cm in size carry the mutation [9]. Activation of the *ras* oncogene may be the initiating event in a subset of tumors and may lead to progression in others.

The deletion of a portion of chromosome 17q has been found in more than 75% of colorectal carcinomas [10,11], but such loss is infrequent in adenomas. This region of loss contains the *p53* gene, a tumor suppressor gene involved in regulating the cell cycle [12]. In addition, point mutations have been reported in the remaining allele in several tumors [12,13]. Therefore, both *p53* alleles may be inactivated in a majority of tumors.

The second most common area of loss is on chromosome 18q. This deletion is found in 50% of dysplastic adenomas and 70% of carcinomas [10,11]. Expression is reduced or absent in all tumors [14]. A candidate suppressor gene named *DCC* (deleted in colon carcinoma) has been identified. This gene is homologous to those encoding cell adhesion molecules [15], and its loss may contribute to tumorigenesis and invasiveness by altering cell-cell or cell-matrix interactions. Deletions of chromosome 5q have been observed in 30% of adenomas and in 20% to 50% of carcinomas [10,16], although the affected gene has not been identified.

From those data, a picture emerges of early adenoma formation mediated by the activation of *ras* and deletions at chromosome 5q or 18q. The tumor progresses as more genetic alterations occur, and loss of the *p53* gene on 17p is associated with only advanced carcinoma. Both the activation of oncogenes and the inactivation of tumor suppressor genes play a role, and mutations in at least four to five genes are required. A similar schema is beginning to emerge for the development of astrocytomas.

CHROMOSOMAL ABNORMALITIES

Common chromosomal abnormalities are either structural or numerical. Structural alterations include translocations, deletions, inversions, and amplifications of regions of chromosomes. Numerical alterations include losses and duplications of whole chromosomes.

Among the gliomas, glioblastoma has the highest frequency of chromosomal alterations. Of approximately 20 low-grade astrocytoma karyotypes reported [17•,18•], all but one has been normal. Similarly, most anaplastic astrocytomas studied have had either a normal or 45 XO karyotype, although in a few cases, trisomy 7 and double minute chromosomes were noted [17•,19•,20••]. Double minute chromosomes are small, spherical structures that occur in pairs; they are the cytogenetic equivalent of gene amplification [21]. Glioblastomas, however, show many abnormalities. Several hundred banded karyotypes have been published [17•–19•,20••,22,23]. Abnormalities noted include polysomy 7 (50% to 80%), loss of chromosome 10 (30% to 60%), and deletions or translocations of chromosome 9p (approximately 30%). Other abnormalities noted, with a smaller frequency, include the loss of chromosome 22 and deletions or unbalanced translocations involving 1p, 6q, 7q, 8p, 11q, 13q, and 19p. In addition, about 10% of tumors showed numerous cells with double minutes, and another 20% to 30% showed occasional double minutes [19•]. With most glioblastomas, the double minutes contain amplification of the epidermal growth factor receptor gene (*erb*-B) [24,25]. Homogeneously staining regions (areas of gene amplification noted within chromosomes) have not been observed. Up to 20% of glioblastoma karyotypes contain predominantly normal metaphase spreads. (For an excellent review, see Bigner *et al.* [26••].)

Such information gathered from cytogenetic studies can be confirmed and extended using restriction fragment length polymorphism (RFLP) analysis. RFLP analyses can show the deletion of a small region of the chromosome, possibly indicating the loss of one of two alleles (called loss of heterozygosity), even when a deletion is not detectable cytogenetically. With this method, loss of heterozygosity at chromosome 10 is detected in the majority of glioblastomas studied. Reported series note a loss of heterozygosity in 28 of 29 glioblastomas, with no losses in 22 astrocytomas of lower grade [27•]; in 10 of 13 glioblastomas, with no losses in four patients with anaplastic astrocytoma [28•]; and in 38 of 53 glioblastomas, but again with intact heterozygosity in the lower grade tumors [29•]. These results show a higher percentage of DNA loss on chromosome 10 than the cytogenetic studies, suggesting that many deletions are too small to be detected microscopically. They may, nonetheless, be functionally significant.

Chromosome 17 is also frequently involved. Fults and colleagues [27•] reported loss of heterozygosity in 17p in 40% of 20 glioblastomas. More intriguing is their finding of loss of heterozygosity in 40% of 15 anaplastic astrocytomas as well. Other studies corroborate the significant association of 17p in astrocytomas, including anaplastic astrocytomas [30•–32•]. An analysis of 41 astrocytomas (26 glioblastomas multiforme, 15 anaplastic astrocytomas) using DNA markers for every chromosome noted loss of heterozygosity in every autosome except chromosome 21 [32]. Chromosomes 10p, 10q, and 17p showed loss of heterozygosity in more than 38%; chromosomes 5q,

7p, 11p, 14q, and 15q showed loss of heterozygosity in 16% to 21%; and the rest showed loss of heterozygosity in less than 14%. As in many other studies, loss of heterozygosity at chromosome 10 was the most common abnormality; it existed in glioblastoma (53%) at a higher frequency than in anaplastic astrocytoma (15%). In addition, this study also noted 17p loss in seven of 10 anaplastic astrocytomas as well as in six of 22 glioblastomas.

Among the multitude of abnormalities noted in these tumors, many experiments based on karyotypic and on RFLP analyses note the most frequent changes to be trisomy 7, the presence of double minutes, and deletions at 10 and 17p. Deletion of chromosome 10 is observed in most glioblastomas but not in anaplastic astrocytomas. Trisomy 7 and double minutes were also noted in glioblastomas only. Similar to the loss of the *p53* gene in colorectal carcinoma, these alterations may characterize the change from anaplastic astrocytoma to glioblastoma.

In contrast to colorectal carcinoma, few changes are noted in anaplastic astrocytomas. The only karyotypic change is the loss of a sex chromosome, which may or may not be important in oncogenesis. With the more sensitive RFLP studies, it has been noted that a significant portion of anaplastic astrocytomas had loss of heterozygosity at 17p.

Protooncogenes

The epidermal growth factor receptor, encoded by the *erb*-B gene on chromosome 7, is a 170 kD transmembrane cell surface receptor. It has an external domain that binds either epidermal growth factor or transforming growth factor α, and a cytoplasmic domain with tyrosine kinase activity that becomes activated in response to that binding. Although the exact mechanism is unknown, tyrosine kinase activity stimulates DNA synthesis in responsive cells [33–36].

The cytogenetic evidence suggests the involvement of *erb*-B in astrocytomas. Not only are double minutes noted in up to 40% of tumors, but trisomy 7 may also represent increased *erb*-B expression. Indeed, the predominant oncogene involved in gliomas is *erb*-B, and its amplification has been widely reported. The highest incidence occurs with glioblastoma, in which 40% to 50% of examined tumors show amplification [25,29•,37–39]. In addition, Bigner and colleagues [37] reported amplification in two of six anaplastic astrocytomas. In 30 grade I to III astrocytomas, Ekstrand and colleagues [39] detected *erb*-B amplification in only one tumor but noted increased levels of mRNA (increased gene expression) in another 14 tumors. Therefore, increased production of the epidermal growth factor receptor may be involved in a significant percentage of both glioblastomas and lower grade astrocytomas. These same studies reported only infrequent amplification of other known protooncogenes, ie, N-*myc*, C-*myc*, and *gli*.

All tumors with *erb*-B amplification had mRNA levels at least 10 times higher than normal brain, with at least 2 times the normal levels of the receptor [40]. When the level of the epidermal growth factor receptor is elevated, enhanced cellular proliferation could occur if a ligand is present. In fact, expression of epidermal growth factor and transforming growth factor α has been noted in gliomas [39]. In addition to this possible autocrine or paracrine mechanism, mutant receptors may be abnormally active without growth factor binding and may provide an unmodulated stimulus to cell proliferation. Rearrangements of *erb*-B have been observed, both with and without amplification [25,39–42]. Three abnormalities are commonly found: an internal deletion in the 3´ region essential for down-regulation, a deletion of 248 base-pairs in domain IV that results in a receptor with elevated autophosphorylating activity, and an 801 base-pair deletion in the 5´ region that produces proteins lacking 267 amino acids in the cell-surface domain. These mutant proteins may provide targets for immunotherapy. In fact, antibodies specific for the mutant epidermal growth factor receptor have been generated [43].

Another protooncogene that has been implicated in glioma oncogenesis is the c-*sis* gene, which encodes the B chain of the platelet-derived growth factor (PDGF)—an important regulator of glial proliferation and differentiation. In the embryonic optic nerve, type 1 astrocytes that proliferate in response to epidermal growth factor or fibroblast growth factor secrete PDGF [44]. PDGF delays the differentiation and sustains the proliferation of O-2A precursor cells, which differentiate into oligodendrocytes and type 2 astrocytes. Several studies show that aberrant expression of PDGF induces transformation. Simian sarcoma virus, which carries v-*sis*, a derivative of c-*sis*, produces glial tumors in animals. A cloned c-*sis* gene from a human tumor is transforming when linked to an appropriated initiation site and retroviral promoter. In addition, antagonists of PDGF, such as trapidil, reduce the rate of astrocytoma cell division [45–47].

Thus, *in vitro* studies seem to show that alteration or overexpression of c-*sis* is oncogenic. Searches for gene rearrangements or amplification in tumors, however, have been generally unsuccessful. Increased expression of PDGF (without gene amplification) has been reported in 16 glioma cell lines and three glioblastomas [48,49], but it remains to be established whether this expression is a fundamental causative feature of tumorigenesis or merely an epiphenomenon of rapid cell division.

TUMOR SUPPRESSOR GENES

Cytogenetic and RFLP analyses point to chromosomes 10 and 17p as possible sites of tumor suppressor gene loss. We do not know which genes may be involved with chromosome 10 loss for two reasons: the deletion involves the whole chromosome, and none of the current candidate tumor suppressor genes localizes to this region [4]. There is a strong possibility, however, that the tumor suppressor gene involved in the 17p deletion is the *p53* gene. Mapping data reveal that the region of 17p loss is between p11.2 and pter [27•]. The *p53* gene has been localized to p13.1 [50]. There may be other tumor suppressor genes in this region: RFLP analyses in medulloblastomas showed a consistent loss of heterozygosity at 17p13.3 not involving the *p53* gene [51]. Several lines of evidence suggest, however, that the *p53* gene is significant in gliomas.

The loss of *p53* gene activity is the most common cancer-related genetic event observed. It has already been implicated as a causal event in tumors of the bladder, liver, breast, lung, colon, and others [52]. Point mutations resulting in amino acid substitutions are noted in a variety of tumors, including four of five glioblastomas [13]. These mutations can affect the function of the p53 protein [53] and are noted both in tumors that have loss of heterozygosity at 17p and in tumors that do not [13]. Further, a survey of 40 gliomas showed mutant *p53* in 37% of tumors without 17p deletions and in 64% of tumors with loss of heterozygosity [54]. An analysis of three recurrent tumors, which were classified as grades I and II at presentation and grade IV at recurrence, showed that progression was associated with increased frequency of *p53* mutation. A smaller percentage of cells from the low-grade tumors had a mutant allele (<50% on average). At recurrence, nearly 100% of cells carried the mutation [55•]. Lastly, there is a germline mutation involving the *p53* gene. Patients from families with the Li-Fraumeni syndrome have normal karyotypes but point mutations within the highly conserved region IV, which is the most common site of mutation in sporadic tumors [56,57]. These patients are heterozygous (mutant/wild-type) in somatic tissues and homozygous (mutant/mutant) in tumor tissues. The spectrum of cancers noted in this syndrome is broad and includes brain tumors, breast and adrenocortical carcinomas, soft tissue sarcomas, and leukemia.

Similar to the retinoblastoma gene, *p53* encodes a nuclear phosphoprotein that preferentially binds certain DNA sequences [58]. Two recent studies [59••, 60••] proved that the *p53* gene is intimately involved in the regulation of the cell cycle and plays a role in

the control of gene amplification. In those investigations, cultured fibroblasts from patients with Li-Fraumeni syndrome were compared with normal controls using agents that arrest the cell cycle. N-phosphonacetyl-L-aspartate (PALA) is a specific inhibitor of *de novo* uridine synthesis and causes cell cycle arrest at G1. The only recognized mechanism by which resistant clones arise is the amplification of the *CAD* gene. The *CAD* gene encodes the trienzyme complex (carbamoyl-P-synthetase, aspartate transcarbamylase, and dihydroorotase) that is the target of PALA. Consequently, the frequency at which PALA-resistant clones arises provides an accurate measure of *CAD* gene amplification.

Livingstone and colleagues [60••] reported that cells with one mutant *p53* gene behaved like normal cells, but cells with two mutant genes did not. They failed to stop cycling when placed in PALA and displayed an ability to amplify at high levels. The *p53* mutation is causally related to these changes. Using a retroviral vector, Yin and colleagues [59••] introduced a wild-type *p53* into PALA-resistant clones with two mutant genes. Transformed cells with low levels of wild-type *p53* expression did not change, but with high levels of expression G1 arrest under PALA was restored, and the level of gene amplification returned to undetectable levels.

CONCLUSIONS

The genesis of cancer involves multiple genetic events with both the inactivation of tumor suppressor genes and the activation of protooncogenes. As the colorectal carcinoma model makes clear, tumor progression involves a changing genetic profile that leads to more aggressive phenotypes (Figure 1.1). Elucidation of these changes provides the best hope for the rational design of new therapies and improved control of tumor growth.

The most common genetic abnormalities noted in glioblastoma are trisomy 7, loss of chromosome 10, loss of heterozygosity at chromosome 17, and amplification of the *erb*-B gene. In that trisomy 7 and loss of chromosome 10 are observed only in glioblastoma, these aneuploid changes may mediate the progression from lower grade tumors to glioblastoma.

What may constitute the more basic events in astrocytoma oncogenesis is less clear. The cytogenetic studies are unremarkable, and no abnormalities are noted with any consistency in the few grade I and II tumors examined. With anaplastic astrocytoma, there are reports of *erb*-B amplification or increased levels of its mRNA. Thus, the epidermal growth factor receptor may have a role in the development of these tumors. In addition, loss of heterozygosity at chromosome 17p is reported in as many as 40% of anaplastic astrocytomas. The deleted region includes the location of the *p53* gene, and several lines of evidence suggest that this gene is fundamentally involved in astrocytoma formation. As we have indicated, patients with Li-Fraumeni syndrome develop brain tumors, and progression to a more aggressive tumor is associated with an increased *p53* mutation rate. Further, there is now proof that the *p53* gene plays a crucial role in cell cycle regulation and the control of gene amplification [59••,60••].

Although it is clear that we have gained many insights into the genetic basis of astrocytoma development, the type of characterization achieved with colorectal carcinoma has not been attained. Some deletions are too small to be detected by karyotypic analyses and may be missed with RFLP analyses. Inactivated single base-pair mutations are particularly difficult to identify. Similarly, increased expression of a gene can occur without the amplification of that gene. A further difficulty is that primary genetic changes initiate a series of events. Yin and colleagues [59••] have proposed that loss of the *p53* gene causes genetic instability, and other genes amplify as a result. This hypothesis is consistent with the finding that many tumor suppressor genes encode nuclear phosphoproteins that may have a role in transcriptional control. Therefore, even a commonly noted genetic change like *erb*-B amplification may be the result of a more basic event. We must distinguish between fundamental changes and their consequences. Indeed, a recent study suggests that a deletion at chromosome 10 precedes the amplification of *erb*-B. When von Deimling and colleagues [29•] examined loss of heterozygosity on chromosome 10 and *erb*-B amplification in the same tumors, they found that all tumors with *erb*-B amplification had loss of chromosome 10, but not all tumors with a chromosome 10 deletion had *erb*-B amplification. It is possible that the loss of a tumor suppressor gene on chromosome 10 leads to *erb*-B amplification.

The current challenge is to understand fully the genetic changes that lead to glioma formation. As a better understanding is gained, it may be possible to delineate the basic changes common to all gliomas. Or it may become evident that *astrocytomas* include several genetic subtypes with a common histopathologic morphology. It is well known that glioblastomas arise in several ways: from lower grade astrocytomas, from oligodendrogliomas and ependymomas (rarely), and from brain with no prior evidence of tumor [61]. Without a doubt, genetic characterization provides benefits—first permitting more accurate classification and improved prognosis and then novel treatments. In the petri dish, tumor lines can be transformed to a normal appearance and behavior by the replacement of deleted genes [62,63]. Gene therapy, and treatments currently unimagined, may be the result.

REFERENCES AND RECOMMENDED READING

Papers of particular interest, published within the annual period of review, have been highlighted as:
• Of special interest
•• Of outstanding interest

1. Bishop JM: The molecular genetics of cancer. *Science* 1987, 235:305–311.

2. Weinberg R: Oncogenes, antioncogenes, and the molecular bases of multistep carcinogenesis. *Cancer Res* 1989, 49:3713–3721.

3. Sager R: Tumor suppressor genes: the puzzle and the promise. *Science* 1989, 246:1406–1412.

4. Weinberg R: Tumor suppressor genes. *Science* 1991, 254:1138–1146.

5. Knudson AG Jr: Mutation and cancer: statistical study of retinoblastoma. *Proc Natl Acad Sci U S A* 1971, 68:820–823.

6. Bos J, Fearon E, Hamilton S, *et al.*: Prevalence of *ras* gene mutations in human colorectal cancers. *Nature* 1987, 327:293–297.

7. Forrester K, Almoguera C, Han K, *et al.*: Detection of high incidence of K-*ras* oncogenes during human colon tumorigenesis. *Nature* 1987, 327:298–303.

8. Vogelstein B, Fearon E, Kern S, *et al.*: Allelotype of colorectal carcinomas. *Science* 1989, 244:207–211.

9. Farr C, Marshall C, Easty D, *et al.*: A study of *ras* gene mutations in colonic adenomas from familial polyposis coli patients. *Oncogene* 1988, 3:673–678.

10. Vogelstein B, Fearon E, Hamilton S, *et al.*: Genetic alterations during colorectal-tumor development. *N Engl J Med* 1988, 319:525–532.

11. Delattre P, Olschwang S, Law D, *et al.*: Multiple genetic alterations distinguish distal from proximal colorectal cancer. *Lancet* 1989, 2:353–356.

12. Baker S, Fearon E, Nigro J, *et al.*: Chromosome 17 dele-

tions and *p53* gene mutations in colorectal carcinoma. *Science* 1989, 244:217–221.

13. Nigro J, Baker S, Preisinger A, *et al.*: Mutations in the *p53* gene occur in diverse human tumour types. *Nature* 1989, 342:705–707.

14. Fearon E, Vogelstein B: A genetic model for colorectal tumorigenesis. *Cell* 1990, 61:759–767.

15. Edelman G: Morphoregulatory molecules. *Biochemistry* 1988, 27:3533–3543.

16. Sasaki M, Okamoto M, Sato C, *et al.*: Loss of constitutional heterozygosity in colorectal tumors from patients with familial polyposis coli and those with non-polyposis colorectal carcinoma. *Cancer Res* 1989, 49:4402–4406.

17. • Jenkins R, Kimmel D, Moertel C, *et al.*: A cytogenetic study of 53 human gliomas. *Cancer Genet Cytogenet* 1989, 39:253–279.
Paper presents good data on glioma karyotypes.

18. • Rey J, Bello M, de Campos J, *et al.*: Chromosomal patterns in human malignant astrocytomas. *Cancer Genet Cytogenet* 1987, 29:201–221.
Paper presents good data on glioma karyotypes.

19. • Bigner S, Mark J, Burger P, *et al.*: Specific chromosomal abnormalities in malignant human gliomas. *Cancer Res* 1988, 48:405–411.
Paper presents good data on glioma karyotypes.

20. •• Thiel G, Losanowa T, Kintzel D, *et al.*: Karyotypes in 90 human gliomas. *Cancer Genet Cytogenet* 1992, 58:109–120.
Paper presents good data on glioma karyotypes.

21. Gebhart E, Bruderlein S, Tulusan A, *et al.*: Incidence of double minutes, cytogenetic equivalents of gene amplification, in human carcinoma cells. *Int J Cancer* 1984, 34:369–373.

22. Rey J, Bello M, de Campos J, *et al.*: Chromosome studies in two human brain tumors. *Cancer Genet Cytogenet* 1983, 10:159–165.

23. Lindstrom E, Salford L, Heim S, *et al.*: Trisomy 7 and sex chromosome loss need not be representative of tumor parenchyma cells in malignant glioma. *Genes Chromosom Cancer* 1991, 3:474–479.

24. Bigner S, Wong A, Muhlbaire L: Relationship between gene amplification and chromosomal deviations in malignant human gliomas. *Cancer Genet Cytogenet* 1987, 29:165–170.

25. Libermann T, Nusbaum H, Razon N, *et al.*: Amplification, enhanced expression and possible rearrangement of EGF receptor gene in primary human brain tumors of glial origin. *Nature* 1985, 313:144–147.

26. •• Bigner S, Mark J, Bigner D: Cytogenetics of human brain tumors. *Cancer Genet Cytogenet* 1990, 47:141–154.
An excellent review with good data on glioma karyotypes.

27. • Fults D, Tippets R, Thomas G, *et al.*: Loss of heterozygosity for loci on chromosome 17p in human malignant astrocytoma. *Cancer Res* 1989, 49:6572–6577.
Paper presents an RFLP analysis of gliomas.

28. • Fujimoto M, Fults D, Thomas G, *et al.*: Loss of heterozy-

gosity on chromosome 10 in human glioblastoma multiforme. *Genomics* 1989, 4:210–214.
An RFLP analysis of gliomas.

29. • von Deimling A, Louis DN, von Ammon K, *et al.*: Association of epidermal growth factor receptor gene amplification with loss of chromosome 10 in human glioblastoma multiforme. *J Neurosurg* 1992, 77:295–301.
Paper presents an RFLP analysis of gliomas.

30. • El-Azouzi M, Chung R, Farmer G, *et al.*: Loss of distinct regions on the short arm of chromosome 17 associated with tumorigenesis of human astrocytomas. *Proc Natl Acad Sci U S A* 1989, 86:7186–7190.
An RFLP analysis of gliomas.

31. • James C, Carlbom E, Dumanski J, *et al.*: Clonal genomic alterations in glioma malignancy stages. *Cancer Res* 1988, 48:5546–5551.
Paper presents an RFLP analysis of gliomas.

32. • Fults D, Pedone C, Thomas G, *et al.*: Allelotype of human malignant astrocytoma. *Cancer Res* 1990, 50:5784–5789.
Paper presents an RFLP analysis of gliomas.

33. Hunter T: The epidermal growth factor receptor gene and its product. *Nature* 1984, 311:413–415.

34. Lin CR, Chen WS, Lazar CS, *et al.*: Expression cloning of human EGF receptor complementary DNA: gene amplification and three related messenger RNA products in A431 cells. *Science* 1984, 224:843–848.

35. Ullrich A, Coussens L, Hayflick JS, *et al.*: Human epidermal growth factor receptor cDNA sequence and aberrant expression of the amplified gene in A431 epidermoid carcinoma cells. *Nature* 1984, 309:418–425.

36. Riedel H, Massoglia S, Schlessinger J, *et al.*: Ligand activation of over-expressed epidermal growth factor receptors transforms NIH 3T3 mouse fibroblasts. *Proc Natl Acad Sci U S A* 1988, 85:1477–1481.

37. Bigner SH, Burger PC, Wong AJ, *et al.*: Gene amplification in malignant human gliomas: clinical and histopathologic aspects. *J Neuropathol Exp Neurol* 1988, 47:191–205.

38. Diedrich U, Soja S, Behnke J, *et al.*: Amplification of the *c-erbB* oncogene is associated with malignancy in primary tumours of neuroepithelial tissue. *J Neurol* 1991, 238:221–224.

39. Ekstrand AJ, James CD, Cavenee W, *et al.*: Genes for epidermal growth factor receptor, transforming growth factor α, and epidermal growth factor and their expression in human gliomas in vivo. *Cancer Res* 1991, 51:2164–2172.

40. Malden LT, Novak U, Kaye AH, *et al.*: Selective amplification of the cytoplasmic domain of the epidermal growth factor receptor gene in glioblastoma multiforme. *Cancer Res* 1988, 48:2711–2714.

41. Wong A, Bigner S, Bigner D, *et al.*: Increased expression of the EGFR gene in malignant gliomas is invariably associated with gene amplification. *Proc Natl Acad Sci U S A* 1988, 84:6899–6903.

42. Wong A, Ruppert J, Bigner S, *et al.*: Structural alterations of the epidermal growth factor receptor gene in human gliomas. *Proc Natl Acad Sci U S A* 1992, 89:2965–2969.

43. Humphrey P, Wong A, Vogelstein B, *et al.*: Anti- synthetic peptide antibody reacting at the fusion junction of deletion mutant EGFR in human glioblastoma. *Proc Natl Acad Sci U S A* 1990, 87:4207–4211.

44. Raff M: Glial cell diversification in the rat optic nerve. *Science* 1989, 242:1450–1455.

45. Gazit A, Igarishi H, Ciu I, *et al.*: Expression of the normal sis/PDGF-2 coding sequence induces cellular transformation. *Cell* 1984, 39:89–97.

46. Lens P, Altena B, Nusse R: Expression of c-sis and PDGF in in vitro transformed glioma cells from rat brain tissue transplacentally treated with ethyl nitrosourea. *Mol Cell Biol* 1986, 6:3537–3540.

47. Kuratsu J-I, Ushio Y: Antiproliferative effect of trapidil, a platelet-derived growth factor antagonist, on glioma cell line in vitro. *J Neurosurg* 1990, 73:436–440.

48. Harsh GR, Keating MT, Escobedo JA, *et al.*: Platelet derived growth factor (PDGF) autocrine components in human tumor cell lines. *J Neurooncol* 1990, 8:1–12.

49. Hermansson M, Nister M, Bersholtz C, *et al.*: Endothelial cell hyperplasia in human glioblastoma: co-expression of mRNA for PDGF B chain and PDGF receptor suggests autocrine growth stimulation. *Proc Natl Acad Sci U S A* 1988, 85:7748–7752.

50. McBride O, Merry D, Givol D: The gene for human *p53* cellular tumor antigen is located on chromosome 17 short arm. *Proc Natl Acad Sci U S A* 1986, 83:130–134.

51. Cogen PH, Daneshvar L, Metzger AK, *et al.*: Involvement of multiple chromosome 17p loci in medulloblastoma tumorigenesis. *Am J Hum Genet* 1992, 50:584–589.

52. Vogelstein B: Cancer: a deadly inheritance. *Nature* 1990, 348:681–682.

53. Hollstein M, Sidransky D, Vogelstein B, *et al.*: *p53* Mutations in human cancers. *Science* 1991, 253:49–53.

54. Frankel RH, Bayona W, Koslow M, *et al.*: *p53* Mutations in human malignant gliomas: comparison of loss of heterozygosity and mutation frequency. *Cancer Res* 1992, 52:1427–1433.

55.• Sidransky D, Mikkelsen T, Schwechheimer K, *et al.*: Clonal expansion of *p53* mutant cells is associated with brain tumour progression. *Nature* 1992, 355:846–847.
Implicates the role of the *p53* gene in gliomas.

56. Malkin D, Li FP, Strong LC, *et al.*: Germ line *p53* mutation in a familial syndrome of breast cancer, sarcomas, and other neoplasms. *Science* 1990, 250:1233–1250.

57. Srivastava S, Zou Z, Pirollo K, *et al.*: Germ-line transmission of a mutated *p53* gene in a cancer prone family with Li-Fraumeni syndrome. *Nature* 1990, 348:747–749.

58. Bischoff JR, Friedman PN, Marshak DR, *et al.*: Human p53 is phosphorylated by p60-cdc2 and cyclin B-cdc2. *Proc Natl Acad Sci U S A* 1990, 87:4766–4770.

59. •• Yin Y, Tainsky MA, Bishoff FZ, *et al.*: Wild-type *p53* restores cell cycle control and inhibits gene amplification in cells with mutant *p53* alleles. *Cell* 1992, 70:937–948.
Excellent paper discussing recent work on the *p53* gene.

60.•• Livingstone LR, White A, Sprouse J, *et al.*: Altered cell cycle arrest and gene amplification potential accompany loss of wild type *p53*. *Cell* 1992, 70:923–935.
An excellent study of the function of the *p53* gene.

61. Harsh GR IV, Wilson CB: Neuroepithelial tumors of the adult brain. In *Neurological Surgery*. Edited by Youmans JR. Philadelphia: WB Saunders; 1990:3040–3146.

62. Huang HJS, Yee JK, Shew JY, *et al.*: Suppression of the neoplastic phenotype by replacement of the RB gene in human cancer cells. *Science* 1988, 242:1563–1566.

63. Steck PA, Hadi A, Pershouse MA, *et al.*: Cellular and molecular consequences of re-insertion of chromosome 10 in glioblastoma multiforme [abstract]. *Proc Am Assoc Cancer Res* 1992, 33:2318.

Chapter 2

Cranial Base Meningiomas

Donald C. Wright
Laligam N. Sekhar

Intracranial meningiomas constitute approximately 18% to 22% of all intracranial tumors, the majority (56%) of which occur over the convexity (34%) and parasagittal regions (22%). Cranial base locations (35% to 50%) are characterized by difficult surgical access, greater morbidity, and higher recurrence rates compared with lesions of the cranial vault. Meningiomas are generally histologically benign tumors originating from arachnoidal cells of the leptomeninges. Atypical or malignant forms occur in approximately 6% of patients, and local invasion and encasement of neurovascular structures (particularly the cavernous carotid artery and trigeminal nerve) are unfortunate features of cranial base meningiomas associated with production of clinical morbidity. They are potentially curable tumors if completely removed, and the relative survival rate of symptomatic meningiomas (all types) is 71% at 15 years following diagnosis. Significant advances in the treatment of cranial base meningiomas have occurred in the last decade; patients with extensive or critically located basal tumors have increasing likelihood of complete excision with reduced morbidity, whereas improved measures for detection and treatment of recurrent tumors offer improved long-term control of atypical and malignant types. We review a series of selected scientific and clinical papers on meningiomas that are potential preludes to future management approaches.

Increasingly the scientific study of meningiomas provides us with prognostic markers in the prediction of recurrence and ultimately may contribute to treatment methods with less risk and reduced morbidity.

SCIENTIFIC COMMUNICATIONS

A number of diagnostic, prognostic, and treatment strategies have emerged in the therapy of meningiomas based on tumor cell receptors and gene regulation of various growth factors. Demonstration of high-density, high-affinity progesterone-binding receptors in meningiomas is the basis of current antiprogestin therapy, whereas a large body of data is developing in cell kinetics, cytogenetic analysis of gene aberrations, and identification of regulatory segments in protooncogenes.

Progesterone receptors, cerebral edema, and proliferative potential

A high percentage of meningiomas (60% to 70%) exhibit progesterone receptor sites on their cell membrane and lack estradiol receptors, which is opposite the ratio found in breast cancers. Similar to breast carcinoma, hormonal manipulation of patients with meningiomas via sex steroid receptors has potential therapeutic benefit. Perrot-Applanat and colleagues [1•] reported on their extensive study of the relationship of progesterone-binding activity, histology, proliferative index (Ki67 antigen), and clinical profile of 36 patients with meningiomas. They describe a new technique for intracellular localization of receptors, using monoclonal antibodies directed against progesterone or estrogen receptor sites, and compared the results with those of established enzyme immunoassay techniques. They found that 72% of meningiomas had specific progesterone staining (none with estrogen staining); the receptors were localized to the nucleus and restricted to arachnoidal cells. There was a correlation in receptor-binding and histologic subtypes: reduction in progesterone receptors with increasing anaplastic features. There was a general increase in receptors in transitional and meningothelial types as compared with fibroblastic forms. There was no correlation between progesterone receptors and histologic features such as mitoses, pleomorphism, or dural or parenchymal invasion, or in degree of Ki67 binding (proliferative index). They found no correlation between progesterone-binding and clinical parameters (sex, age, menopausal states) or whether these tumors were recurrent. The authors describe the advantages of the monoclonal antibody

assay and suggest that other indices of cellular proliferation are more reliable indicators of invasive, recurrent, or anaplastic growth.

Meixensberger and colleagues [2•] attempted to elaborate on a prior study finding a correlation between progesterone receptor sites and degree of peritumoral cerebral edema (assessed by diagnostic scanning) in meningiomas. Using receptor-binding assays (18 of 28 positive for progesterone receptor), they found no correlation in progesterone receptor binding activity and tumor size, location, histologic subtype, menopausal status, or peritumoral edema patterns. They noted that 10 of 28 patients with little or no evidence of progesterone receptors had variable degrees of cerebral edema, whereas four of the five tumors with no surrounding edema were positive for progesterone-binding sites. They speculate that meningiomas produce cerebral edema via a secretory-excretory mechanism unrelated to progesterone receptors, and antiprogestin therapy has no role in management of cerebral edema.

Somatostatin receptors

Koper and colleagues [3•] reported on somatostatin in meningiomas, drawing on clinical experience in the use of somatostatin receptor analogs in endocrine-active tumors. They were generally unable to demonstrate inhibition of in vitro meningioma cells using somatostatin except in a specific (forskalin-stimulation), mitogen-induced form of growth and thus were unable to duplicate a prior report of tumor inhibition by somatostatin and somatostatin analogs. They conclude that somatostatin has low likelihood of a clinical role in medical therapy as a direct antitumor agent, although there may be a role in blocking the autocrine secretion of growth factors elaborated by meningiomas, which might indirectly affect proliferation. They also comment on the possible role of somatostatin in the treatment of peritumoral edema incited by meningioma.

Dopamine D$_1$ receptors

Schrell and colleagues [4•] added to their extensive literature characterizing various aspects of receptor physiology in meningiomas in their report on dopamine receptors. The D$_1$ receptor is known to be coupled to a cAMP/adenlyate cyclase enzyme system, whereas the D$_2$ receptor is involved in various responses that inhibit this enzyme. Although the function of the D$_1$ receptor site is unknown, it is postulated to be involved in the site of action of various neuroleptic drugs. Their interest was based on the inhibitory effects by dopamine and D_1 agonists on *in vitro* cell proliferation and the widespread distribution of dopamine receptors in a variety of tumor types. Using a receptor-binding assay (labeled D_1 and D_2 antagonists), the authors demonstrate the presence of dopamine D_1 receptor sites in meningiomas and the absence of D_2 receptors. They postulate that medical therapy may be feasible using selective D_1 agonists in patients with resistant meningiomas.

Insulin-like growth factors

Insulin-like growth factors (IGFs) are polypeptide mitogens (sharing a close structural relationship to proinsulin) with growth-promoting effects, including cell proliferation, and thus a potential target for exerting control over tumor growth. Autocrine or paracrine production of mRNA coding for such factors as interleukins (IL-1B and IL-6), epidermal and platelet-derived growth factors, basic fibroblast growth factor, and IGFs is elaborated by various tumors, including meningiomas and gliomas. Lichtor and colleagues [5•] studied the geneic expression in various tumors (including two meningiomas) of IGF I and II by Northern blot and DNA probe analysis and immunofluorescence (monoclonal antibody directed against IGF II). They found substantial amounts of mRNA encoding the IGF II protein, which is normally present in fetal leptomeninges and choroid plexus. The physiologic role and functional significance of IGF to tumors is unknown. The authors postulate that certain growth factors such as IGF II have specific mitogenic effects on tumors.

Cytogenic studies

The majority (50% to 60%) of (sporadic) meningiomas manifest a deletion in the long arm of chromosome 22, near the c-*sis* gene. Several tumor suppressor regions have been identified in this region, and one has been implicated in the development of heritable tumors found in bilateral acoustic neurofibromatosis. The c-*sis* gene encodes for a polypeptide making up chemical forms of platelet-derived growth factor, found in normal tissues and certain malignant tumors (eg, glioblastoma). Smidt and colleagues [6•] reported on additional work involving the c-*sis* gene in sporadic meningiomas, as a complementary study to an earlier paper on a familial meningioma population. They found no similarity between the familial meningioma deletion (in the fifth intron of the *Alu* sequence) and the chromosomal aberrations of 86 sporadic meningiomas. They further determined that the *Alu* sequence is not involved in the regulation of the platelet-derived growth factor protein. In a related study, Sanson and colleagues [7•] also used DNA typing (Southern blot DNA probes to chromosome 22) correlated with histologic features of 34 patients with meningiomas. They assigned a tumor score based on six histologic criteria of atypical or malignant features (mitosis, vascularity, sheeting of tumor cells, nuclear pleomorphism, prominent nucleoli, and micronecrosis). They found 17 of 34 patients with a chromosomal abnormality of all or part of the allele on chromosome 22 and a correlation with three of the six histopathologic criteria (mitosis, nucleolar prominence, and pleomorphism). Tumor scores greater than or equal to 8 were associated with chromosomal 22 deletion, whereas scores less than or equal to 7 rarely had the allele abnormality. Two of the patients recurred during the follow-up period of 2 years, both with tumor scores greater than 8 and monosomy 22. Arnoldus and colleagues [8•] described cytogenetic methods (in situ DNA hybridization using specific DNA cosmid probes directed to the interphase nucleoli of chromosome 22) to investigate the biologic behavior of tumors (eg, growth rate, genetic abnormalities) and applied these methods to 63 patients, with a subpopulation of 30 meningiomas. Seventy percent of the meningiomas showed the monosomy 22 deletion, and 10 of 30 had other aberrations, including five tumors that were recurrent or atypical histopathologic types. Two malignant meningiomas had deletions in chromosome 10 (also reported in glioblastoma). The authors present convincing data that interphase cytogenetic methods offer rapid assessment of chromosomal aberrations in tumors, and this data may foster identification of prognostic factors for the clinical behavior of tumors.

Cell cytokinetics, prognosis, and recurrence

Hoshino and colleagues [9•] and a companion paper by the same group [10••] described their continuing work in cell kinetics of various tumors, including 178 meningiomas (in the latter study) using *in vivo* bromodeoxyuridine (BUdR) and a double-labeling technique (in the former paper). Both papers evaluate the labeling index (LI), or percentage of cells in S phase of meningiomas. Hoshino and colleagues [9•] reviewed the prognostic value of proliferative measures of meningiomas and also commented on the ethical aspects and clinical risk of administering halogenated pyrimidines (BUdR/IUdR) to tumor patients. Shibuya and colleagues [10••] performed a detailed analysis of 53 of the 178 patients in whom atypical or malignant features were noted. They developed a mathematical model for the risks of recurrence based on the LI. Patients with an LI greater than 5% had 100% recurrence; the two groups with LIs of 3% to 5% and 1% to 3% had 55% and 30% recurrence rates, respectively (Table 2.1, Figure 2.1). They also correlated the data with the extent of surgical resection. They conclude that malignant tumors had higher proliferative potential as measured by the LI, and the overall recurrence rate for tumors with LIs greater than or equal to 1% was 88%, whereas those with LIs less than or equal to 1% was 22%.

Demographic, Pathologic, and Diagnostic Reports

Epidemiologic and demographic data

Several large series of patients with meningiomas are reviewed, giving some insight into the demographics, true incidence, and risk factors associated with mortality arising from these tumors. Valuable data are given on the mortality risk incurred by patients with incomplete excision, a problem common to basal meningiomas. In companion papers [11••,12•], data from the Finnish Cancer Registry are analyzed to examine the risk factors determining the excess mortality associated with intracranial meningiomas in a stable population with longitudinal follow-up data. Sankila and colleagues [11••] analyzed 1986 patients from 1954 through 1984 and compared the 15-year *observed* survival rates with the expected survival

derived from a matched general population. Eighty-six percent (1711 patients) underwent surgery, and the histology of a subgroup of 936 tumors was classified (using the World Health Organization schema for meningiomas) into atypical (4.7%), anaplastic (1%), and benign (94.3%) subtypes. They defined *excess mortality* attributable to meningioma as the difference in mortality between the tumor patient group and the comparable general population. They found a mean difference of 14% (3.4 years) between observed and expected survival. The short-term excess mortality (17.7%) in the tumor group occurred primarily in the first year of diagnosis, reflecting the hazards of surgery and associated risk factors. The relative survival rates were 83%, 79%, 74%, and 71% at 1, 5, 10, and 15 years, respectively. They conclude that the *observed* survival rates should not be used alone in meningioma studies, as the impact of mortality due to other (nontumor) causes imparts a low estimate of survival. Kallio and colleagues [12•] examined the risk factors involved in this same group (Finnish study) of patients. They listed poor preoperative condition, advanced age, negative history of seizure, complications (*eg*, postoperative hematoma, pulmonary embolus), and incomplete tumor removal as the principal risk factors. The extent of surgery was the most significant factor associated with long-term excess mortality; patients with incomplete removal had a 4.2-fold relative increase in risk of death. Recurrence was strongly correlated with histologic subtype: 5-year recurrence rates for benign (3%), atypical (38%), and

Table 2.1

Early postoperative recurrence and extent of surgical resection in 53 patients with meningiomas with a bromodeoxyuridine labeling index of 1% or more*

Extent of surgical resection	Recurrence according to the bromodeoxyuridine labeling index, n/n (%)			
	≥5	3%–5%	1%–3%	Total
Subtotal	10/14 (71.4)	4/9 (44.4)	7/24 (29.2)	21/47 (44.7)
Gross total	3/4 (75.0)	3/5 (60.0)	7/24 (29.2)	13/33 (39.4)

*Adapted from Shibuya *et al.* [10••]; with permission.

malignant (78%) meningiomas reflect this; malignant meningiomas carry a 4.6-fold increased risk of death compared with benign tumors. They conclude that meningiomas, traditionally regarded as benign and curable tumors, cause both considerable operative mortality and long-term excess mortality when patients are elderly, are in poor clinical condition, or had tumors that could not be completely removed.

Clinicopathologic correlation

Predicting clinical behavior based on the histopathologic features of meningiomas was the aim of a scholarly retrospective of 1739 surgical specimens by Maier and colleagues [13••] (Table 2.2). These authors extensively reviewed clinicopathologic features and evaluated a subset of these tumors using argyrophilic nucleolar organizer region protein patterns (Ag-NOR) as a measure of proliferative potential. They proposed

incorporation of an intermediate meningioma subtype for atypical tumors to bridge the current classification of classic meningiomas (meningothelial, transitional, and fibroblastic) and anaplastic tumors. This atypical group was characterized by increased cellularity and greater than or equal to 5 mitotic figures per high power (*eg*, 400 × magnification) field. Hemangiopericytomas and papillary meningiomas are considered a fourth category in their classification. They also analyzed a subgroup of 252 tumors with respect to clinical data (size, location, extent of surgery), histopathologic classification, and proliferative potential using Ag-NOR staining (analysis done on 112 tumors), with emphasis on recurrent, atypical, and anaplastic lesions. In this subgroup of 252 tumors, they noted that complete removals were slightly more common in the classic meningioma types (73%) than in atypical (62.9%) and anaplastic (60%) forms. They found an increasing number of Ag-

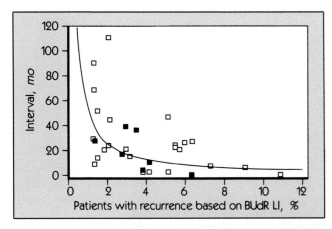

Figure 2.1

Time to reoperation after gross total or subtotal resection in 34 patients. Logarithmic regression line representation of data. *Open boxes* indicate tumor recurrence at the bromodeoxyuridine (BUdR) study; *solid boxes* indicate recurrence after the BUdR study. LI—labeling index. (*From* Shibuya *et al.* [10••]; with permission.)

Table 2.2
Histologic subtype in 1582 meningioma patients with and without tumor recurrence*

Meningioma subtype	Total, n	Nonrecurrent tumors, n(%)	Recurrent tumors, n (%)
Classic†	1423	1324(93.0)	99(7.0)
Atypical	104	68(65.3)	36(34.6)
Anaplastic	33	9(27.3)	24(72.7)
Hemangiopericytic and papillary	22	7(31.8)	15(68.2)
All types	1582	1408(89.0)	174(11.0)

Adapted from Maier *et al.* [13••]; with permission.
†Consists of benign meningothelial, transitional, and fibroblastic types.

NOR (mean) counts (Figure 2.2) across the spectrum from classic to atypical and anaplastic meningiomas. They summarize their findings as follows: 1) the proposed classification is based on simple and reproducible criteria of increased cellularity and mitotic activity; 2) primary atypical and anaplastic tumors have high recurrence rates, even after complete resection; 3) extent of surgical resection is the principal determinant of the clinical course; and 4) mean Ag-NOR counts correlate with the three-step scale of classic, atypical, and anaplastic tumors, but the prognostic value is limited owing to the wide range of counts seen in all three groups.

Surgery in the elderly

A final survey paper by Umansky and colleagues [14•] examined the question of risk of major intracranial surgery for meningiomas in the elderly population, which is particularly germane to the often lengthy and complex procedures associated with cranial base lesions. They reported on 37 patients of advanced age (mean, 74 years; range, 70 to 85 years) with symptomatic intracranial meningiomas (tumors >3 cm). Thirty-five of the 37 patients were followed up for a mean period of 29 months and analyzed as to outcome. There were two perioperative deaths (5.4% mortality), one attributed to aspiration pneumonia in a foramen magnum tumor) and another to epidural hematoma. An overall morbidity of 37% (15 of 35 surviving patients) was noted (20 major complications, nine minor complications) and was not related to the age of the patient. The average Karnofsky score improved from a mean of 59 preoperatively to a mean of 80 postoperatively. They review their approach to careful preoperative evaluation in this group and conclude that "age alone is not a contraindication for surgery" [14•].

Neuroophthalmologic features in cavernous sinus meningiomas

Golnik and colleagues [15•] reviewed 24 patients with meningiomas and documented the progression and severity of neuroophthalmologic signs in a group of patients with cavernous sinus involvement by meningioma. Their aim was to document the neuroophthalmic progression of cavernous sinus meningiomas and determine if a more aggressive approach was indicated. Eighteen of 24 patients had subtotal resec-

tion (two of 18 were also treated with radiation), and six of 24 were followed up without therapy. The most common signs were optic neuropathy (67%), proptosis (50%), and ocular motor nerve palsy (40%). They found no evidence of tumor progression or change in neurologic examination in either group. Six patients (25%) worsened during the observation period (mean follow-up, 47 months). The authors conclude that cavernous sinus meningiomas produced variable rates of progression of signs and symptoms and must be contrasted with potential morbidity and mortality of aggressive surgery for cavernous sinus meningiomas [16•].

Magnetic resonance appearance and histologic subtyping of meningioma

Preoperative data on tumor vascularity, consistency, encasement of neurovascular structures, and local invasion are of great value in appraising patients of treatment risk and in planning surgical strategy. Several papers attempting to correlate magnetic resonance (MR) imaging features with meningioma histologic subtypes and tumor character are reviewed. Demaerel and colleagues [17•] employed a five-point scoring system using signal intensity of meningiomas on T_1-, proton-density, and T_2-weighted images to assess 50 surgically verified meningiomas. They also evaluated peritumoral edema, calcification, and cystic changes (no contrasted images were included) and were unable to distinguish meningioma histologic subtypes based on their chosen criteria. Their study was in contrast to that of Kaplan and colleagues [18•], who were able to predict meningioma subtypes based on similar criteria. They reviewed 24 patients with biopsy-proven meningiomas by signal intensity pattern on T_1-, intermediate, and T_2-weighted images; mass effect; and gadolinium contrast enhancement. They correlated imaging patterns with the histologic subtype (fibroblastic, meningothelial, transitional, and angioblastic), tumor cellularity, collagen content, and calcification. They found two patterns: meningothelial and angioblastic tumors had persistent signal hyperintensity on T_2-weighted images, whereas fibroblastic and transitional types had a relative drop or hypointensity of signal on T_2-weighted images. They attributed these differences in signal intensity patterns to cellularity and collagen content of the tumor and were able to predict meningioma subtypes correctly in 80% of cases on signal intensity patterns alone. On using ancillary imaging characteristics (mass effect, necrosis, cyst formation, and contrast enhancement), their accuracy improved to 96%.

Dural tail sign

An intriguing phenomenon of enhanced MR images is the so-called dural tail sign, which has been associated with meningiomas and is a common feature of basal tumors involving the lateral wall of the cavernous sinus and tentorium. Two reports dealt with the possible pathophysiology responsible for this observation. Larson and colleagues [19•] reported on two cases of meningiomas with dural tail signs that proved to be positive for tumor cells within the surrounding dural excised at surgery. Tien and colleagues [20•] added three cases to a retrospective review of 16 patients with this sign and found 13 of 16 to be associated with meningioma. The three nonmeningioma patients with this phenomenon had chloroma, lymphoma, and sarcoidosis, suggesting lymphocytic infiltration as an explanation of the dural enhancement. Both papers review the proposed mechanisms advanced to explain this peculiar enhancement pattern. The dural tail sign has a high association with meningioma (particularly patients without prior therapy) but is not pathognomonic.

Magnetic resonance imaging of embolized tumors

Preoperative embolization is a valuable adjunct to successful surgical excision of basal meningiomas. Terada and colleagues [21•] described MR changes in meningiomas following superselective embolization of hypervascular meningiomas with either Gelfoam (Upjohn, Kalamazoo, MI) or polyvinyl alcohol particles. Extensively embolized tumors showed decreased contrast enhancement on MR and reduced signal void, suggesting obliteration of neoplastic vessels. They also described prolongation of T_1 and T_2 signal in the majority of patients and confirmed previously reported observations of pooling of contrast in Gelfoam-embolized tumors. Further studies are needed to assess the risks and complications associated with superselective embolization of basal meningiomas.

SURGICAL REPORTS

Techniques and refinement of surgical approaches to cranial base lesions

Vascular reconstruction

Sen and Sekhar [22••] updated their experience using vein graft reconstruction of the cervical, petrous, and cavernous portions of the internal carotid artery in patients with cranial base tumors. These authors advocate excision of diseased portions of the internal carotid artery in highly selected patients and perform vascular reconstruction using saphenous vein grafts where indicated. Thirty patients with basal tumors (17 meningiomas) and cerebrovascular lesions were reviewed from the standpoint of indications for vascular reconstruction, value of preoperative testing, and technical aspects of vein grafting. They stratified patients into three risk groups based on results of clinical balloon test occlusion (BTO) and quantitative cerebral blood flow (CBF) measurement using the

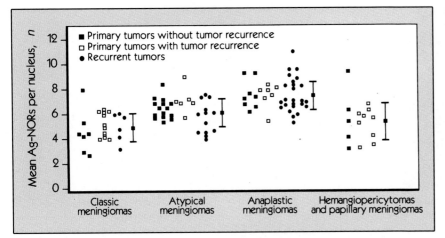

Figure 2.2

Scattergram showing silver-stained nucleolar organizer region protein (Ag-NOR) counts in primary and recurrent tumors of classic, atypical, and anaplastic meningiomas, and of hemangiopericytomas and papillary meningiomas, with mean values and respective standard deviations of all cases shown for each histologic group. (*From* Maier *et al.* [13••]; with permission.)

xenon–computed tomography method. The carotid-carotid bypass procedures (Figures 2.3 and 2.4) consisted of either *short* grafts (petrous to supraclinoid or infraclinoid carotid) or *long* grafts (cervical carotid to supraclinoid carotid), depending on the anatomic site of carotid involvement. They reported no late graft occlusions, stenoses, or pseudoaneurysm formations, with an overall 86% patency rate (mean follow-up interval, 18 months). They analyze the reasons underlying early (< 24 hours) graft occlusions (*n* = 4) and discuss the complications they encountered. The results are presented according to the preoperative assessment of risk (BTO/CBF). They conclude that direct vein graft reconstruction is safe and has a patency rate approaching 90%.

Extended frontal approach

Sekhar and colleagues [23•] present a technical description and surgical experience in 49 patients (four basal meningiomas) using an extended frontal approach. This refinement of the transbasal approach (described by Derome) employs a bilateral orbitofrontoethmoidal osteotomy (Figure 2.5A) and extensive bony removal to gain additional exposure and reduce working distance. Temporary removal of the orbital

rims and nasion, combined with resection of the posterior portion of the superomedial orbital walls and complete removal of ethmoidal air cells, allows wide exposure of the basisphenoid and midline clival regions to the level of the foramen magnum. Further removal of the planum, tuberculum, and optic foramen (as necessary) affords wide exposure of the sella, clinoidal, and cavernous carotid artery to the petrous apex (Figure 2.5B, C) and the anterior-medial cavernous sinus. This exposure can be readily combined with lateral (subtemporal-infratemporal) approaches for greater access to cavernous sinus, middle, and posterior fossa lesions. The practical limits of the approach are the foramen magnum inferiorly, hypoglossal and Dorello's canals laterally (unless combined with lateral approaches), and the internal carotid artery at the sphenoidal level. Enophthalmos and exophthalmos have not been noted despite the extensive orbital bony removal; this is attributed to incorporating a generous portion (approximately 2 cm) of the orbital roof with the frontoorbital osteotomy and careful preservation of the periorbita. The authors emphasize the importance of pericranial vascularized graft reconstruction to avoid septic complications (Figure 2.5D). The authors have used this

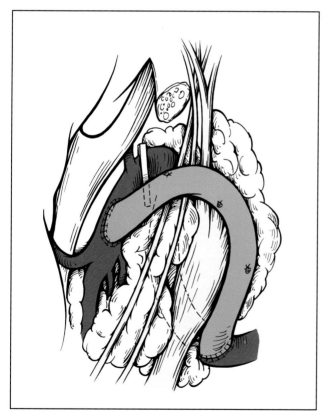

Figure 2.3

Short-vein graft from the petrous internal carotid artery. End-to-side anastomosis with supraclinoid internal carotid artery. (*From* Sen and Sekhar [22••]; with permission.)

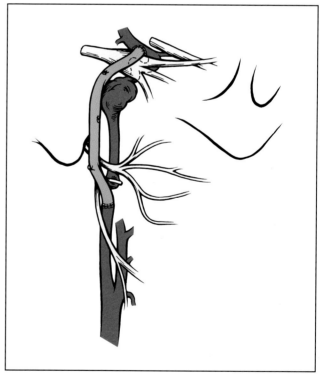

Figure 2.4

Cervical-to-supraclinoid internal carotid artery vein graft; the vein passes through the preauricular subcutaneous tissue. (*From* Sen and Sekhar [22••]; with permission.)

approach for intradural and extradural tumors of the anterior cranial base or predominantly extradural lesions of the middle and lower clivus. They discuss their experience with complications, results, and limitations of the approach.

Lateral transcondylar approach

Two articles are reviewed describing this valuable addition to the various surgical approaches designed to reach anterior and anterolateral lesions of the craniocervical junction. This technique is suited for

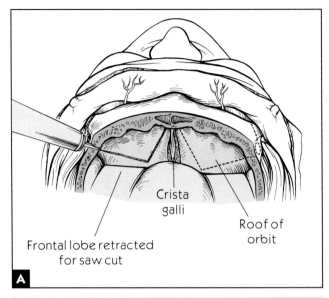

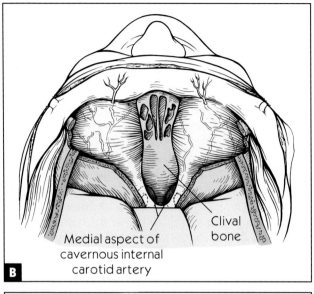

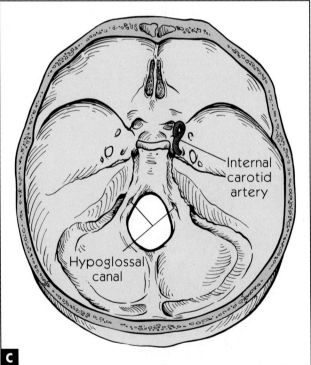

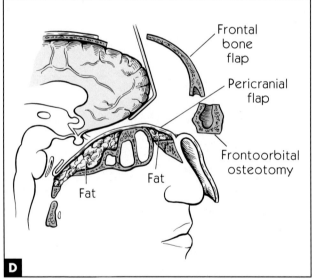

Figure 2.5

A, Orbitofrontoethmoidal osteotomy. Note the preservation of the orbital roof bilaterally. **B,** Orbitofrontoethmoidal craniotomy and osteotomy for a tumor of the middle or posterior skull base. The optic nerves have been unroofed along with the orbits. Bone medial and inferior to the optic nerve has been removed to uncover the medial aspect of the anterior cavernous internal carotid artery. **C,** The potential exposure of the extended sub-frontal approach. The sphenoidal and clival exposure is limited by the internal carotid artery, Dorello's canal, and the hypoglossal canal on each side. **D,** Example of the reconstruction methods required following the extended subfrontal approach. Note the pericranial flap is positioned below the frontoorbital osteotomy, separating this osteotomy segment from the paranasal sinuses. (*From* Sen and Sekhar [30]; with permission.)

intradural and extradural tumors of the mid to lower clivus located anterior to the lower brain stem and upper cervical cord and is also suitable for vascular lesions of the distal vertebral artery and vertebrobasilar junction. Bertaliniffy and Seeger [24•] describe a dorsolateral-transcondylar approach used in six patients (three meningiomas) with intradural, ventrally placed lesions at the craniocervical junction. Sen and Sekhar [25•] update their experience using a similar approach in nine patients (three meningiomas). This approach, as described by the latter authors, is a direct lateral route with partial (one half to two thirds) removal of the condyle (and upper cervical hemilaminae, as necessary). Mobilization and transposition of the extradural-intradural course of the vertebral artery from the transverse (C-1 and C-2) foramen to the vertebral-basilar junction are possible by using a ringlike circumferential dural incision around the entrance point of the vertebral artery (Figure 2.6). Additional superior exposure is gained by using a mastoidectomy to obtain extradural and intradural control of the neurovascular structures of the jugular foramen and hypoglossal canal (Figure 2.7); a transjugular approach is possible when venous crossflow allows ligation of the sigmoid sinus. In a similar manner, lower to mid clival lesions are accessible up to the level of the internal auditory meatus. Careful reconstruction and duraplasty are required for extensive tumors with dural involvement

(eg, meningiomas). Single-stage stabilization by occipital-cervical arthrodesis is feasible, if necessary. Cerebrospinal fluid fistulae and septic complications associated with approaches that transgress the aerodigestive tract (eg, transoral, transpalatal, transmaxillary) are avoided. Despite the complexity of the approach, excellent exposure of the ventral aspect of the craniocervical junction is possible without requiring retraction of the brain stem.

Cranial nerve reconstruction

Sekhar and colleagues [26•] reported on 14 patients with cavernous sinus tumors (12 meningiomas) requiring reconstruction of cranial nerves following tumor resection. Fibrous, adherent tumors encasing cranial nerves, prior surgery, and radiation were most commonly associated with nerve injury. Generally with intraoperative injury or section of cranial nerves (III, V, and VI), reconstruction was attempted in those patients with good preoperative function. The authors describe technical details in 16 reconstructions with direct resuture performed in five patients and interposition nerve graft in 11. Donor grafts were taken from the sural (eight), great auricular (two), or supraorbital (one) nerves. Partial or complete recovery occurred in 13 of 16 patients (cranial nerves III, two of two; IV, one of one; V, four of four; VI, six of nine) within a follow-up interval of 10 to 60 months. A useful ocular motility

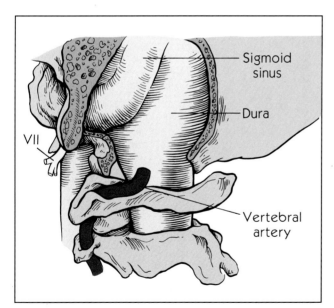

Figure 2.6

Extent of bony removal for predominantly suboccipital tumor (cervical tumors require resection of the lateral mass of C-1 or C-2). Note that the occipital condyle has been partially removed to provide access to the anterior rim of the foramen magnum. (*From* Sen and Sekhar [25•]; with permission.)

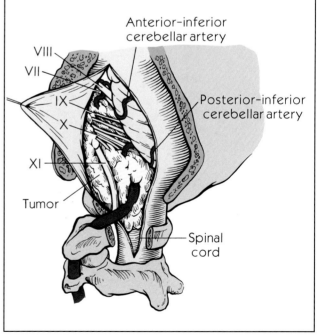

Figure 2.7

Complete mobilization of the vertebral artery in its extradural and intradural course facilitates its dissection from the tumor. (*From* Sen and Sekhar [25•]; with permission.)

classification system is introduced in the clinical assessment of binocular function. The authors emphasize the functional impact of various cranial nerve palsies, particularly those involving the third nerve (*eg*, aberrant regeneration, the cosmetic impact of ptosis) and neurotrophic keratitis associated with fifth nerve injury.

NONSURGICAL THERAPY

Focused beam irradiation: radiosurgery

Meningiomas are considered to be an ideal tumor type for radiosurgery, being distinct from normal brain; being accurately localized by computed tomography and MR scanning; and growing slowly, allowing time for cytotoxic and obliterative vascular effects to develop following radiation. Kondziolka and Lunsford [27•] updated their experience using stereotactic radiosurgical techniques (single-fraction, multiple photon beam irradiation) in 65 selected patients. They review their guidelines for therapy (size, < 35 mm average diameter; 5-mm clearance from optic nerve and chiasm) and present results and follow-up data from 3 to 36 months. They report a *growth control* rate of 95% for 2 years and reduction in tumor size in 13 of 25 (52%) patients with 12 to 34 months of follow-up. Two patients with poorly demarcated tumor borders had progressive growth beyond the irradiated field. A loss of central contrast enhancement (signifying necrosis) was seen in nine of 25 patients. Temporary deficits were reported in three patients, which resolved with a course of steroid therapy. The authors conclude that radiosurgery is an effective and safe form of therapy for selected patients with residual or recurrent meningiomas and an alternative primary treatment in patients in whom advanced age, medical condition, or high-risk tumor location preclude microsurgical resection.

Antiprogestin therapy

Meningiomas tend to be hormonally dependent, although not uniformly so. Progesterone acts to stimulate the mitogenic effect of various growth factors, and tumors with large numbers of progesterone receptors are potentially susceptible to modulation. Modulation of progesterone receptors (or the receptor protein) has been shown to inhibit tumor growth both *in vitro* and *in vivo*. Previous studies of hormonal manipulation in meningiomas using estrogen antago-

nists (tamoxifin), medroxyprogesterone (agonist and antagonist), and luteinizing hormone–releasing hormone analogues showed some effect, prompting further studies. Mifepristone (RU486), the first clinically available antiprogesterone agent, has been used by several investigators in stage II trials of efficacy. Grunberg and colleagues [28•] reported their experience using RU486 in the treatment of 14 patients with unresectable meningiomas. Five of 13 assessed patients had subjective and objective improvement, the latter involving clinical improvement (*eg*, ocular motility) or minor reduction in tumor volume as measured on diagnostic images (computed tomography and MR scanning). Three of the 13 patients had progressive growth during therapy, with two of these patients harboring malignant meningiomas. Side effects of the drug were well tolerated (consisting primarily of antiglucocorticosteroid effects), and 12 of 14 patients completed greater than or equal to 6 months of therapy. The authors conclude that long-term therapy with oral mifepristone is feasible and well tolerated by patients. They comment on the tendency of atypical and malignant meningiomas to have reduced, inactive, or absent progesterone receptors and to be unlikely to benefit from this form of therapy. They plan future studies to correlate clinical response with tumor pathology and progesterone receptor density. Lamberts and colleagues [29•] treated 10 patients (all women) with oral doses (200 mg/d) of mifepristone and were able to show symptomatic improvement in four of 10 patients but only minor effects on tumor growth. Three of 10 had a decrease in tumor volume (one only transiently); three of 10 were stable during the study period; and four of 10 had progressive growth (two patients died during therapy). They also note that aggressively growing recurrent tumors appear less susceptible to antiprogestin therapy.

CONCLUSIONS

Although surgical methods and perioperative management for basal meningiomas continue to improve results in patients with benign tumors, further substantive progress outside the surgical sphere awaits the development of new therapeutic methods for patients with recurrent tumors. Evidence is accumulating that despite the narrow histologic spectrum of meningiomas, inherent differences in proliferative indices, cytogenetic abnormalities, and cell receptors for the atypical and malignant meningioma forms offer clues to future management.

REFERENCES AND RECOMMENDED READING

Papers of particular interest, published within the annual period of review, have been highlighted as:
• Of special interest
•• Of outstanding interest

1. • Perrot-Applanat M, Groyer-Picard MT, Kujas M: Immunocytochemical study of progesterone receptor in human meningioma. *Acta Neurochir* 1992, 115:20–30.

This study of 36 patients with meningiomas (five of 36 were anaplastic) correlates proliferation (measured by Ki67 antigen) and progesterone receptors with clinical parameters and recurrence patterns.

2. • Meixensberger J, Caffier H, Naumann M, *et al.*: Sex hormone binding and peritumoural oedema in meningiomas: is there a correlation? *Acta Neurochir* 1992, 115:98–102.

Authors evaluate progesterone steroid receptor in 28 patients and correlate findings with peritumoral edema patterns using computed tomography and MR scanning. They found no significant association between edema patterns and progesterone receptor binding.

3. • Koper JW, Markstein R, Kohler C, *et al.*: Somatostatin inhibits the activity of adenylate cyclase in cultured human meningioma cells and stimulates their growth. *J Clin Endocrinol Metab* 1992, 74:543–547.

Authors find slight growth-stimulating effect of somatostatin (and analogues) on cultured meningiomas in contrast to a prior report of growth inhibition. They caution against use of somatostatin in meningiomas until further studies clarify the biologic effect *in vivo*.

4. • Schrell UM, Nomikos P, Fahlbusch R: Presence of dopamine D_1 receptors and absence of dopamine D_2 receptors in human cerebral meningioma tissue. *J Neurosurg* 1992, 77:288–294.

Authors report their continuing investigation of various receptors present in meningiomas; they describe their assay methods, confirm the presence of dopamine receptors, and postulate the physiologic role of this receptor in tumor growth.

5. • Lichtor T, Kurpakus M, Gurney M: Differential expression of IGF II in human meningiomas. *Neurosurgery* 1991, 29:405–410.

The authors investigate the geneic expression of IGF II in 10 tumors, reporting increasing expression in meningiomas (absent in gliomas), and discuss the physiologic role of this receptor in tumor biology.

6. • Smidt M, Dumanski JP, Collins VP, *et al.*: Structure and expression of the c-*sis* gene and its relationship to sporadic meningiomas. *Cancer Res* 1991, 51:4295–4298.

A brief report on 86 sporadic meningiomas evaluated for the c-*sis* protooncogene. The authors failed to demonstrate a previously described gene deletion associated with familial meningiomas.

7. • Sanson M, Richard S, Delattre O, *et al.*: Allelic loss on chromosome 22 correlates with histopathological predictors of recurrence of meningiomas. *Int J Cancer* 1992, 50:391–394.

The authors correlate the chromosomal aberrations in 22 meningiomas with histopathologic features and clinical recurrence.

8. • Arnoldus EP, Wolters LB, Voormolen JH, *et al.*: Interphase cytogenetics: a new tool for the study of genetic changes in brain tumors. *J Neurosurg* 1992, 76:997–1003.

The authors describe newer methodologies to investigate genetic aberrations of various tumors with the ultimate goal of identifying prognostic tumor markers and specific gene defects. The advantages of the in situ hybridization technique include ease and rapidity of analysis (2 days), no hazard to patients, and no requirement for tissue culture.

9. • Hoshino T, Ito S, Asai A, *et al.*: Cell kinetic analysis of human brain tumors by in situ double labeling with bromodeoxyuridine and iododeoxyuridine. *Int J Cancer* 1992, 50:1–5.

The authors describe their use of double-label proliferative index measures of meningiomas. A good discussion of the utility of the LI in predicting recurrence and the hazards of administration of halogenated pyrimidines in human subjects is given.

10. •• Shibuya M, Hoshino T, Ito S, *et al.*: Meningiomas: clinical implications of a high proliferative potential determined by bromodeoxyuridine labeling. *Neurosurgery* 1992, 30:494–497.

Excellent review and companion paper to Hoshino *et al.*'s update of the LI in 178 meningiomas (Hoshino *et al. Int J Cancer* 1992, 50:1–5). The report correlates the histologic findings and LI with recurrence and extent of surgery.

11. •• Sankila R, Kallio M, Jaaskelainen J, *et al.*: Long-term survival of 1986 patients with intracranial meningioma diagnosed from 1953 to 1984 in Finland: comparison of the observed and expected survival rates in a population-based series. *Cancer* 1992, 70:1568–1576.

Authors report further analysis of an extensive database on meningiomas collected by the Finnish Cancer Registry regarding long-term survival in 1986 patients to determine the excess mortality associated with intracranial meningiomas. Analysis compares the expected and observed 15-year survival using matched population controls.

12. • Kallio M, Sankila R, Hakulinen T, *et al.*: Factors affecting operative and excess long-term mortality in 935 patients with intracranial meningioma. *Neurosurgery* 1992, 31:2–12.

Companion paper to Sankila *et al.* (*Cancer* 1992, 70:1568–1576) identifying risk factors and relative mortality associated with intracranial meningiomas in 935 patients. They analyze short-term and long-term relative survival of patients undergoing surgical therapy.

13. •• Maier H, Öfner D, Hittmair A, *et al.*: Classic, atypical, and anaplastic meningioma: three histopathological subtypes of clinical relevance. *J Neurosurg* 1992, 77:616–623.

Excellent review correlating proliferative indices and meningioma histologic subtypes with clinical profiles, treatment methods, and recurrence patterns. They found that extent of removal and histologic subtypes were the most important factors predicting potential recurrence.

14. • Umansky F, Ashkenazi E, Gertel M, *et al.*: Surgical outcome in an elderly population with intracranial meningioma. *J Neurol Neurosurg Psychiatry* 1992, 55:481–485.

Authors review clinical outcome of 37 patients with a mean age of 74 undergoing surgery for symptomatic meningiomas; they conclude that age is not a significant factor determining outcome in selected patients.

15. • Golnik K, Miller N, Long D: Rate of progression and severity of neuroophthalmologic manifestations of cavernous sinus meningiomas. *Skull Base Surg* 1992, 2:129–133.

A longitudinal follow-up of patients with cavernous sinus tumors emphasizing the saltatory nature of ophthalmic signs that argues for a conservative approach in patients with stable visual neuropathy.

16. • Lindblom B, Truwit CL, Hoyt WF: Optic nerve sheath meningioma: definition of intraorbital, intracanalicular, and intracranial components with magnetic resonance imaging. *Ophthalmology* 1992, 99:560–566.

A careful review of the pathoanatomic forms of sheath meningiomas demonstrated by MR imaging.

17. • Demaerel P, Wilms G, Lammens M, *et al.*: Intracranial meningiomas: correlation between MR imaging and histology in fifty patients. *J Comput Assist Tomogr* 1992, 15:45–51.

A review describing the mixed results of attempts to classify meningiomas based on MR signal intensity.

18. • Kaplan R, Coons S, Drayer B, *et al.*: MR characteristics of meningioma subtypes at 1.5 Tesla. *J Comput Assist Tomogr* 1992, 16:366–371.

The authors present data on the accurate prediction of meningioma subtypes based on MR appearance correlated with histopathologic features.

19. • Larson JJ, Tew JJ, Wiot JG, *et al.*: Association of meningiomas with dural "tails": surgical significance. *Acta Neurochir* 1992, 114:59–63.

Authors describe the dural tail phenomenon in two patients and correlate MR images with histologic findings.

20. • Tien R, Yang P, Chu P: "Dural tail sign": a specific MR sign for meningioma? *J Comput Assist Tomogr* 1991, 15:64–66.

Retrospective review of 16 patients, including three new patients; the authors discuss the pathophysiology and causes associated with the dural tail sign.

21. • Terada T, Nakamura Y, Tsuura M, *et al.*: MRI changes in embolized meningiomas. *Neuroradiology* 1992, 34:162–167.

Authors describe decreased signal voids, loss of enhancement, and increased T_1 signal in meningiomas subjected to interventional techniques.

22. •• Sen C, Sekhar L: Direct vein graft reconstruction of the cavernous and upper cervical internal carotid artery: lessons learned from 30 cases. *Neurosurgery* 1992, 30:732–743.

The authors detail their experience in 30 direct vein bypass grafts for cranial base tumors (17 meningiomas). Excellent review of technique, indications, and analysis of complications.

23. • Sekhar L, Nanda A, Sen C, *et al.*: The extended frontal approach to tumors of the anterior, middle, and posterior skull base. *J Neurosurg* 1992, 76:198–206.

A detailed description of the authors' modification of the transbasal approach used in 49 patients. They review their indications, complications, and patient outcome in a variety of basal tumors.

24. • Bertalaniffy H, Seeger W: The dorsolateral, suboccipital, transcondylar approach to the lower clivus and anterior portion of the craniocervical junction. *Neurosurgery* 1992, 29:815–821.

A descriptive review of the authors' approach applied to meningiomas; their larger experience using the procedure in other lesions is referenced.

25. • Sen C, Sekhar L: Surgical management of anteriorly placed lesions at the craniocervical junction: an alternative approach. *Acta Neurochir* 1991, 108:70–77.

The authors describe their experience in nine cases using the lateral-transcondylar approach, a valuable surgical technique for a difficult and hazardous tumor location.

26. • Sekhar LN, Lanzino G, Sen CN, *et al.*: Reconstruction of the third through sixth cranial nerves during cavernous sinus surgery. *J Neurosurg* 1992, 76:935–943.

A brief report describing reconstruction methods and results in 14 patients with cavernous sinus tumors. Thirteen of 16 nerves had partial or complete recovery.

27. • Kondziolka D, Lunsford LD: Radiosurgery of meningiomas. *Neurosurg Clin North Am* 1992, 3:219–230.

The authors analyze results of radiosurgery in 65 patients (57 of 65 with basal meningiomas), 19 of whom received radiation as primary treatment. They report a tumor control rate of 95% at 2 years and review their observed complications using this treatment method.

28. • Grunberg S, Weiss M, Spitz I, *et al.*: Treatment of unresectable meningiomas with the antiprogesterone agent mifepristone. *J Neurosurg* 1991, 74:861–866.

The authors report on the generally positive initial results of antiprogestin (RU486) therapy of 14 patients with unresectable meningiomas, including two patients with malignant tumors.

29. • Lamberts S, Koper JW, Reubi JC, *et al.*: Endocrine aspects of the diagnosis and treatment of primary brain tumours: review. *Clin Endocrinol* 1992, 37:1–10.

The authors describe the mixed results of antiprogestin therapy in 10 patients, showing limited or transient benefit in six of 10 patients and progressive growth in four of 10. Their population of patients had aggressive tumors, including a patient with neurofibromatosis, and they discuss their analysis of the limited response to therapy.

30. Sen C, Sekhar L: Extended subfrontal approach to the skull base. In *Neurosurgical Operative Atlas*, vol 2, no 2. Edited by Rengachary S, Wilkins R. Baltimore: Williams & Wilkins; 1992:97–106.

Chapter 3

Cavernous Sinus Surgery

Kyu Man Shin
Ossama Al-Mefty

As early as 1895, Krogius [1] operated directly on the cavernous sinus to remove an endothelioma. Nearly 70 years later, Parkinson [2] first reported using a direct surgical approach to the cavernous sinus for a carotid cavernous fistula, laying the foundation for the modern era of cavernous sinus surgery based on a comprehensive study of surgical anatomy. Parkinson's surgery was performed on a hypothermic patient with cardiac arrest, however, and his technique did not gain wide acceptance. Consequently, the cavernous sinus remained a formidable area for surgeons who feared injuring the carotid artery or cranial nerves and profuse bleeding from the venous sinus. Dolenc [3], however, reported directly repairing intracavernous lesions with an acceptable rate of operative morbidity and mortality.

With the advent of direct intracavernous surgery, neoplastic and vascular lesions of the cavernous sinus are now amenable to direct surgical approaches [4–9]. Unfortunately, no conclusive data exist concerning the effectiveness, morbidity, and long-term results of the various therapeutic means available for cavernous lesions, whether conservative, surgical, endovascular, or irradiation modalities. Consequently, treatment is currently tailored according to factors related to the patient, the lesion, and the surgeon's expertise [4].

PATIENT SELECTION

Patient selection is the most crucial and highly debatable issue concerning direct surgery of the cavernous sinus. A direct operative approach to the cavernous sinus is indicated when it is anticipated that the lesion can be removed. Parkinson and West [8] believe that a preoperative diagnosis of only aneurysms, meningiomas, or neurofibromas justifies a direct surgical approach to the cavernous sinus. Zozulia and colleagues [10] reported on 247 tumors involving the cavernous sinus (160 meningiomas and 80 pituitary tumors) and concluded that tumors involving only the lateral wall of the sinus could be removed surgically.

The major risk of cavernous sinus surgery arises from injury to the carotid artery and subsequent cerebral ischemia. Frequently, patient selection depends heavily on the preoperative confirmation of adequate collateral circulation to prevent ischemia if the intracavernous carotid artery is occluded. This preoperative evaluation includes a balloon carotid occlusion test with measurement of cerebral blood flow. Patients who clinically tolerate the occlusive test and maintain blood flow above 35 mL/100 g/min are considered likely to tolerate permanent carotid occlusion [9]. The authors give more weight to the patient's benefit from cavernous sinus surgery, however, than the mere grading of surgical risk. At present, we do not perform or advocate direct surgery of the cavernous sinus for patients with highly malignant tumors such as nasopharyngeal carcinoma and squamous carcinoma of the paranasal sinus. We have limited experience with en bloc resection including the cavernous sinus area [11•]. A longer follow-up period and greater experience are necessary before a conclusion can be reached about this technique. Less aggressive lesions, such as chordomas and chondrosarcomas, are recommended for surgical removal [9,12].

Among benign tumors, schwannomas warrant aggressive surgical removal and yield the best results (Demonte F, Al-Mefty O: Surgery of benign tumors of the cavernous sinus. Paper presented at the First International Skull Base Congress, Hannover, Germany, 1992). Although some authors have reservations about the successful removal of meningiomas [6,13], we pursue their aggressive removal (Figure 3.1), acknowledging that some meningiomas lack intervening dissecting planes and adhere directly to the carotid adventitia. In patients with this type of tumor, total removal may not be possible [14••]. Prolactinomas involving the cavernous sinus may be best treated initially with bromocriptine. Other pituitary tumors require thorough evaluation to compare the long-term outcome of direct surgery with the effects of radiation therapy.

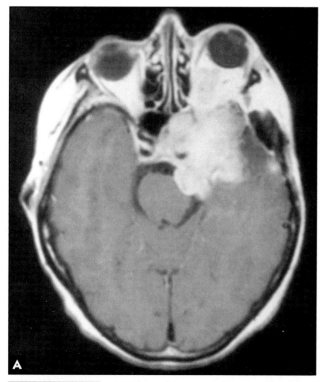
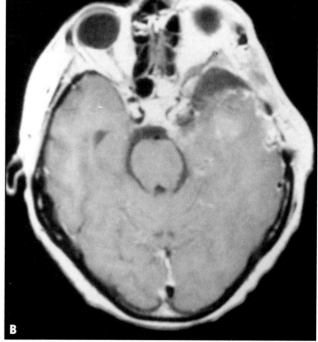

Figure 3.1

A, Preoperative magnetic resonance image of a meningioma invading the cavernous sinus. **B,** Image after total removal.

Craniopharyngiomas, myxochondrofibromas, and hemangiomas are indications for a surgical approach; frequently, however, the diagnosis is made during surgery. Juvenile angiofibromas and other rare lesions invade the cavernous sinus but remain extradural and may be approached extradurally [15•]. Direct clipping of ophthalmic aneurysms has become routine because of better knowledge about anatomy and advancements in cavernous sinus surgery [16,17]. In patients with giant intracavernous aneurysms, the surgeon stands at a crossroads in selecting the optimal treatment from the competitive modalities of endovascular techniques [18–20], direct aneurysmal reconstruction, or a venous bypass graft [21,22]. Benign bilateral lesions and asymptomatic tumors require an individualized decision.

PREOPERATIVE EVALUATION

After preoperative clinical evaluation, including neurologic, ophthalmologic, and endocrinologic assessment, patients are studied using thin-section computed tomography with soft tissue and bony windows in axial and coronal planes. Three-dimensional recon-struction is useful for assessing bony lesions and is employed for certain patients. Magnetic resonance (MR) images with and without gadolinium enhancement are obtained in axial, coronal, and sagittal planes in all patients. These images show the precise location of the tumor and identify structures around the sinus. Because meningiomas frequently have a low signal, the injection of gadolinium can help define the tumor [23••]. The relationship between the internal carotid artery and an enhanced meningioma is superbly recognized after the use of contrast medium [24]. Enhancement of the pituitary gland can partially obscure borders the gland might share with tumors. Although the internal carotid artery is easily seen on MR images, detailed study using angiography is still necessary for planning the surgical approach.

Cerebral angiography with cross-compression studies defines the anatomy of the cerebral circulation and assesses potential collateral circulation and the vascularity of a tumor. Clinical and physiologic evaluations are obtained with a carotid balloon occlusion test and concomitant evaluation of cerebral blood flow (Figure 3.2). To avoid the ischemic complications of a balloon occlusion test, an alternative method of evaluation using carotid compression with transcra-

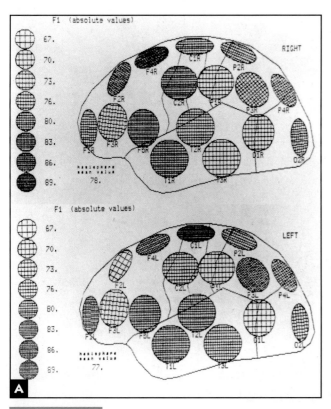 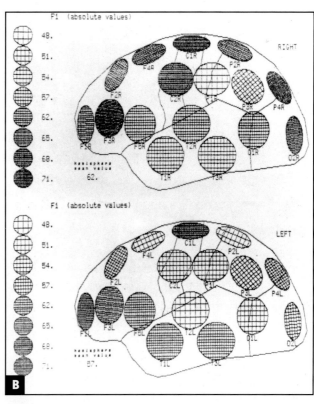

Figure 3.2

Evaluation of cerebral blood flow. **A,** Baseline measurements. **B,** Measurement during carotid compression shows decreased blood flow. Circular patterns represent location of the brain probes; corresponding numbers indicate the flow measured in mL/100 g/min.

nial Doppler studies and concomitant scans of single-photon emission computed tomography is currently under investigation. The purpose of this collateral evaluation is to make the surgeon and the patient aware of the degree of risk involved and what the surgeon can and cannot do to the carotid artery. It should not, however, be the sole reason to proceed with or to deny the patient direct cavernous sinus surgery.

SURGICAL APPROACHES

The cavernous sinus is easily reached through several cranial approaches, the subtemporal [8], the pterional [3], and the transsphenoidal. The transsphenoidal approach, however, offers only restrictive exposure and does not allow proximal and distal control of the

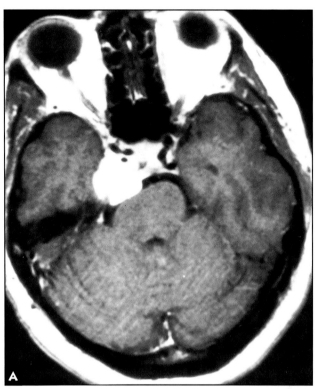

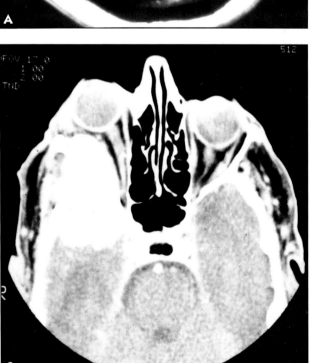

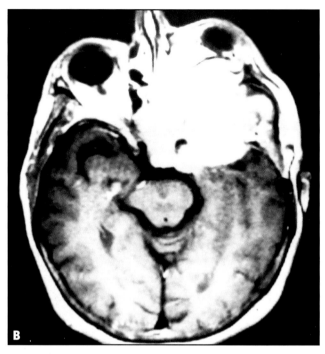

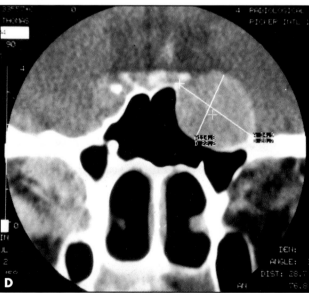

Figure 3.3

A through **C,** Magnetic resonance images of a meningioma in the cavernous sinus. **C,** Computed tomographic scan of a schwannoma. These lesions are best exposed through the cranioorbital zygomatic approach.

internal carotid artery. The authors use one of the skull base approaches, depending on the nature and extent of the lesion.

The cranioorbital zygomatic approach provides superb access to vascular and neoplastic lesions of the cavernous sinus [7,25]. Figure 3.3 shows an example of lesions optimally exposed through this approach. Occasionally tumors extending into the petroclival area and posterior fossa are better exposed through the petrosal approach [26••]. The zygomatic approach [27] is suitable for tumors located in the infratemporal fossa and involving the cavernous sinus. With this approach, dissection can be entirely extradural for some tumors, such as angiofibromas involving the cavernous sinus. Over the past 8 years, we have used the cranioorbital zygomatic approach predominantly because of its advantages of minimal brain retraction and easy dissection through the subfrontal, transsylvian, and subtemporal areas. The single bone flap includes the superior and lateral orbital rim attached to the frontal and temporal bones.

SURGICAL TECHNIQUE

Cranioorbital zygomatic flap

For the cranioorbital zygomatic approach, the patient is placed supine, and a spinal drainage needle is inserted. The patient's head is rotated 30° to 40° to the opposite side, dropped toward the floor, tilted 5° to 10°, and fixed in the Mayfield head rest.

A bicoronal incision is made behind the hairline, extending from the zygomatic arch on the side of the lesion to the superior temporal line on the opposite side (Figure 3.4). The scalp is turned, preserving the superficial temporal artery. The two layers of superficial fascia of the temporal muscle are cut parallel to the zygomatic arch (subfascial incision) and dissected from the muscle fiber. This maneuver preserves the frontal branches of the facial nerve, which are superficial to this fascial plane and are kept along with the fat pad and skin flap.

The pericranium is incised as posteriorly as possible; the large pericranial flap is reflected forward over the scalp flap. Its intact base is dissected free from the roof and lateral wall of the orbit. This vascularized flap is crucial for repairing the floor of the frontal fossa and covering the frontal and ethmoidal sinuses at closure to avoid leakage of cerebrospinal fluid. The zygomatic arch is dissected in a subperiosteal fashion and is incised at its most anterior and posterior ends. The cuts are made obliquely so the zygomatic arch can be anchored during attachment. The zygoma is displaced downward with its masseter attachment. The temporalis muscle is detached from its insertion anteriorly down to the zygomatic arch. The muscle is then retracted posteriorly and inferiorly, exposing the junction of the zygomatic, sphenoidal, and frontal bones.

Three entry holes are required to remove the

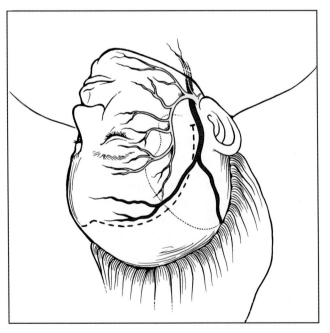

Figure 3.4

The patient's position and the skin incision (*dotted line*) in relation to the superficial temporal artery and branches of the facial nerve. (*From* Al-Mefty [14••]; with permission.)

supraorbital-pterional flap (Figure 3.5). The first and most important hole placed is the keyhole. This is made in the temporal fossa just medial to the frontozygomatic suture. The upper half of the bur hole should expose the dura mater of the frontal fossa, while the lower half exposes the periorbita. These two membranes are separated by the roof of the orbit. From this vantage point, an osteotomy is made in the orbital roof, extending medially. Then, while protecting the periorbita with a brain spatula, an osteotomy is made through the lateral wall of the orbit, extending from the keyhole to the level of the inferior orbital fissure. The inferior extension of this osteotomy is then connected to an osteotomy extending through the lateral orbital margin just superior to the malar prominence.

At this point, a second hole is placed in the inferior-posterior portion of the squamous temporal bone just superior to the base of the zygomatic arch. Using a high-speed drill with a foot attachment, an osteotomy is made extending anteriorly along the base of the temporal fossa to the sphenoid ridge. The bone of the sphenoid ridge is removed using a high-speed drill.

The last hole is placed in the frontal bone immediately above the superior orbital rim, slightly lateral to the midline. For cosmetic reasons, this hole should be kept small. In adults, the frontal sinus is almost certainly entered, and its anterior and posterior walls must be perforated.

Extending from this hole and through both walls of the frontal sinus, an osteotomy is carried inferiorly and medially into the orbital roof. The posterior-inferior temporal bur hole is then connected to the frontal hole using the foot attachment of the drill, passing 4 cm above the supraorbital rim. At this point, the flap is freed by controlled fracture of the remaining portion of the orbital roof. The mucosa of the frontal sinus is exenterated, and the sinus is cranialized (the posterior wall is removed) and plugged with muscle. All instruments used to handle the sinus mucosa are disposed of, and the surgical team redresses.

The orbital flap then is created with two cuts. The first is a medial cut in the roof of the orbit, extending posteriorly along the ethmoid but without entering the ethmoid sinus. The second cut is made at the base of the lateral wall along the inferior orbital fissure. The two cuts are then connected (Figure 3.6). The orbital flap is reattached to the cranial flap at the end of the procedure to reconstruct the bony orbit and avoid enophthalmos or pulsating exophthalmos.

UNLOCKING THE CAVERNOUS SINUS

With rare exception, safe surgery in the cavernous sinus is difficult without gaining proximal and distal control of the internal carotid artery. The cavernous sinus thus is "unlocked" through two steps, exposing the intrapetrous carotid and the subclinoid carotid segment. An alternative method of gaining proximal control is to expose the internal carotid artery in the neck.

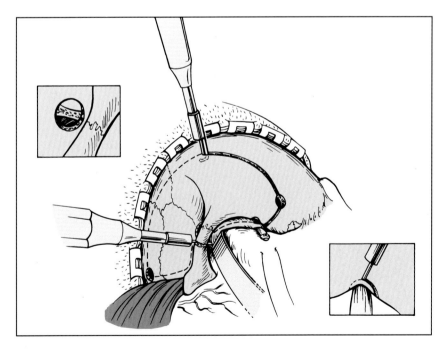

Figure 3.5

The cranioorbital zygomatic approach. A craniotome connects the frontal and posterior temporal bur holes. The line of connection between the temporal and keyhole bur holes is shown, and the bony incision along the roof of the orbit is defined. The lateral orbital rim is incised with a high-speed drill. **Left inset,** The position of the keyhole. **Right inset,** The supraorbital nerve is freed from its foramen. (*From* Al-Mefty [14••]; with permission.)

EXPOSURE OF THE INTRAPETROUS CAROTID ARTERY

Glasscock's triangle is the important landmark [28] in which the intrapetrous carotid artery is exposed to obtain proximal control. Starting posteriorly and working forward, the dura of the temporal fossa is elevated from the floor. The foramen spinosum is identified, and the middle meningeal artery is coagulated and sectioned. The greater and lesser superficial petrosal nerves are identified and sectioned with microscissors, preventing traction that could paralyze the facial nerve. The horizontal portion of the petrous internal carotid artery is deep, parallel to the greater superficial petrosal nerve, and posterior to the mandibular division of the trigeminal nerve (Figure 3.7).

The internal carotid artery is unroofed for a length of 1 to 1.5 cm with a diamond drill. The artery is mobilized and prepared for temporary clipping when necessary. In perhaps one half of patients [29], the bony canal is deficient and only the artery is covered with periosteum; this portion of the internal carotid artery is exposed when the dura is elevated. The geniculate ganglion of the facial nerve, lying just posterolateral to the exposed area, should be spared injury. The eustachian tube lies lateral to the intrapetrous carotid artery under the tensor tympani muscle. This tube may be opened to expose the lateral aspect of the

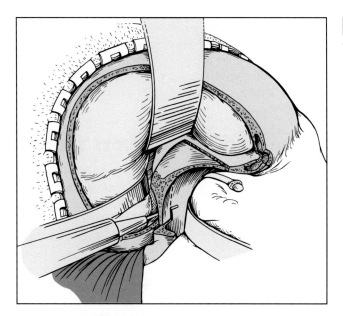

Figure 3.6

The steps to remove the orbital flap.

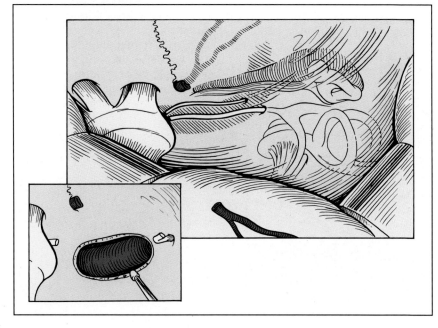

Figure 3.7

The anatomic relationship during surgical exposure of the intrapetrous carotid artery in Glasscock's triangle. The course of the carotid artery, facial nerve, tensor tympani muscle, eustachian tube, and the middle and inner ear are outlined. The epidural landmarks are clearly seen. **Inset,** The greater petrosal nerve is cut, and the bone is drilled to expose the horizontal segment of the carotid artery.

artery better. If it is opened, the eustachian tube is closed with a piece of fascia at the end of the operation to avoid leakage of cerebrospinal fluid. A myringotomy may be necessary during the patient's postoperative course.

EXPOSING THE SUBCLINOID SEGMENT OF THE INTERNAL CAROTID ARTERY

The subclinoid segment of the internal carotid artery is exposed by drilling away the anterior clinoid process, the optic canal, and the remainder of the superior orbital fissure, using the diamond bit of a high-speed air drill (Figure 3.8). This can be performed epidurally [16,30••], or after opening the dura and directly visualizing the optic nerve and carotid artery [7,31]. We prefer the extradural removal for patients with tumors.

Removing an orbital bone flap leaves only a small area over the optic canal and a rim of bone at the superior orbital fissure to be opened. The optic nerve is prepared for mobilization by drilling the bony roof of the optic canal. Because it can be damaged by the heat generated during drilling, the nerve must be protected with constant irrigation. The superior orbital fissure also is opened by drilling the rim of bone from the lesser sphenoid wing, exposing the dura of the superior orbital fissure. The anterior clinoid process is removed by drilling the inferior strut of the lesser sphenoid wing beneath the optic nerve. The subcli-

noid segment of the internal carotid artery is extradural and also outside the cavernous sinus; it is marked by the proximal and distal carotid rings, which correspond to the exit point of the carotid artery from the cavernous sinus and its entry into the intradural space, respectively (Figure 3.8).

DURAL OPENING

The dural incision is centered on the pterion and extended in a semicircular fashion. The frontal and temporal lobes are separated by opening the sylvian fissure. Thus, the parasellar area and the roof of the cavernous sinus are exposed. The dural sheath of the optic nerve is incised along the length of the optic nerve from the falciform fold to the entire length of the canal (Figure 3.9). This permits further visualization of the superior aspect of the cavernous sinus and the internal carotid artery and exposes the ophthalmic artery and the anterior portion of the cavernous sinus.

ENTRY INTO THE CAVERNOUS SINUS

An understanding of the relationships among the anatomic structures of the cavernous sinus gives the surgeon a better understanding of the surgical approaches. The surgical anatomy of the skull base

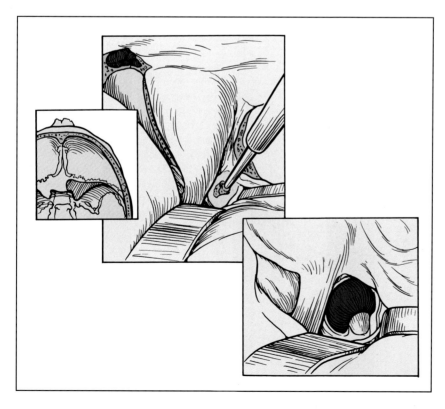

can be illustrated by the anatomic relationships of dural, osseous, neural, and vascular structures, identifying 10 triangles in the three subregions [6]. The parasellar region has four triangles: the anteromedial, paramedial, oculomotor, and Parkinson's. The middle cranial fossa also has four triangles: the anterolateral, lateral, posterolateral (Glasscock's), and posteromedial (Kawase's). The paraclival region has two triangles: the inferomedial and inferolateral (trigeminal).

The cavernous sinus can be entered through any of the windows or triangles mentioned, depending on the anatomic variation of the patient and the nature and location of the lesion. In most operative procedures, however, lateral and superior avenues through a cranial approach are the two main paths of entry to the sinus. These may be extended or combined depending on the nature of the lesion.

Entry through the superior aspect

After mobilizing the optic nerve, the distal dural ring anchoring the carotid artery as it enters the subdural cavity is opened; this opening is extended posteriorly to the third nerve, allowing superb entry to the cavernous sinus through its superior wall (Figure 3.9). Most tumors can be easily removed and dissected from the carotid artery as its course is followed in retrograde fashion. This exposure is enlarged by mobilizing the carotid artery laterally. The posterior clinoid process can be dissected from the dura and removed along with a portion of the dorsum sellae with a diamond drill to expose the upper clivus. This maneuver allows removal of tumors involving the upper petroclival area or large aneurysms of the basilar artery.

Tumors with an intrasellar origin or extension that involves the cavernous sinus, such as pituitary tumors and craniopharyngiomas, can be removed by expanding the superior approach medially. The approach can be expanded by drilling the planum sphenoidale after dissecting the dura over it. The sphenoid mucosa is removed. The pituitary gland and the medial aspect of the carotid artery can be visualized by incising the diaphragm sellae. Opening the sphenoid sinus, however, should be undertaken only when necessary, and full attention must be paid to plugging the sinus with fat, then covering the area with fascia to avoid leakage of cerebrospinal fluid.

Entry through the lateral aspect

The lateral approach to the cavernous sinus is through Parkinson's triangle, which is delineated by the fourth nerve as its medial border, the medial aspect of the first division of the trigeminal nerve as its lateral border, and the dura between these two nerves as its posterior border. This entry is the conventional avenue, especially for a lesion confined to the cavernous sinus. Through this triangle, the lateral surface of the horizontal bend can be exposed.

The free margin of the tentorium and the third and fourth cranial nerves are identified. The position of both nerves in the superior lateral wall of the cavernous sinus is relatively constant, but the fourth nerve is harder to identify because it courses below the third. An incision of about 8 mm both anteriorly and posteriorly is made beneath the projected course of the third nerve, centering on the point where this nerve appears over the horizon of the free margin of the tentorium. The outer layer of the lateral wall of the cavernous sinus is then peeled away from the first and second divisions of the trigeminal nerve. The inner layer of the lateral wall remains intact, and, up to this

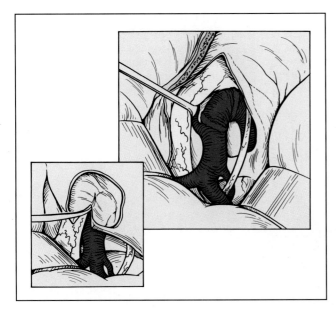

Figure 3.9

Entry through the superior aspect of the cavernous sinus. The optic nerve is mobilized medially. The superior wall is opened and the opening is extended posteriorly from the carotid ring to the third nerve. The carotid artery is followed into the cavernous sinus in retrograde fashion. **Inset,** The dura propria of the optic nerve is opened, as is the distal ring of the carotid artery.

point, venous bleeding is not encountered. A natural gap exists in the inner layer between the fourth nerve and the first division of the trigeminal nerve. This gap can be enlarged to expose the carotid artery and the sixth nerve on the lateral wall of the carotid artery (Figure 3.10) [8,32••]. The sixth nerve may have two divisions and is the only nerve coursing inside the sinus.

The lateral exposure can be enhanced by peeling the outer layer of the lateral wall posteriorly and infe-riorly to expose the third division and the trigeminal ganglion and opening Meckel's cave, allowing expo-sure of the posterior entrance of the carotid artery into the cavernous sinus.

The petrous tip medial to the carotid artery and anterior to the internal auditory meatus (Kawase's tri-angle) is drilled away, providing entry to the posterior fossa and exposing the posterior aspect of the cav-ernous sinus, particularly the sixth nerve's entry and

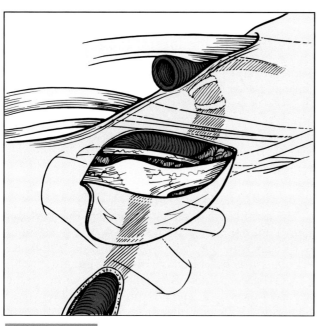

Figure 3.10

Entry into the cavernous sinus through the lateral aspect. The dura is peeled away over Parkinson's triangle between the third and fourth cranial nerves superiorly and V₁ inferiorly. Cranial nerve VI runs within the sinus, lateral to the carotid artery. The mobilized optic nerve (II) and the exposed intrapetrous carotid artery are demonstrated.

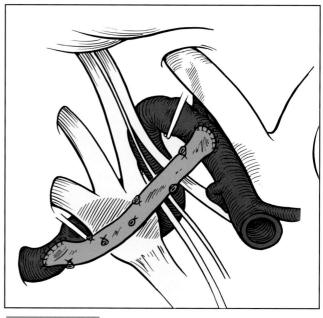

Figure 3.11

The bypass venous graft with end-to-side anastomosis at both ends. The intracavernous carotid artery is isolated between two permanent clips. (*From* Al-Mefty *et al.* [34]; with permission.)

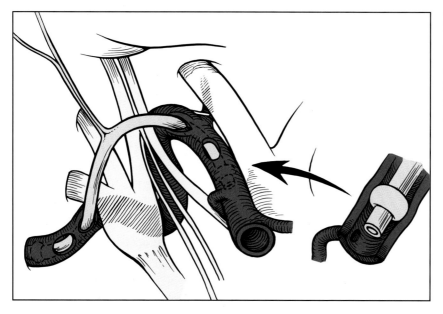

Figure 3.12

An intraluminal shunt with a double bal-loon catheter for a venous bypass graft of the cavernous sinus. The position of the balloons in the intrapetrous and supracli-noid carotid arteries is shown. (*From* Al-Mefty *et al.* [34]; with permission.)

Meckel's cave. To open the entire sinus, the lateral approach can be combined with the superior approach.

NEUROVASCULAR DISSECTION AND MANAGEMENT

A tumor in the cavernous sinus is dissected using the microscope and bipolar cautery along with microdissectors and microscissors. Venous hemorrhage is not encountered until the tumor is nearly removed because the tumor compresses the venous plexus. Profuse venous bleeding is easily controlled by elevating the patient's head and packing the sinus. The sixth cranial nerve should be carefully identified, dissected, and preserved. If any of the cranial nerves are severed during surgery, direct suture or an interpositioned graft should be carried out [32••,33••].

The major risk of cavernous sinus surgery stems from injury to the carotid artery. If the carotid wall is torn during dissection, the surgeon should be prepared to apply a temporary vascular clip of 30 to 40 g/mm^2 of pressure. A tear can be easily repaired through direct suture with 8–0 microsutures. If the injury is beyond direct repair, carotid reconstruction with a venous graft may be considered (Figure 3.11) to avoid the long-term effects of a permanently occluded artery [21]. A bypass shunt (Figure 3.12) used during the grafting procedure has been studied for patients who have poor collateral circulation and who do not tolerate the prolonged temporary occlusion needed for a carotid bypass venous graft [34].

REFERENCES AND RECOMMENDED READING

Papers of particular interest, published within the annual period of review, have been highlighted as:
• Of special interest
•• Of outstanding interest

1. Krogius A: Om operativ behandlund of tumoren i fossa media cranii. *Rev Chir* 1896, 16:434.

2. Parkinson D: A surgical approach to the cavernous portion of the carotid artery: anatomical studies and case report. *J Neurosurg* 1965, 23:474–483.

3. Dolenc VV: Direct microsurgical repair of intracavernous vascular lesions. *J Neurosurg* 1983, 58:824–831.

4. Al-Mefty O, Smith RR: Surgery of tumors invading the cavernous sinus. *Surg Neurol* 1988, 30:370–381.

5. Dolenc VV, ed: *The Cavernous Sinus: A Multidisciplinary Approach to Vascular and Tumorous Lesions.* Wien: Springer-Verlag; 1987.

6. Dolenc VV: *Anatomy and Surgery of the Cavernous Sinus.* Wien: Springer-Verlag; 1989.

7. Hakuba A, Tanaka K, Suzuki T, *et al.*: A combined orbitozygomatic infratemporal epidural and subdural approach for lesions involving the entire cavernous sinus. *J Neurosurg* 1989, 71:699–704.

8. Parkinson D, West M: Lesions of the cavernous plexus region. In *Neurological Surgery*, vol 5, 3rd ed. Edited by Youmans JR. Philadelphia: WB Saunders; 1990:3351–3370.

9. Sekhar LN, Sen CN, Jho HD, *et al.*: Surgical treatment of intracavernous neoplasms: a four-year experience. *Neurosurgery* 1989, 24:18–30.

10. Zozulia YA, Romodanov SA, Patsko YV: Diagnosis and surgical treatment of benign craniobasal tumours involving the cavernous sinus. *Acta Neurochir* 1979, 28(suppl):387–390.

11. • Origitano TC, Al-Mefty O, Leonetti JP, *et al.*: En bloc resection of an ethmoid carcinoma involving the orbit and medial wall of the cavernous sinus. Neurosurgery 1992, 31:1126–1131.
The authors report a successful en bloc resection of an invasive ethmoid carcinoma involving the cavernous sinus in a 46-year-old man.

12. Arnold H, Herrmann HD: Skull base chordoma with cavernous sinus involvement: partial or radical tumour-removal? *Acta Neurochir (Wien)* 1986, 83:31–37.

13. Lesoin F, Jomin M: Direct microsurgical approach to intracavernous tumors. *Surg Neurol* 1987, 28:17–22.

14. •• Al-Mefty O: Clinoidal meningiomas. In *Meningiomas.* Edited by Al-Mefty O. New York: Raven Press; 1991:427–443.
Clinoidal meningiomas were divided into three subgroups according to their relationship to interfacing arachnoid membranes, which influence surgical difficulty, the success of total removal, and the patient's outcome. Unless total removal is achieved, however, detrimental regrowth is expected in most patients.

15. • Anand VK, House JR, Al-Mefty O: Management of benign neoplasms invading the cavernous sinus. *Laryngoscope* 1991, 101:557–564.
The authors summarize their experience with unusual benign extracranial tumors invading the cavernous sinus for which a one-stage combined extracranial-intracranial approach was used.

16. Dolenc VV: A combined epi- and subdural direct

approach to carotid-ophthalmic artery aneurysms. *J Neurosurg* 1985, 62:667–672.

17. Day AL: Aneurysms of the ophthalmic segment: a clinical and anatomical analysis. *J Neurosurg* 1990, 72:677–691.

18. Diaz FG, Ohaegbulam S, Dujovny M, *et al.*: Surgical alternatives in the treatment of cavernous sinus aneurysms. *J Neurosurg* 1989, 71:846–853.

19. Barrow DL, Spector RH, Braun IF, *et al.*: Classification and treatment of spontaneous carotid-cavernous sinus fistulas. *J Neurosurg* 1985, 62:248–256.

20. Linskey ME, Sekhar LN, Hirsch Jr WL, *et al.*: Aneurysms of the intracavernous carotid artery: natural history and indications for treatment. *Neurosurgery* 1990, 26:933–937.

21. Sekhar LN, Sen CN, Jho HD: Saphenous vein graft bypass of the cavernous internal carotid artery. *J Neurosurg* 1990, 72:35–41.

22. Spetzler RF, Fukushima T, Martin N, *et al.*: Petrous carotid-to-intradural carotid saphenous vein graft for intracavernous giant aneurysm, tumor, and occlusive cerebrovascular disease. *J Neurosurg* 1990, 73:496–501.

23. •• Zimmerman RD: MRI of intracranial meningiomas. In *Meningiomas.* Edited by Al-Mefty O. New York: Raven Press; 1991:209–223.

With MR imaging, the signal void produced by flowing blood contrasts highly with the adjacent soft tissue of the tumor. This high contrast, combined with the absence of bone artifact and multiplanar imaging, superbly delineates large vascular structures. Thus, displacement, encasement, narrowing, and occlusion of the carotid artery or its proximal branches or dural venous sinuses can be identified without angiography.

24. Bradac GB, Riva A, Schönner W, *et al.*: Cavernous sinus meningiomas: an MRI study. *Neuroradiology* 1987, 29:578–581.

25. Al-Mefty O: *Surgery of the Cranial Base.* Boston: Kluwer Academic; 1989.

26. •• Al-Mefty O, Smith RR: Clival and petroclival meningiomas. In *Meningiomas.* Edited by Al-Mefty O. New York: Raven Press; 1991:517–537.

The petrosal approach described herein is centered on the petrous bone, allowing exposure of the tumor from the middle fossa to the foramen magnum.

27. Al-Mefty O, Anand VK: Zygomatic approach to skull-base lesions. *J Neurosurg* 1990, 73:668–673.

28. Glasscock III ME: Exposure of the intrapetrous portion of the carotid artery. In *Disorders of the Skull Base Region.* Edited by Hamburger C-A, Wersall J. New York: John Wiley; 1969:135–143.

29. Inoue T, Rhoton AL Jr, Theele D, *et al.*: Surgical approaches to the cavernous sinus: a microsurgical study. *Neurosurgery* 1990, 26:903–932.

30. •• Al-Mefty O: Management of the cavernous sinus and carotid siphon. *Otolaryngol Clin North Am* 1991, 24:1523–1533.

As a guide to treatment of the cavernous sinus and carotid siphon, the author explains the rationale for direct surgery of the cavernous sinus. Patient selection, preoperative evaluation, and operative techniques are described in detail.

31. Patouillard P, Vanneuville G: Les parois du sinus caverneux. *Neurochirurgie* 1972, 18:551–560.

32. •• Al-Mefty O, Ayoubi S: Neurovascular reconstruction during and after skull base surgery. In *Neurosurgeons: Proceedings of the 10th Annual Meeting of the Japanese Congress of Neurological Surgeons.* Edited by Sato K. Tokyo: Japanese Congress of Neurological Surgeons; 1991:286–298.

The authors describe various techniques to protect and reconstruct the neural and vascular structures during surgery of the skull base.

33. •• Sekhar LN, Lanzino G, Sen CN, *et al.*: Reconstruction of the third through sixth cranial nerves during cavernous sinus surgery. *J Neurosurg* 1992, 76:935–943.

The authors analyze the results of 16 reconstructive procedures involving the third through sixth cranial nerves performed in 14 patients. Recovery of function, either partial or complete, was observed in 13 cases. These results suggest that repair of nerves injured during surgery should be attempted in suitable patients.

34. Al-Mefty O, Khalil N, Elwany MN, *et al.*: Shunt for bypass graft of the cavernous carotid artery: an anatomical and technical study. *Neurosurgery* 1990, 27:721–728.

Chapter 4

Recent Advances and Future Directions in Interstitial Brachytherapy

Michael Salcman

Interstitial brachytherapy has emerged as one of the most exciting therapeutic options in the management of benign and malignant brain tumors. Its use in the treatment of malignant gliomas is based on a number of assumptions, which include the greater sensitivity of glial tumors to escalating doses of radiation, the necessity to spare the surrounding brain from the toxic effects of radiotherapy, and the belief that malignant astrocytoma is a local disease in which recurrence is almost always regional. Enthusiasm for brachytherapy also is based on its eminent suitability as a component of combined modality therapy, the extensive clinical experience already available in the use of radiation in the treatment of glial tumors, and the ease of implementing a brachytherapy program with present technology.

Problems raised by the relative radioresistance of some cell compartments within glioblastoma, an aspect of this tumor's extreme biologic heterogeneity, and the relatively few patients who are suitable for implantation have not blunted the optimism of most clinical investigators. Nevertheless, a number of alternative technologies to brachytherapy are already being studied in clinical trials; these include intraoperative endocurietherapy, stereotactic radiosurgery, and fractionated stereotactic radiotherapy. For the time being, however, interstitial radiation in most clinics is now the single most effective rescue therapy in selected patients with recurrent brain tumors; its role in the primary treatment of newly diagnosed patients remains to be defined. This chapter is restricted to recent advances in brachytherapy and a personal perspective on its methodology and future direction.

EXPERIMENTAL STUDIES

Neurosurgical therapies are not infrequently first evaluated in clinical trials without critical information available from laboratory studies, sometimes because of the desperate nature of the disease being treated, often because of the comfort level we have with the modality being employed, and occasionally because of the difficulty involved in replicating the clinical situation in an experimental model. Such has been the case with brachytherapy until recent years, when a few animal and tissue culture studies have provided guidelines on tumor and tissue sensitivity to low dose

rate irradiation. A controlled trial in the avian sarcoma virus tumor model in the rat failed to demonstrate the superiority of brachytherapy to conventional external radiation or teletherapy [1]. Animals receiving interstitial radioactive iodine (^{125}I) seeds that were exposed to a median dose of 7123 cGy did significantly better than animals implanted with dummy seeds or those that were left untreated. The total comparison dose for external radiation, however, was only 3000 cGy. In a study of 9L tumor cells transplanted into F344 rats, the increased survival produced by bischloroethylnitrosourea (BCNU) alone was more impressive than the results obtained with ^{125}I seeds; however, the combination of interstitial radiation and chemotherapy was the most effective treatment of all [2]. Recent *in vitro* studies have shown that radiation combined with hyperthermia, chemotherapy, or both modalities is more effective in the treatment of human and canine glioma cells than radiation alone [3••].

A study of low dose rate radiotherapy in rats implanted with the 9L gliosarcoma confirmed the assumption that tumor control is highly dependent on both the dose rate (*ie*, Gy/h) and the total dose (Gy) delivered to the tumor [4]. The most effective tumor control was observed at 120 cGy/h to a total tumor dose of 40 Gy with acceptable sparing of normal tissues; 40 cGy/h was the threshold dose rate for achieving significant tumor control in 50% of the animals at a total dose of 100 Gy. Of course, as the total dose increased, so did the incidence of harmful effects in normal tissue. Coagulative necrosis is often observed at a total dose of 200 to 300 Gy, and break-

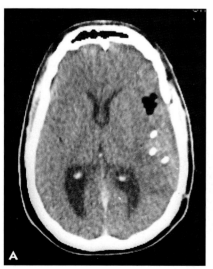 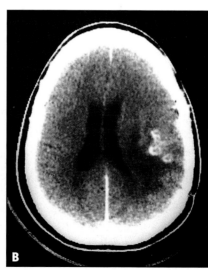

Figure 4.1

Radiographic demonstration of a blood-brain barrier change due to interstitial radiation. **A,** Axial scan performed on the day of surgery shows an L-shaped implantation that was carried out with three after-loading catheters. **B,** Six weeks later, an enhanced axial scan demonstrates breakdown of the blood-brain barrier at each catheter site.

down of the blood-brain barrier has been detected at a total dose of 130 to 165 Gy [5•]. Damage to the blood-brain barrier appears to progress during the first 6 months after implantation and stabilizes or decreases thereafter (Figure 4.1). This time course approximates the median length of time required for the onset of mass effect that requires surgical debulking for radionecrosis in most clinical trials.

TREATMENT OF RECURRENT TUMORS

Interstitial radiation has been used in the treatment of recurrent brain tumors for more than seven decades [6,7]. Although quite extensive, the early experience in some European centers was poorly controlled and the results often difficult to interpret by tumor type and other prognostic factors. Contemporary clinical interest in brachytherapy has been based on the experience of the group at the University of California in San Francisco (UCSF) [8]. In 95 patients with recurrent gliomas, ^{125}I implants were used to deliver a total dose of 5270 to 15,000 cGy at a maximum distance of 0.5 cm outside the enhancing rim. Up to six catheters were employed at a dose rate of 40 to 60 cGy/h to the periphery. The median additional survival for the 50 patients with anaplastic astrocytoma was 81 weeks, with a median of 54 weeks observed in the 45 patients with glioblastoma multiforme. The quality of survival was generally acceptable, and the longest survivals were obtained in those patients who required reoperation for radionecrosis (49%). It is possible that the tumors of reoperated patients were more effectively treated because the patients were

taken to the edge of toxicity; it should also be remembered that reoperation has an independent beneficial effect on the length of survival [9]. The UCSF patients were selected for implantation based on a maximum tumor diameter of less than 6 cm but only if the tumor was not diffuse in nature and did not involve the corpus callosum, the infratentorial space, the subependymal region, or more than one focus. These geometric criteria have largely been adopted by subsequent investigators, and similar results have been obtained with either ^{125}I or iridium (^{192}Ir).

A median survival of 10 months has been observed in patients with glioblastoma multiforme regardless of whether the tumor was treated up front or at recurrence [10]. The median survival was 11 months in the 41 implants carried out with ^{192}Ir in a series of 39 patients who had recurrent anaplastic astrocytoma. The reoperation rate was only 9%. Favorable prognostic criteria included a patient age of less than 50 years, a total dose less than 100 Gy, complete surgical resection before implantation, and non–glioblastoma multiforme histology. When ^{125}I was used to deliver 70 Gy to 18 patients with recurrent gliomas, the median survival was 44 weeks [11•]. The results obtained in our clinic have been similar. The survival curve for 37 patients implanted with ^{192}Ir for recurrent malignant astrocytoma indicates a median additional survival of 34 weeks, or more than 8 months (Figure 4.2).

The list of criteria used in the selection of patients to be entered into clinical trials has been quite extensive. In addition to the geometric factors previously mentioned, some investigators have avoided using implants near the motor strip, along the course of major vessels, or in the floor of the middle cranial

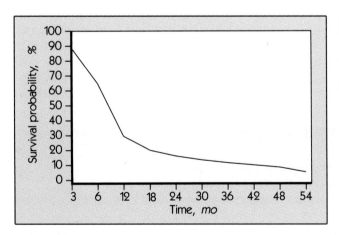

Figure 4.2

Survival curve for 37 patients with malignant astrocytoma who were implanted at recurrence. All patients were treated with ^{192}Ir; survival was calculated from the time of implantation to death. The median additional survival was 34 weeks.

fossa [10], whereas others have required that patients be less than 70 years of age and have a Karnofsky performance status greater than 70 [11•]. Despite every caution, complications have occurred, and reoperations have frequently been necessary (Table 4.1). The impact of patient selection on survival has been examined by comparing matched groups of patients deemed eligible or ineligible for brachytherapy [12••]. It was demonstrated that the total survival of eligible patients was significantly longer than that of ineligible patients (16.6 months vs 9.3 months) and that eligible patients were younger, had undergone larger resections, and had a better functional status. For glioblastoma alone, the survival differences between the two groups were even more striking (13.9 months vs 5.8 months). Because only one fourth to one third of all patients are even eligible for implantation, these results further amplify the necessity for controlled clinical trials in the field of brachytherapy research.

PRIMARY TREATMENT OF BRAIN TUMORS

Despite applicability to relatively few patients, the initial experience with the use of brachytherapy in the management of recurrent malignant astrocytoma has been reasonably favorable and has spurred interest in the use of this modality for the up-front treatment of newly diagnosed patients. In a series of 20 anaplastic astrocytomas implanted with ^{192}Ir, the results with primary therapy were superior to those obtained at recurrence until 28 months postimplantation, after which the two survival curves converged [10]. In another iridium trial, the median survival in 20 glioblastoma multiforme patients after up-front therapy was 14.5 months compared with a median of 15.5 months for nine patients with anaplastic astrocytoma [13]. Increasing the dose from 120 to 160 Gy did not further increase survival or local control, and those patients given a total dose of 16,000 cGy did worse than those receiving a total of 12,000 cGy. Once again,

patients were primarily selected with regard to performance status, age, tumor diameter, and tumor location. Three to eight catheters were employed at a dose rate of 80 to 100 cGy/h. In the largest clinical experience reported to date, 63 patients received 60 Gy of external radiation in combination with hydroxyurea chemotherapy, followed by a focal boost of 50 to 60 Gy from interstitial ^{125}I and six courses of chemotherapy with procarbazine, lomustine, and vincristine [14•]. Survival was clearly related to histology in this series because 29 patients with anaplastic astrocytoma achieved a median survival of 157 weeks compared with the 88-week survival observed in 34 patients with glioblastoma multiforme. The results are difficult to compare with those of other series because of the multiplicity of treatments used in addition to brachytherapy; once again, the best results were observed in those glioblastoma multiforme patients who required reoperation. Patients receiving interstitial radiation up front for newly diagnosed glioblastoma represent a highly selected group because fewer than one fourth of all glioblastoma multiforme patients are eligible; however, their 1- and 2-year survival rates of 87% and 57%, respectively, have been shown to be significantly better ($P < 0.001$) than those of matched controls [15•].

Brachytherapy has been employed on a number of occasions in the treatment of low-grade astrocytomas, especially in Europe. In a series of 89 patients with grade 1 or 2 gliomas of the brainstem, 26 received ^{192}Ir and 29 were implanted with ^{125}I [16]. The 5-year survival rate in the patients receiving ^{125}I was 54.8%, whereas it was only 26.9% after an iridium implant and 14.7% after biopsy alone. Similar results have been obtained in children with more rostral diencephalic tumors [17]. Further, a high degree of radiographic response has been observed in the brainstem gliomas of children permanently implanted with ^{125}I [18]. The clinical experience with nonglial tumors such as meningiomas and cartilaginous neoplasms is much more limited. Thirteen

Table 4.1
Incidence of complications and reoperation after brachytherapy in patients with glioblastoma and anaplastic astrocytoma

Study	Isotope	Patients, n	Dose to edge, cGy/h	Complications, %	Reoperations, %
Lucas et al. [10]	Ir	41	40	12	9
Leibel et al. [8]	I	95	40–60	7.3	49
Bernstein et al. [11•]	I	46	50	21.7	26.1
Salcman et al. [20]	Ir	33	100	NA	0
Chun et al. [13]	Ir	37	80–100	NA	24.3
Gutin et al. [14•]	I	63	40–60	NA	47

patients with skull-base meningiomas were treated with 100 to 500 Gy at a dose rate of 5 to 25 cGy/h with ^{125}I, and nine of the 11 patients without calcification achieved a complete response at a median follow-up of 15 months [19•]. A rare myxoid chondrosarcoma of the falx has been successfully treated with a permanent iodine implant after conventional radiation and reoperation failed to control the tumor [20].

METASTATIC BRAIN TUMORS

Individual cases of metastatic brain tumor have been included in virtually all of the pioneering studies of brachytherapy for recurrent lesions [10,11•]. In a group of 14 patients with progressive metastatic brain tumors, a median survival of 80 weeks has been observed after iodine implantation, even though nine of the patients were treated at recurrence [21].

COMPLICATIONS AND TREATMENT FAILURE

A purely local or regional therapy for a malignant brain tumor must fail if any one of the following conditions is met: 1) an inadequate dose is delivered to the target, 2) the tumor extends beyond the margins of the treatment volume, or 3) too high a dose is delivered to the normal surrounding tissue. Virtually all examples of treatment failure are due to violation of these three cardinal points, unless the tumor is inherently resistant to the modality employed against it. In the case of interstitial brachytherapy, the practical aspects of the principles of treatment failure include the radiation tolerance of the neural parenchyma and its blood supply, the intimate relationship of the infiltrating margins of the tumor to the surrounding brain, and limitations in our ability to image the margin of the lesion for treatment planning. The degree to which a primary glioma in an individual patient can be considered to be a strictly localized disease process is an issue of central importance.

Although the majority of treatment failures in one iridium implant series occurred locally at the treatment site (14 patients), six patients also had evidence of subependymal spread, and two had distant multicentric recurrences [13]. In a mixed group of 53 primary and recurrent glioma patients treated with iodine, eight of 22 failures occurred at the treatment margin, but 10 of the 22 occurred at more distant sites [22••]. The median survival after implantation was 18 months for the group as a whole. This pattern of treatment failure is consistent with what is known about the cytoarchitectonic structure of cerebral gliomas and the results of stereotactic biopsies in newly diagnosed patients [23,24]. Malignant gliomas have a tendency to spread along deep white matter tracts such as the association fibers of a single hemisphere and the corpus callosum contralaterally. Isolated malignant cells are frequently detected several centimeters from the enhancing rim of the tumor. Hence, it is almost never the case that the entire lesion is contained within the target volume.

Outside the target, radiation necrosis obviously occurs when too high a dose has been delivered to normal or to neoplastic tissues, and mass effect from radionecrosis is the most frequent cause of reoperation following implant therapy (Table 4.1). In a series of 20 patients with low-grade tumor specifically selected to study this problem, 40% of patients permanently implanted with iodine developed radionecrosis, a figure similar to that observed after temporary implants [25].

SUGGESTED TECHNIQUE

Patients selected for interstitial brachytherapy should fulfill a number of clinical and radiographic criteria if optimal results are to be obtained. Poor performance status or a neurologic deficit severe enough to disqualify the patient from consideration for other therapies probably should also rule against the use of interstitial radiation. The presence of a scalp infection or a cerebrospinal fluid leak is a sure harbinger of a serious postoperative complication. Devitalized scalp tissue after reoperation, radiation, or chemotherapy is not a contraindication if a stereotactic twist drill technique is employed to introduce the catheters into the brain [26]. Whenever possible, the use of additional linear scalp incisions, especially in segments of the craniotomy flap, and formal bur holes should be avoided in previously operated patients. Attention to the condition of the superficial tissues is especially important whenever the duration of the implant is prolonged by the concomitant use of other treatments such as hyperthermia.

The radiographic appearance of the tumor is critical to the proper selection of patients for brachytherapy. A patient should not be implanted if the tumor has poorly defined margins or does not enhance with contrast, especially if the diameter of the poorly visualized tissue approaches 5 cm or if a sizable portion of the ill-defined area encroaches on an eloquent region of the brain. In general, bilateral tumors, tumors in the corpus callosum, multicentric tumors, and lesions greater than 5 cm in diameter should not be implanted. Brachytherapy is regional therapy and is not appropriate for diffuse or nonlocalized disease. If a tumor cannot be encompassed within a single surgical field, it probably cannot be treated by implant therapy.

Neurosurgeons should not embark on an interstitial brachytherapy program without the full cooperation of a radiation oncologist and radiation physicist who have access to and expertise in volumetric computerized dosimetry and treatment planning. It is essential to have the capacity to transfer the computed tomography (CT) or magnetic resonance (MR) images of the tumor to the treatment planning computer so the outlines of the enhancing margin can be traced and isodose radiation lines superimposed (Figure 4.3). Mechanical and surgical limitations in the operating room usually require that the intercatheter distance be equal to or greater than 1 cm, center to center. This consideration, together with aspects of the local anatomy and the intended angle of approach, usually determines the total number of catheters and seeds in the implant. Limiting the number of catheters reduces mechanical disruption of the brain and simplifies the dosimetric computations. Other factors that influence the number of catheters include the shape of the lesion (ie, how much it varies from a simple spherical geometry), the strength of the seeds available, the type of isotope selected, and the spacing of the seeds within the catheters (generally 0.5 to 1 cm). The physicist and radiation oncologist must adjust these variables in such a way so as to deliver a total dose of 50 to 60 Gy to the outer edge of the enhancing rim or to some arbitrary boundary, usually 0.5 to 1 cm beyond the visible edge of the tumor. The dose rate at this site in an individual patient further depends on the strength of the available seeds in millicuries and determines the total implantation time in hours.

On the day of surgery, the stereotactic frame is applied in the usual manner, and the patient is placed in the CT or MR scanner. Whenever possible, treatment planning should be based on a rectilinear array of catheters with the assumption that implantation will be carried out perpendicular to the skull surface. It is then possible to use the CT or MR slice at the greatest diameter of the tumor as the only intraoperative image needed for target computation. If a regular array can be used (ie, one with a constant dimension between each row and column), it is possible to calculate a *single* (x,y) coordinate pair from the central slice and implant the catheters at regular intervals along each of these two axes. Other investigators have developed similar approaches in which a template centered on a single target is used to implant an entire array of hyperthermia seeds and radiation catheters [27•]. It is important for the radiation oncologist to be present when the surgical targets are selected in order to confirm that the central plane of the planning volume conforms to the central slice used by the surgeon. In addition, the team must review each of the other slices to determine the need for extra seeds or a change in the depth of a particular catheter along the z axis; these are the most critical decisions with regard to

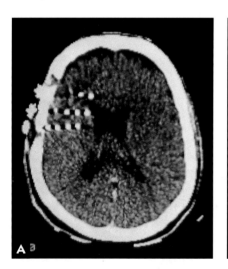 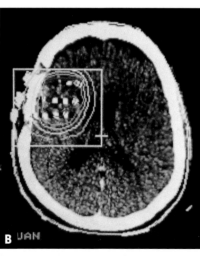

Figure 4.3

Pseudocolor display of isodose curves superimposed on the computed tomographic (CT) image of a malignant astrocytoma. During treatment planning, the patient's CT or magnetic resonance images are transferred to the treatment planning computer and the predicted distribution of radiation can be displayed and adjusted until the desired configuration is achieved. **A,** Axial CT scan demonstrates one row of three catheters with the dummy seeds in place (same patient as in Figure 4.7). **B,** Superimposition of the isodose curves has been performed and can be compared with the predicted preoperative curves already stored in the treatment planning computer.

final adjustments for nonspherical lesions. The radiation oncologist can then prepare a set of dummy seeds and active catheters, while the surgeon returns the patient to the operating theater.

The procedure is usually carried out with the patient in the supine position. The use of a stereotactic drill through the electrode carrier allows the surgeon to make twist drill holes that are perfectly colinear with the intended trajectory of the catheters, thus avoiding binding of the catheters in the skull (Figure 4.4); this technique facilitates the rapid creation of rectilinear arrays [28]. The drill is lowered to the surface of the scalp and 1% lidocaine with epinephrine is infiltrated into the skin. The drill point is hand-twisted through the scalp until it can be felt to turn on bare bone. A safety stop is placed along the shaft of the drill so as to prevent penetration of the brain, and a power

drill is used to make the hole (Figure 4.5A). A Kirschner wire is used to palpate the channel and determine if the dura has been reached. After completion of the hole, the drill is withdrawn from the electrode carrier and the Kirschner wire used to penetrate the dura and the underlying pia-arachnoid. A catheter of standard length is then fitted with a metal stylet and introduced through the electrode carrier. Before the catheter reaches the surface of the scalp, a metal disk is placed over the nose of the catheter, and the latter is driven down into the brain according to the z coordinate. When the proper depth is reached, a crimping tool is used to crush the collar of the metal cap around the catheter (Figure 4.5B). The collar of the metal cap contains holes for sutures, and a single 4-0 or 3-0 nylon suture is used to fix the catheter to the scalp. The stylet is carefully withdrawn and the excess

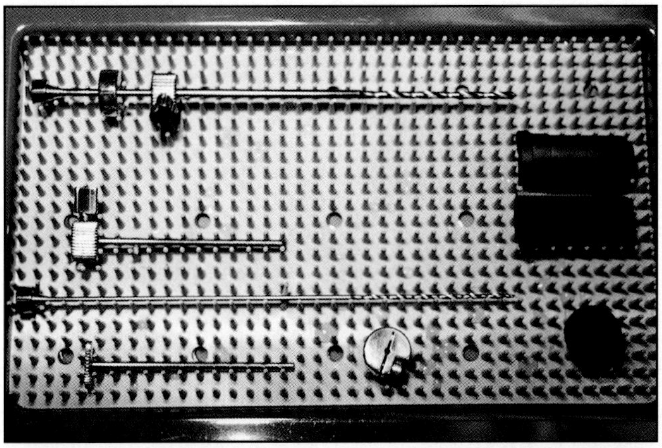

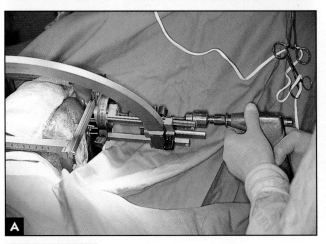

Figure 4.4

Stereotactic drill kit for the Leksell frame. The tray includes drills of two diameters (3/32 and 1/8 in), matching stops and outer cannulas, an extra large electrode carrier insert, a converter tube for small probes or catheters, and two Kirschner wires. (*From* Salcman *et al.* [46]; with permission.)

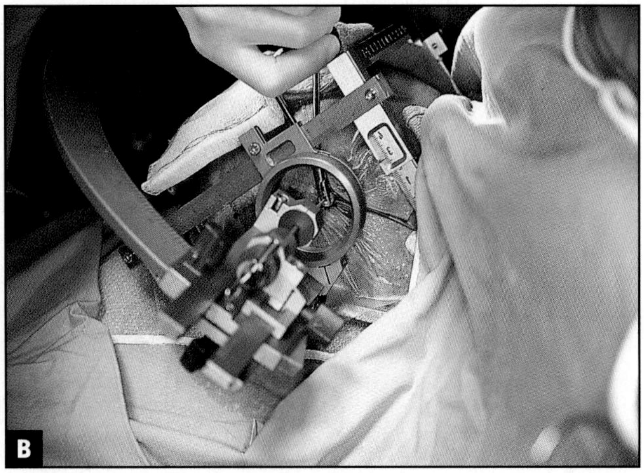

Figure 4.5

A, Stereotactic drill in use. The power drill holds a hexagonal wrench and the drill is directed perpendicular to the temporal bone through the lateral ring of the electrode arc. (*From* Salcman *et al.* [46]; with permission.) **B,** Use of the crimping tool beneath the plane of the lateral ring to fix the metal flange to the catheter.

catheter trimmed until 2 cm of tubing is left above the surface of the scalp. The electrode arc is then moved a regular distance to the next x or y coordinate, and the process is repeated (Figures 4.6 and 4.7A).

After all catheters have been implanted, the dummy seeds are introduced and the patient taken for a CT check scan to confirm that all catheters have reached their intended target points (Figure 4.3A). This is also a good time to make sure that no unsus-

pected intracerebral bleeding has been produced by the procedure. Once again, the image is transferred to the treatment planning computer and the postoperative isodose profiles are compared with the preoperative plan. Some radiation oncologists like to obtain a pair of orthogonal skull films against a measured grid as a quick way of determining comparability; such studies also illustrate the life-size scale of the treatment field (Figure 4.7B). In the unlikely event of a

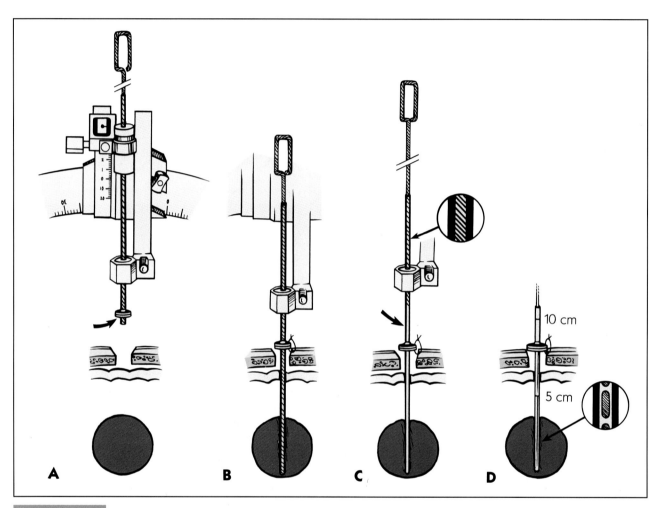

Figure 4.6

Steps in the insertion of the afterloading catheter. **A,** The flange (*arrow*) is slipped onto the front end of the catheter after the latter has been pushed through the electrode carrier. **B,** After insertion of the probe into the brain, the flange is sutured to the scalp with the stylet still in place. **C,** When the stylet is withdrawn, the catheter can be trimmed to the appropriate height (*curved arrow*) and the excess pulled out of the carrier. **D,** The inner catheter with the dummy seeds (**inset**) is then inserted into the afterloading catheter. (*From* Salcman *et al.* [28]; with permission.)

misplaced catheter, the flange can be uncrimped and the catheter adjusted along the axis of penetration until the desired depth is achieved.

In the intensive care unit, the patient is nursed in an isolated room with appropriate environmental protection for the nursing staff [29]. Radiation safety, shielding (Figure 4.8), and duty rosters for the staff are more complicated to arrange for a hot source such as iridium than they are for the shallower penetration of a low-energy β emitter such as iodine. In the intensive care unit, the radiation oncologist removes the dummy seeds and introduces the active inner catheters; this afterloading concept allows the preceding steps in the operating room and the radiology suite to be carried out in an unhurried and safe manner. At the end of the calculated implant time, all catheters are removed by the surgeon, and the twist-drill holes are closed with a single 4-0 nylon suture.

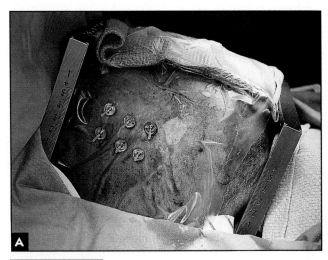
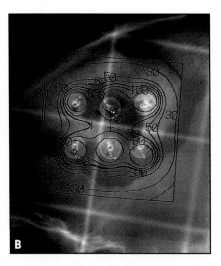

Figure 4.7

A, The rectangular array of six afterloading catheters implanted after calculation of a single target point. Catheters are affixed to the scalp by the metal flanges and sutures; no incisions are visible. (*From* Salcman *et al.* [46]; with permission.) **B,** Postoperative localizing radiograph with superimposed isodose curves. The grid consists of 3-cm squares superimposed on the immediate postoperative lateral skull film of the implant array shown in Figure 4.5A. Note the complex interaction of the sources in the six different catheters, the 80 to 100 cGy/h dose rates around each site and in the center of the array, and the rapid fall-off with distance to less than 30 cGy/h at the periphery.

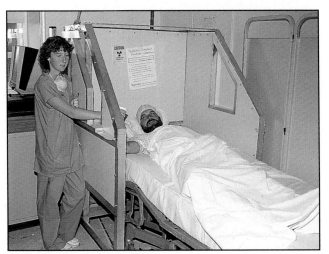

Figure 4.8

Example of a portable lead shield for use in the intensive care unit. Sliding windows in the side walls permit nursing care to be delivered to iridium implant patients with minimal radiation exposure to personnel. The entire assembly can be rolled (with effort) from one location in the unit to another and fits around the head of the bed.

When microwave-induced hyperthermia is combined with radiation, the microwave antennas are introduced into the afterloading catheters before the active radiation sources and 45° C is administered for 60 minutes (Figure 4.9). The antennas are then withdrawn, the radiation sources introduced for the required number of hours (usually 50 to 80), and the hyperthermia treatment repeated for 1 hour at the conclusion of brachytherapy [30••]. Many investigators recommend a lower total radiation dose to the periphery when using hyperthermia in combination with brachytherapy. Treatment planning for combined therapy is somewhat simplified by the fact that the intercatheter spacing for hyperthermia delivered by microwave antennas operating at 915 mHz (about 1 to 1.5 cm) is easily covered by most commonly used radiation sources.

Although the emphasis in this chapter has been on closed or stereotactic techniques for interstitial radiation, it is possible for the surgeon and the radiation oncologist to load low-energy sources safely into the resection cavity at the time of craniotomy. This approach is most useful for relatively slow-growing tumors such as meningiomas and cartilaginous

lesions that present as narrow-aspect targets in difficult locations. For example, it is almost impossible to implant stereotactically a meningioma en plaque along the skull base or to place safely parasagittal catheters in contact with the falx or around the great veins in the pineal region (Figure 4.10). A total dose of more than 200 Gy (20,000 rad) can be administered over the course of several months by permanent implantation of ^{125}I seeds. The latter can be stitched into polyethylene terephthalate (Dacron, DuPont, Wilmington, DE) sheets or polytetrafluoroethylene (Teflon, DuPont) blocks so as to prevent migration into the ventricular system or subarachnoid space. The relative frequency of both open and closed implants within the context of a busy neurooncology program is demonstrated in Table 4.2.

STRATEGIES FOR THE FUTURE

Delivery of an adequate dose to the target volume depends on appropriate radiobiologic planning, accurate dosimetry, and careful surgical implementation. Definition of the target volume is based on neu-

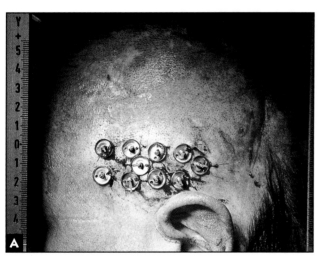

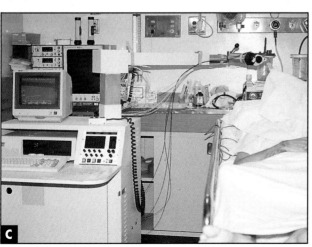

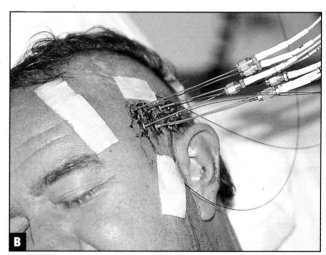

Figure 4.9

Example of a combined interstitial radiation and hyperthermia implant. The operative photograph (**A**) demonstrates three rows of catheters. The top and bottom rows contain a total of eight catheters, each of which was used for afterloading with ^{192}Ir and a microwave antenna. The closeup picture from the intensive care unit (**B**) shows the antennas loaded into the catheters and connected to their power cables. Note the relatively small size of the computer-controlled microwave generator used to power all eight antennas (**C**).

roimaging even though arbitrary decisions are usually made about the tumor margin since it may exist beyond the visible boundary of the lesion as visualized by CT and MR imaging. The target volume should never be thought of as being equivalent to the tumor volume because it almost always underestimates the latter. Dosimetric planning attempts to place the highest, most effective, and most homogeneous dose within the target volume without exposing normal tissues outside it to unacceptable radiobiologic toxicity. Some radiation sources are anisotropic and do not produce the same isodose profiles in all directions. A homogeneous source simplifies computation of the predicted isodose profiles and facilitates comparison of predicted with experimentally measured doses [28,31]. The isodose distributions of different isotopes have recently been compared and published [32]. For both ^{125}I and ^{192}Ir, the homogeneity of the dose delivered improved as the number of catheters was increased. The dose gradient more than 1 cm outside the target volume also depended on the geometry of the implant and the type of isotope used.

A number of new treatment planning programs and hardware systems have been developed to improve visualization of three-dimensional dose configurations [27•,33•]. A simple and effective technique that we have used is to transfer the digitized CT or MR imaging slices of the lesion's image to the radiation treatment planning computer and to trace by hand with a tracker ball the outline of the enhanced margin on each slice. The slices can then be stacked. Various computational systems can be used to interpolate the shape of the tumor between slices, or the slice thickness can be assumed to be equal to the straight-line edge between the cuts. Once the numbers of seeds and catheters has been determined, the computer program can display the predicted isodose profiles on any selected CT or MR imaging slice (Figure 4.3). New methods for selecting seed configuration have also been recently described [34,35].

Finally, the radiobiologic impact of a given dose of brachytherapy can be increased by chemical or thermal potentiation of its subcellular effects. In theory, if the same or greater cell killing can be achieved by a lower dose of radiation, improved sparing of surrounding normal tissues should be possible, especially if the chemical agent is selectively taken up by neoplastic cells, or the thermal dose at the edge of the lesion is below threshold for damage or injury to normal tissues. Etanidazole has been piloted in 42 brain tumor patients as a chemical potentiator for interstitial radiation [36••]. Its mechanism of action is similar to that of misonidazole and metronidazole, agents that proved ineffective in improving survival after conventional external radiation. A more interesting approach is to use thymidine analogues such as IUdR in combination with ^{192}Ir because a 5% replacement of native thymi-

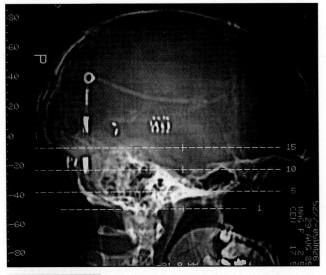

Figure 4.10

Example of an open implant performed for a pineal tumor. The lateral radiograph demonstrates a rectangular array of closely spaced ^{125}I seeds in the pineal region. The seeds were loaded into four rectangular blocks of polytetrafluoroethylene (Teflon, DuPont, Wilmington, DE) and the latter were manually packed into the resection cavity with the aid of the operating microscope and a transoccipital approach.

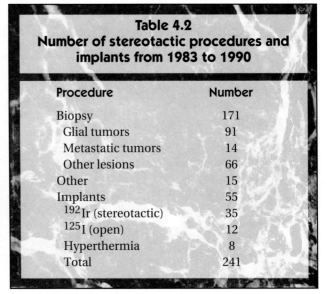

Table 4.2 Number of stereotactic procedures and implants from 1983 to 1990	
Procedure	**Number**
Biopsy	171
Glial tumors	91
Metastatic tumors	14
Other lesions	66
Other	15
Implants	55
^{192}Ir (stereotactic)	35
^{125}I (open)	12
Hyperthermia	8
Total	241

dine in DNA can double the effectiveness of ionizing radiation [37•]. It is also possible to generate a sufficient flux of neutrons through the use of the isotope californium (Cf) such that boron neutron capture therapy might become a practical reality via ^{252}Cf brachytherapy [38•]. Another new approach involves the use of cesium as the source in a remote afterloading system; this technique requires the surgeon to implant a single large catheter into the resection cavity and the transcutaneous use of remote afterloading technology in the postoperative period [39].

A number of centers have initiated clinical trials of combined interstitial radiation and interstitial hyperthermia based on the ability of relatively low levels of heat to potentiate significantly the cell killing of ionizing radiation and the direct cell killing effect of hyperthermia itself [30••,40]. In 13 recurrent glioblastoma patients implanted with ^{125}I and microwave antennas, a 41-week median survival has been achieved; 16 other patients with anaplastic astrocytoma and cerebral metastases have also been treated [41•]. Pilot series that combine microwave antenna hyperthermia with ^{192}Ir implants have also been reported, but survival data are not available [30••,42]. Ferromagnetic seeds have been used to deliver heat in 14 glioma patients implanted with ^{192}Ir [43]; four patients required reoperation, and three were alive 16 to 19 months after diagnosis. When Curie point ferromagnetic seeds have been used without interstitial radiation, the response rate was 34.8% in a series of 25 patients, including 13 with malignant gliomas and seven with cerebral metastases [44•]. Better methods are needed to produce a more homogeneous deposition of heat in tissue, either by changing catheter materials to improve the electrical match of microwave frequencies to the dielectric properties of the catheter and brain [45] or through improved knowledge of cerebral blood flow and its impact on thermal dose planning [46]. In any case, temperatures do not need to be exactly the same throughout the target volume but must exceed some effective threshold to achieve radiopotentiation.

Whether chemical or physical agents can ever be shown to increase the clinical effectiveness of interstitial brachytherapy successfully remains to be seen because brachytherapy, similar to surgery and hyperthermia, is a purely regional modality and is unlikely to be the ultimate answer for many patients with glioblastoma or other intracranial tumors. Regional therapies are severely limited by our inability to visualize precisely the tumor volume as well as the impossibility of restricting the side effects of treatment to only the tumor when an attempt is made to encompass it in its entirety. Nevertheless, aggressive local therapies will continue to play an important clinical role for the foreseeable future, especially in combination with new blood-borne agents developed on molecular biologic principles.

REFERENCES AND RECOMMENDED READING

Papers of particular interest, published within the annual period of review, have been highlighted as:
• Of interest
•• Of outstanding interest

1. El-Hennawi Y, Gillespi GY, Mahaley MS, *et al.*: A controlled study of efficacy of interstitial or external irradiation in a virus-induced brain-tumor model in rats. *J Neurosurg* 1989, 71:898–902.

2. Gutin PH, Bernstein M, Sano Y, *et al.*: Combination therapy with 1,3-bis (2-chloroethyl)-1-nitrosourea and low dose rate radiation in the 9L rat brain tumor and spheroid models: implications for brain tumor brachytherapy. *Neurosurgery* 1984, 15:781–786.

3. •• Salcman M, Ebert PS: In vitro response of human glioblastoma and canine glioma cells to hyperthermia, radiation, and chemotherapy. *Neurosurgery* 1991, 29:526–531.
Important demonstration of treatment interactions in glioma cell lines *in vitro*.

4. Kim JH, Alfieri AA, Rosenblum M, *et al.*: Low dose rate radiotherapy for transplantable gliosarcoma in the rat brain. *J Neurooncol* 1990, 9:9–15.

5. • Bernstein M, Marotta T, Stewart P, *et al.*:Brain damage from ^{125}I brachytherapy evaluated by MR imaging, a blood-brain barrier tracer, and light and electron microscopy in a rat model. *J Neurosurg* 1990, 73:585–593.
Clinical time course and appearance of radiation damage confirmed by laboratory study.

6. Frazier CH: The effects of radium emanations upon brain tumors. *Surg Gynecol Obstet* 1920, 31:236–239.

7. Sachs E: The treatment of glioblastomas with radium. *J Neurosurg* 1954, 11:119–121.

8. Liebel SA, Gutin PH, Wara WM, *et al.*: Survival and the quality of life after interstitial implantation of removable high-activity iodine-125 sources for the treatment of patients with recurrent malignant gliomas. *Int J Radiat Oncol Biol Phys* 1989, 17:1129–1139.

9. Salcman M: Epidemiology and factors affecting survival. In *Malignant Cerebral Glioma.* Edited by Apuzzo MLJ. Park Ridge, IL: American Association of Neurological Surgeons; 1990:95–109.

10. Lucas GL, Luxton G, Cohen D, *et al.*: Treatment results of stereotactic interstitial brachytherapy for primary and metastatic brain tumors. *Int J Radiat Oncol Biol Phys* 1991, 21:715–721.

11. • Bernstein M, Laperriet N, Leung P, *et al.*: Interstitial brachytherapy for malignant brain tumors: preliminary results. *Neurosurgery* 1990, 26:371–380.

Early experience with up-front therapy is detailed in addition to confirmatory data on recurrent gliomas.

12. •• Florell RC, MacDonald DR, Irish WD, *et al.*: Selection bias, survival, and brachytherapy for glioma. *J Neurosurg* 1992, 76:179–183.

Important study detailing the selection bias involved in brachytherapy trials, including those of the authors.

13. Chun M, McKeough P, Wu A, *et al.*: Interstitial iridium-192 implantation of malignant brain tumors. Part II: clinical experience. *Br J Radiol* 1989, 62:158–162.

14. • Gutin PH, Prados MD, Philips TL, *et al.*: External irradiation followed by an interstitial high-activity iodine-125 implant "boost" in the initial treatment of malignant gliomas: NCOG study 6G-82-2. *Int J Radiat Oncol Biol Phys* 1991, 21:601–606.

Up-front use is less successful in glioblastoma than in malignant astrocytoma.

15. • Loeffler JS, Alexander III E, Wen PY, *et al.*: Results of stereotactic brachytherapy used in the initial management of patients with glioblastoma. *J Natl Cancer Inst* 1990, 82:1918–1921.

Another report detailing selection bias and eligibility criteria in the use of brachytherapy.

16. Mundinger P, Braus DF, Krauss JK, *et al.*: Long-term outcome of 89 low-grade brain-stem gliomas after interstitial radiation therapy. *J Neurosurg* 1991, 75:740–746.

17. Etou A, Mundinger F, Mohadjer M, *et al.*: Stereotactic interstitial irradiation of diencephalic tumors with iridium 192 and iodine 125: 10 year follow-up and comparison with other treatments. *Child Nerv Syst* 1989, 5:140–143.

18. Voges J, Sturm V, Berthold F, *et al.*: Interstitial irradiation of cerebral gliomas in childhood by permanently implanted 125-iodine: preliminary results. *Klin Paediatr* 1990, 202:270–274.

19. • Kumar PP, Patil AA, Leibrock LG, *et al.*: Brachytherapy: a viable alternative in the management of basal meningiomas. *Neurosurgery* 1991, 29:676–680.

Detailed report of brachytherapy for unresectable benign tumors.

20. Salcman M, Scholtz H, Kristi D, *et al.*: Extraskeletal myxoid chondrosarcoma of the falx. *Neurosurgery* 1992, 31:344–348.

21. Prados M, Leibel S, Barnett CM, *et al.*: Interstitial brachytherapy for metastatic brain tumors. *Cancer* 1989, 63:657–660.

22. •• Loeffler JS, Alexander III E, Hochberg FH, *et al.*: Clinical patterns of failure following stereotactic interstitial radiation for malignant gliomas. *Int J Radiat Oncol Biol Phys* 1990, 19:1455–1462.

Important study of tumor recurrence patterns, confirming earlier reports based on conventional radiation.

23. Schiffer D: Patterns of tumor growth. In *Neurobiology of Brain Tumors.* Edited by Salcman M. Baltimore: Williams & Wilkins; 1991:85–136.

24. Kelly PJ, Daumas-Duport C, Kispert DB, *et al.*: Imaging-based stereotactic serial biopsies in untreated intracranial glial neoplasms. *J Neurosurg* 1987, 66:865–874.

25. Wowra B, Schmitt HP, Sturm V: Incidence of late radiation necrosis with transient mass effect after interstitial low dose rate radiotherapy for cerebral gliomas. *Acta Neurochir (Wein)* 1989, 99:104–108.

26. Salcman M, Corradino G, Moriyama E, *et al.*: Cerebral blood flow and the thermal properties of the brain: a preliminary analysis. *J Neurosurg* 1989, 70:592–598.

27. • Lulu BA, Lutz W, Stea B, *et al.*: Treatment planning of template-guided stereotaxic brain implants. *Int J Radiat Oncol Biol Phys* 1990, 18:951–955.

Common-sense technique for coordinated planning of combined radiation and hyperthermia implants.

28. Salcman M, Sewchand W, Amin P, *et al.*: Technique of stereotactic irradiation for primary brain tumors. *J Neurooncol* 1986, 4:141–149.

29. Sewchand W, Drzmal RE, Amin P, *et al.*: Radiation control in the ICU for high-intensity iridium-192 brain implants. *Neurosurgery* 1987, 20:584–588.

30. •• Salcman M: Hyperthermia. In *Neurobiology of Brain Tumors.* Edited by Salcman, M. Baltimore: Williams & Wilkins; 1991:359–373.

Most current review of the biology and application of hyperthermia for brain tumor treatment.

31. Sewchand W, Amin P, Salcman M, *et al.*: Removable high intensity iridium-192 brain implants: techniques and *in vivo* measurements in canine brain. *J Neurooncol* 1984, 2:177–186.

32. Saw CB, Suntharalingam N, Ayyangar KM, *et al.*: Dosimetric considerations of stereotactic brain implants. *Int J Radiat Oncol Biol Phys* 1989, 17:887–891.

33. • Weaver K, Smith V, Lewis JD, *et al.*: A CT-based computerized treatment planning system for I-125 stereotactic brain implants. *Int J Radiat Oncol Biol Phys* 1990, 18:445–454.

Useful example of computerized treatment planning for implementation in multiple centers.

34. Rosenow UF, Wojcicka JB: Clinical implementation of stereotaxic brain implant optimization. *Med Phys* 1991, 18:266–272.

35. Wu A, Chun M, Kasdon D, *et al.*: Interstitial iridium-192 implantation for malignant brain tumors. Part I: techniques of dosimetry planning. *Br J Radiol* 1989, 62:154–157.

36. •• Coleman CN, Noll L, Riese N, *et al.*: Final report of the phase I trial of continuous infusion etanidazole (SR 2508): a radiation therapy oncology group study. *Int J Radiat Oncol Biol Phys* 1992, 22:577–580.

Another negative study on electron-affinic compounds for the potentiation of radiotherapy.

37. • Goodman JH, Gahbauer RA, Kanellitsas C, *et al.*: Theoretical basis and clinical methodology for stereotactic interstitial brain tumor irradiation using iodeoxyuridine as a radiation sensitizer and 145 Sm as a brachytherapy source. *Stereotact Funct Neurosurg* 1990, 54-55:531–534.

Thymidine analogues may prove to be excellent radiopotentiators.

38. • Beach JL, Schroy CB, Ashtari M, *et al.*: Boron neutron capture enhancement of 252Cf brachytherapy. *Int J Radiat Oncol Biol Phys*1990, 18:1421–1427.

Innovative combination of two technologies to produce focal boron neutron capture therapy.

39. Ashpole RD, Snyman H, Bullimore JA, *et al.*: A new technique of brachytherapy for malignant gliomas with cesium-137: a new method utilizing a remote afterloading system. *Clin Oncol* 1990, 2:333–337.

40. Salcman M, Samaras GM: Hyperthermia for brain tumors: biophysical rationale. *Neurosurgery* 1981, 9:327–335.

41. • Sneed PK, Stauffer PR, Gutin PH, *et al.*: Interstitial radiation and hyperthermia for the treatment of recurrent brain tumors. *Neurosurgery* 1991, 28:206–215.

A model clinical trial using combined therapy, confirming earlier observations.

42. Roberts DW, Coughlin CT, Wong TZ, *et al.*: Interstitial hyperthermia and iridium brachytherapy in treatment of malignant glioma: a phase I clinical trail. *J Neurosurg* 1985, 64:581–587.

43. Stea B, Cetas TC, Cassady JR, *et al.*: Interstitial thermoradiotherapy of brain tumors: preliminary results of a phase I clinical trial. *Int J Radiat Oncol Biol Phys* 1991, 19:1463–1471.

44. • Kobayashi T, Kida Y, Tanaka T, *et al.* Interstitial hyperthermia of malignant brain tumors by implant heating system: clinical experience. *J Neurooncol* 1991, 10:153–163.

Pioneer study of an alternative technology for producing hyperthermia in the brain.

45. Farraro FT, Salcman M, Broadwell RD, *et al.*: Alumina ceramic as a biomaterial for use in afterloading radiation catheters for hyperthermia. *Neurosurgery* 1989, 25:209–213.

46. Salcman M, Bellis EH, Sewchand W, *et al.*: Technical aids for the flexible use of the Leksell stereotactic system. *Neurol Res* 1989, 11:89–96.

Chapter 5

Stereotactic Radiosurgery for Brain Tumors

Douglas Kondziolka
L. Dade Lunsford

Stereotactic radiosurgery is the closed-skull destruction of a precisely defined intracranial target using ionizing beams of radiation, delivered during a single session. To define an intracranial tumor for radiosurgery, neuroimaging is used to visualize the normal and abnormal anatomy. Leksell [1] initiated the radiosurgical technique in 1951 by coupling an orthovoltage x-ray tube to a stereotactic guiding device. For the next 25 years, the use of stereotactic radiosurgery was dependent on whether the tumor could be defined with angiography, encephalography, or skull roentgenography. Although first used to create lesions in normal brain targets for functional neurosurgery, radiosurgery subsequently was used most often to manage mass lesions localized by angiography (*eg*, arteriovenous malformations) or by contrast cisternography (*eg*, a tumor near the skull base) [2]. Imaging was unsatisfactory for the radiosurgical management of most intra-axial lesions. Stereotactic computed tomography (CT) and magnetic resonance (MR) imaging overcame these inadequacies by providing high-resolution information on the shape, volume, and location of brain tumors. In this chapter, we discuss indications, techniques, and results in the management of 500 patients with benign and malignant brain tumors using gamma knife radiosurgery.

TECHNIQUE

Either photon or charged-particle irradiation can be used to provide focal single-session destruction of an intracranial target using stereotactic guidance. The Gamma unit (model U; Elekta Instruments, Atlanta) consists of a permanent 18,000-kg shield surrounding a primary hemispheric array of 201 sources of ^{60}Co [3]. The central beam of radiation is fixed at an angle of 55° to the horizontal plane, with the other beams arranged in an arc, all reaching a focal point 403 mm from the sources. A secondary collimator helmet with beam channel diameters of 4, 8, 14, or 18 mm is used to vary the volume of prescribed radiation (Figure 5.1). The model B unit currently used in Europe and Asia has the radiation sources arranged in a donut-shaped array. The stereotactic frame is suspended within the secondary collimator helmet to ensure that the center of the radiation volume (the target isocenter) is held at the focal point of the 201 cobalt sources. A second system for photon irradiation uses a modification of a standard linear accelerator (LINAC) [4–8]. A cyclotron is necessary to accelerate heavy-charged particles toward an intracranial target with steep radiation fall-off. The Bragg peak of protons, helium ions, or carbon ions can be used to provide focal radiation [9,10]. This technique is available at only a limited number of centers.

At our institution, gamma knife radiosurgery in adult patients is performed using local anesthesia supplemented with mild intravenous sedation. Chil-dren under the age of 14 years undergo radiosurgery using general endotracheal anesthesia [11•]. After application of the stereotactic coordinate frame to the patient's head, CT or MR imaging is used to define the tumor. Although initially we used contrast-enhanced CT for stereotactic targeting, we now use contrast-enhanced stereotactic MR imaging as the sole imaging modality in almost all cases. MR imaging provides better tumor visualization and nonreformatted imaging in all three planes and is accurate [12••]. The recti-linear (X, Y, and Z) stereotactic coordinates of the planned irradiation isocenters are determined. Two- or three-dimensional multiplanar isodose plots are integrated with the MR images. The goal of radiosurgical dose planning is to enclose the lesion margin as closely as possible within the 50% isodose line or greater in order to maintain a steep fall-off of radiation dose beyond the lesion margin [13••]. After determination of the appropriate number of isocenters required, the tumor dose is selected jointly by the neurosurgeon and radiation oncologist.

Dose selection depends on tumor pathology, location, volume, and prior therapy. To help choose radiosurgical doses for our first patients with brain tumors, we used an integrated logistic formula, originally developed for the treatment of arteriovenous malformations [14]. This formula predicts the dose likely to be associated with an approximate 3% risk of permanent delayed radiation-induced complications. Location of the tumor in a critical region near or in the brain (*eg*, the cavernous sinus or adjacent to the brainstem) did not in itself lead to a reduction in

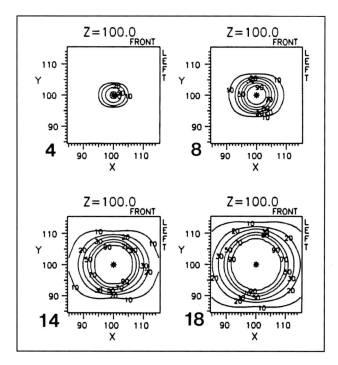

Figure 5.1

Axial plots of isodose lines produced by the 4-, 8-, 14-, and 18-mm collimators of the gamma unit. The steep radiation fall-off is maintained from the 90% to 10% isodose lines.

radiosurgical dose. For parasellar tumors, the tumor margin should be at least 4 mm from the optic chiasm. We believe that the optic apparatus is radiosensitive, and thus limit the dose received by the optic chiasm to 8 Gy.

Immediately after radiosurgery, patients receive a single 40-mg intravenous dose of methylprednisolone, and for those at risk for seizures, 90 mg of pentobarbital. Patients are discharged from the hospital the morning after radiosurgery. We recommend that patients with benign tumors have follow-up clinical and imaging examinations at 6-month intervals; patients with malignant tumors should undergo follow-up imaging studies beginning 6 to 12 weeks after radiosurgery. Contrast-enhanced MR or CT scans are used to monitor tumor volume and to detect possible complications.

BENIGN TUMORS

Acoustic tumors

Microsurgical removal is considered the standard approach for healthy patients with unilateral acoustic nerve sheath tumors. However, alternatives to conventional surgery may be important to consider for patients who have tumors on the side of their only ear with hearing, for elderly patients, for those whose medical problems make microsurgery unacceptably dangerous [15•], and for those who refuse microsurgery. In such patients, stereotactic radiosurgery of small- to moderate-sized acoustic tumors offers an effective management option.

The goal of radiosurgery in the treatment of acoustic tumors is to arrest growth, preserve cranial nerve function, and prevent further neurologic deficits. Whereas microsurgery enables tumor removal in many patients, only recently have attempts at preserving facial and even auditory function been possible [16•]. Furthermore, although current microsurgical techniques have reduced the incidence of early postoperative meningitis, cerebrospinal fluid leakage, and stroke, such complications never occur after radiosurgery. To study the efficacy of radiosurgery in arresting tumor growth and maintaining cranial nerve function, we reviewed our experience in 187 patients with acoustic tumors. Radiosurgery was recommended when one or more of the following criteria existed: 1) the patient had significant concomitant medical illness, 2) the patient was elderly, 3) the tumor was recurrent after microsurgery, 4) the tumor was on the side of the patient's only ear with hearing, 5) the patient had bilateral acoustic tumors with at least unilateral hearing preservation, or 6) the patient refused surgical removal.

The 187 patients varied in age from 14 to 83 years (mean, 56 years). Twenty-one patients had bilateral tumors in the setting of neurofibromatosis type II. Microsurgery had been performed at least once in 47 patients (25%); 14 patients had had gross total removal and 33 had had subtotal resections.

In the majority of patients, the irregular shape of the tumor required the use of multiple irradiation isocenters (range, two to 11). At least one isocenter was placed in the extracanalicular portion of the tumor and one was placed in the intracanalicular portion (Figure 5.2). Tumor volumes varied from 225 to 28,000 mm^3 (mean, 6110 mm^3). To maintain a sharp fall-off in the specified radiation dose the 50% or greater isodose line was used to encircle the tumor margin in most patients. The mean dose delivered to the center of the tumor was 32.7 Gy (range, 24 to 50 Gy); the dose to the tumor margin varied from 12 to 20 Gy (mean, 16.7 Gy).

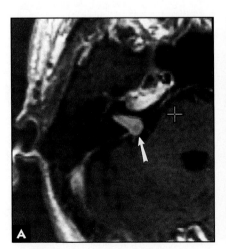
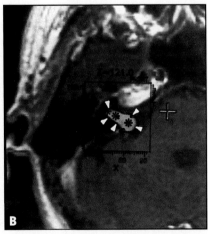

Figure 5.2

A, Axial gadopentetate dimeglumine–enhanced magnetic resonance image showing a small acoustic neurinoma (*arrow*). **B,** One 8-mm and two 4-mm isocenters were used to construct the radiosurgical plan (*arrowheads*).

Tumor response

The biological effect by which radiosurgery arrests tumor growth probably is related to direct tumor cytotoxicity followed by delayed vascular obliteration [17•]. Relatively high rates of central tumor necrosis and delayed shrinkage indicate that the effect of radiosurgery on benign tumors is considerable [18••]. In our first 136 patients, we defined a 4-year actuarial tumor control rate of 89.2% ± 6.0% (Figure 5.3). Tumor growth occurred in four patients after radio-surgery. Regression in tumor volume was noted in 42% of patients evaluated 24 months or more after radiosurgery. Successful local control was not significantly related to tumor volume, the presence or absence of neurofibromatosis, or minimum and maximum tumor doses.

Cranial nerve preservation

The 2- and 4-year actuarial rate for preservation of preradiosurgery useful hearing function was 34.4% ± 6.6% (defined by pure tone audiogram and speech discrimination scores). Preservation of some degree of hearing as measured by pure tone audiometry occurred in 71% of patients who had preoperative hearing present. The presence of neurofibromatosis correlated significantly with later decreased hearing and complete hearing loss.

The risks of postradiosurgery facial or trigeminal neuropathy increased with increasing transverse tumor diameter (a measure of the length of nerve irradiated), but decreased with increasing number of isocenters used. This latter observation likely indicates our increased experience, which led to the use of narrower radiation beams and better conformal dose planning. The 4-year actuarial incidences of facial and trigeminal neuropathies after radiosurgery were 29.0% ± 4.4% and 32.9% ± 4.5%, respectively, in our initial experience. For patients with pons-petrous tumor diameters less than 20 mm and those who were treated with four or more isocenters, the risk of facial neuropathy was less than 10%. Patients with intracanalicular tumors had a risk of less than a 5%. Radiation effects usually occurred between 6 and 18 months after radiosurgery; no patient developed a neuropathy after 21 months. In most patients, cranial neuropathies subsequently improved; 86% ± 9% of patients had improved by one or more House-Brack-mann classes 2 years after onset. Of 122 patients who had grade 1 to 3 facial nerve function before radio-surgery, only two had grade 4 to 6 function at the time of this review; both complete deficits were attributed to microsurgical tumor resection after radiosurgery.

Radiosurgery has proven to be a safe and effective surgical alternative for carefully selected patients with acoustic tumors. The incidence of postradiosurgery cranial neuropathy has been lowered by the increased use of multiple irradiation isocenters and by the early management of small tumors.

Meningiomas

Because meningiomas usually are well demarcated and rarely invade the brain, the steep radiation fall-off achieved by radiosurgery can be directed at the tumor margin. Meningiomas are easily visible on MR or CT images used for targeting and dose planning and now can be recognized even when small (< 30 mm in diameter). Their dural blood supply can be included within a high isodose in an attempt to achieve vascular obliteration. In many patients, radiosurgery can

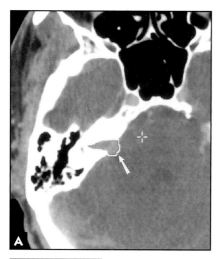 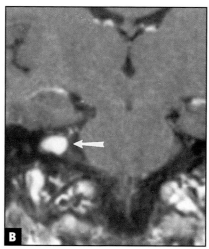 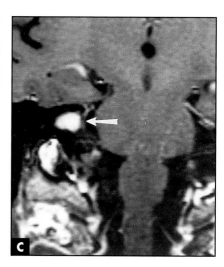

Figure 5.3

Contrast-enhanced computed tomographic image at radiosurgery (**A**) showing a small acoustic neurinoma (*arrow*). Coronal magnetic resonance images 11 months (**B**) and 51 months (**C**) after radiosurgery show no change in tumor size with preservation of all cranial nerve function (*arrows*).

reduce the risks associated with cranial base micro-surgical resection. Despite these potential advantages, for most patients surgical removal is the ideal goal. Long-term disease-free survival can be achieved after surgical resection of the tumor and its dural base [19,20]. However, delayed tumor recurrence after surgery, neurologic morbidity, surgical mortality (especially in elderly patients), and the lack of consistent benefit provided by fractionated radiotherapy have led to stereotactic radiosurgery increasingly being considered for primary or adjuvant management in selected high-risk meningioma patients.

We used radiosurgery in 103 patients with meningiomas (aged 14 to 82 years). Patients were accepted for radiosurgery only if the tumor was less than 35 mm in average diameter. Radiosurgery was not recommended if the tumor was amenable to open surgical resection with acceptable risk or was within 4 mm of the optic chiasm [21••]. Contrast-enhanced CT or MR imaging revealed a well-demarcated dural-based or intraventricular tumor in all patients; 89% of patients had basal meningiomas, and 66% had undergone at least one prior surgical procedure (28 of 66 patients had multiple resections).

Multiple isocenters of irradiation were necessary in most patients to create irregular isodose configurations that closely corresponded to the tumor volumes (Figure 5.4) [22•]. An irregular tumor contour was present if a previous resection had been performed. Dose plans were more difficult to devise for cavernous sinus or parasellar tumors because of the tendency of these tumors to extend into multiple intracranial and extracranial compartments. The presence of major vessels (*eg*, the internal carotid or anterior cerebral arteries) within the tumor did not cause us to reduce the delivered dose below an anticipated therapeutic level.

We evaluated CT or MR scans performed 6 to 60 months after radiosurgery in the first 85 patients. Fifty-five patients had no tumor growth documented in follow-up, 24 patients had decreased tumor size, and six patients had an increase in tumor size (Figure 5.5). Of these latter six patients, two had malignant meningiomas, three had tumor growth outside the radiosurgical volume, and two had undergone three prior craniotomies. Loss of central contrast enhancement (an imaging finding we believe to be consistent with intratumoral necrosis) was noted in 12 patients and was related to the occurrence of subsequent

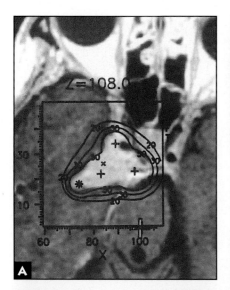
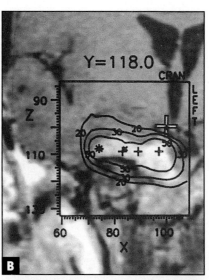

Figure 5.4

Axial (**A**) and coronal (**B**) magnetic resonance images showing a residual right cavernous sinus meningioma after prior microsurgery. Multiple irradiation isocenters were used to construct this irregular isodose configuration to fit the tumor margin at the 50% isodose line.

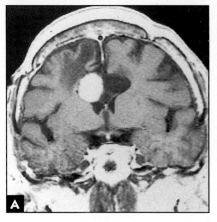
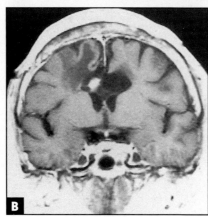

Figure 5.5

A, Coronal magnetic resonance image at the time of radiosurgery for a recurrent intraventricular meningioma. **B,** Twenty months after radiosurgery, the tumor was significantly reduced in volume.

tumor shrinkage ($P < 0.001$). Of 21 patients with more than 36 months of follow-up, 10 had no change in tumor size and 11 had tumor shrinkage.

Clinical evaluation 6 to 60 months after radio-surgery in 89 patients found that 72 remained clinically stable, 10 had improved, two had worsened deficits that appeared permanent, and two had died (death unrelated to tumor status). Three patients, currently classified as neurologically stable, developed temporary deficits 6 to 12 months after radiosurgery that subsequently improved. Three patients had later surgical resection of their tumors within 6 months of radiosurgery; all had no change in tumor size.

Further follow-up is necessary to evaluate the benefits of radiosurgery in providing long-term curative control of meningiomas. The low morbidity seen in patients with basal tumors has been followed by the increasing use of radiosurgical techniques for these difficult neoplasms.

Pituitary adenomas

We consider radiosurgery to be an adjuvant strategy for pituitary adenomas recurrent or residual after sur-gical resection and a primary strategy for patients whose advanced age or medical condition militates against surgery. Multimodality management is required for many patients and includes surgery, pharmacologic and hormonal treatment, and conventional radiation therapy. In contrast to the treatment of acoustic tumors and meningiomas, conventional fractionated radiation therapy has proven valuable in the treatment of pituitary tumors [23]. The total fractionated dose is limited by the amount of radiation that can be delivered safely to adjacent critical structures.

The initial radiosurgical efforts in the treatment of pituitary tumors began in the 1950s with the use of charged particles. Linfoot and Lawrence [24] reported on 781 patients who received charged-particle single-fraction irradiation to the pituitary gland. Kjellberg and Abe [9] subsequently described the Bragg peak stereotactic proton irradiation of 1125 pituitary adenomas. Their series included patients with acromegaly, Cushing's disease, Nelson's syndrome, prolactinoma, thyrotropin-secreting adenomas, and nonfunctioning adenomas. In most of the patients with acromegaly, they found that clinical features and elevated growth

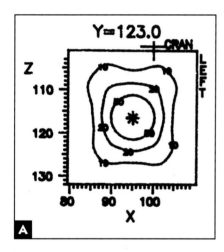

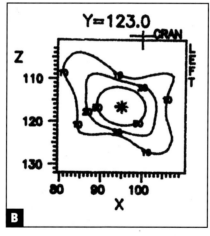

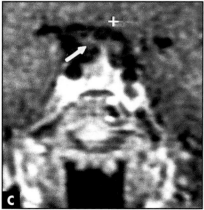

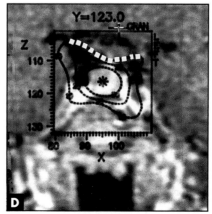

Figure 5.6

A, Coronal isodose plan using one 8-mm isocenter of irradiation with all 201 ^{60}Co beams used. **B,** Using a selective beam-blocking pattern, the superior isodose curves can be modified to minimize the dose delivered to the optic chiasm (*arrow* in **C**). The 10% isodose line is seen below the optic chiasm, while the 50% isodose line is contoured to the tumor margin (**D**).

hormone levels began to abate 3 to 6 months after treatment. However, normalization of growth hormone levels occurred slowly; at 2 years, 28% of patients had attained levels less than 5 ng/mL, and at 5 years, 75% of patients had reached this level. Of the patients with Cushing's disease, 55% had no adrenocortical production of hormone 2 years after treatment. This rate improved to 80% at 5 years and 90% at 20 years. The investigators noted a 10% rate of delayed hypopituitarism and a 13% incidence of delayed visual field disturbances.

The results of gamma knife radiosurgery at the Karolinska Institute in Stockholm have been reported for patients with Cushing's disease [25,26] and acromegaly [27•]. Normalization of urinary cortisol levels was seen in more than 75% of patients within the first 3 years after treatment. In most of these patients, multiple radiosurgical procedures were required to achieve disease control. Pituitary insufficiency developed in 55% of patients.

In our series, we performed radiosurgery in 36 patients with pituitary adenomas. Transsphenoidal or transcranial tumor resection had been performed previously in 22 patients. Prior fractionated radiation therapy had failed in eight patients. Mean follow-up was 19 months (range, 3 to 48 months). Imaging follow-up was available in 26 patients. Tumor volumes were unchanged in 13 patients, decreased in six, increased in one, and absent in six. Two patients had repeat radiosurgery for persistent hormonal elevation. No patient had a prolactinoma. Two patients with Cushing's disease had subsequent surgical resection because of persistent adrenocorticotrophic hormone production (14 and 27 months after radiosurgery).

At other centers, initial radiosurgical efforts in treating pituitary adenomas were directed toward ablation of the sellar contents. With high-resolution imaging, we believe that the tumor alone, if possible, should be identified and treated. Proper selection of radiosurgical candidates with pituitary tumors depends on imaging. First, the tumor must be distinct from the gland, a feature best demonstrated by contrast-enhanced coronal MR imaging. Coronal images also provide important information on the relationship of the tumor to the optic nerves and chiasm; treatment is prohibited if the tumor-chiasm distance is less than 5 mm. Selective radiation beam blocking permits the lower isodoses to be moved away from the optic apparatus (Figure 5.6) [28•]. Lateral tumor invasion of the cavernous sinus is not a contraindication to radiosurgery.

The availability of successful medical treatment has virtually eliminated the use of radiosurgery for prolactinomas. The role of radiosurgery is more important in Cushing's disease, because the rate of hormonal relapse can be high after microsurgery [29]. We are currently evaluating multiple radiosurgical procedures in patients with Cushing's disease who have persistent cortisol hypersecretion 12 to 24 months after radiosurgery. Radiosurgery seems best reserved for the adjuvant management of residual or recurrent pituitary tumors after microsurgery. It can be considered as a primary approach for small tumors in elderly or medically infirm patients and for patients with tumors that laterally involve the cavernous sinus.

MALIGNANT TUMORS

Brain metastases

Based on the hypothesis that stereotactic radiosurgery could replace the benefit provided by surgical resection for solitary brain metastases, we began a phase I/II trial of "boost radiosurgery" in 1987 [15•]. We anticipated that small solitary brain metastases (that appear to be well circumscribed on CT or MR scans) might also respond similarly to small circumscribed benign tumors. Although some centers use radiosurgery alone for brain metastases [30], we use radiosurgery to enhance, not replace, fractionated radiotherapy. Due to the possibility of remote microscopic metastases not revealed by neuroimaging studies and the risk for local tumor infiltration beyond the contrast-enhanced imaging margin, we believe that fractionated whole-brain irradiation remains necessary [31••].

Modern neuroimaging techniques enable the earlier detection of metastatic brain tumors, including those in asymptomatic patients. However, despite earlier diagnosis and a variety of management options, results have not improved significantly. The best management results to date were demonstrated by a randomized study that compared surgical excision plus radiotherapy with radiotherapy alone; this study found increased survival (median, 10 months) and improved quality of life in the surgical arm [32••].

Initially, we used stereotactic radiosurgery to manage small (< 3 cm), solitary metastatic tumors. Most patients had active systemic disease. Recently, several patients with multiple metastases (up to four) had radiosurgery. Our goal was to equal the rate of tumor control provided by surgical excision. Radiosurgery would then obviate craniotomy, reduce the length and cost of hospitalization, and lessen the potential morbidity associated with surgical resection [30,33]. At our center, 79 patients had radiosurgery. Tumor pathologies included malignant melanoma (35%), non–small cell lung carcinoma (32%), renal cell carcinoma (13%), breast carcinoma, colorectal carcinoma, choriocarcinoma, oropharyngeal carcinoma, and adenocarcinoma of unknown origin (all in the latter group were biopsy proven). Mean tumor diameter was 16 mm. The mean dose delivered to the tumor margin was 16 Gy. Fractionated radiotherapy consisted of 30 Gy to the whole brain. The majority of patients improved clinically after radiosurgery, usually in association with CT or MR evidence of a reduction in the amount of cerebral edema surrounding the tumor. Of the first 60 patients followed up with solitary tumors, four (7%) had a later tumor resection. Local control was provided in 91% of patients. There was no change in tumor size in 53%, a decrease in size in 29%, and complete tumor disappearance in 9% (Figure 5.7). Mean survival after metastatic brain tumor diagnosis was 12.4 months (after utilization of combined treatments). Mean survival after radiosurgery was 9.3 months, at which time 17 patients were still living (actuarial postradiosurgery survival was 10 months).

Loeffler and colleagues [34••] reported their results in 18 patients with 21 recurrent brain metastases treated by LINAC radiosurgery. All patients had previously received conventional radiotherapy to total doses of 30 to 49 Gy. Local tumor control was achieved within the prescribed radiation field in every patient, but two tumors recurred at the treatment margin. As in our series, most patients showed evidence of clinical improvement, often accompanied by a reduction in the amount of surrounding cerebral edema.

Radiosurgery offers two attractive surgical features for solitary brain metastases. First, because a stereotactic technique is used, the problem of locating subcortical or deep, small tumors during craniotomy is avoided. Second, radiosurgery offers potential treatment to patients with tumors in locations associated with a high risk for neurologic deficit after conventional surgery [31••]. It is unlikely that the eight brainstem tumors in this series would have been amenable to conventional resection. Radiosurgery offers satisfactory local control for patients with solitary brain metastases less than 3 cm in diameter that appears similar to the reported survivals after surgical removal. Multicenter randomized trials will evaluate the usefulness of radiosurgery in patients with multiple metastases.

Glial tumors

Uncontrolled local growth eventually leads to the death of patients with primary malignant brain tumors [35]. In an attempt to control local growth, interstitial brachytherapy had been used to deliver a radiation boost to selected, well-circumscribed supratentorial malignant gliomas less that 5 cm in diameter [36•,37]. We have used radiosurgery as an alternative strategy to boost the fractionated radiation dose delivered to biopsy-proven gliomas less than 3 cm in diameter [38•].

We used radiosurgery as an adjuvant to fractionated external-beam radiation therapy or chemotherapy in 19 patients with biopsy-proven glioblastoma multiforme. One patient had also received brachytherapy. Prior craniotomy and resection was performed in 10 patients. Patient age varied from 4 to 63 years. The mean dose delivered to the tumor margin was 15.2 Gy (range, 12 to 20 Gy). During follow-up, which ranged from 3 to 28 months after radiosurgery (mean, 12 months), no imaging or clinical evidence of cerebral radiation injury was seen. The median survival after initial diagnosis was 27 months; 11 patients were still alive 34, 52, 31, 10, 16, 21, 5, 35, 38, 27, and 39 months, respectively, after diagnosis. Median survival after radiosurgery (for the first 14 patients treated with greater than 7 months' follow-up) was 16 months.

Fifteen patients with anaplastic astrocytoma also had radiosurgery after first receiving external-beam fractionated radiation. Mean survival after tumor

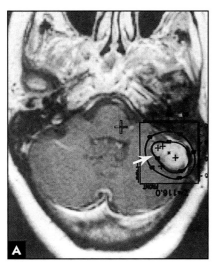
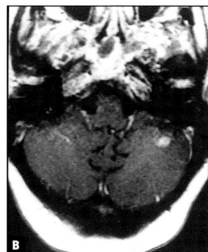

Figure 5.7

Contrast-enhanced magnetic resonance image of a metastatic lung carcinoma in the lateral left cerebellum of a 69-year-old woman. The 50% isodose line (*arrow*) is superimposed on the tumor margin (**A**). Six weeks after radiosurgery, the tumor is markedly decreased in size (**B**).

diagnosis using multimodality therapy was 24.5 months. Nine patients are still alive. There were no cases of radiation injury. Complete disappearance of tumor after radiosurgery was noted in two patients.

Radiosurgery was used as an alternative, rather than an adjunct, to fractionated irradiation in 12 patients with astrocytomas (pilocytic and nonpilocytic). Tumor locations included midbrain ($n = 3$), pons ($n = 2$), cerebellum ($n = 2$), intraventricular ($n = 2$), hypothalamus ($n = 1$), thalamus ($n = 1$), and frontal lobe ($n = 1$). A mean dose of 16 Gy was delivered to the tumor margin (12 to 20 Gy). Three months after radiosurgery, one patient with a midbrain tumor had imaging evidence of radiation-induced blood-brain barrier disruption around the tumor. Marked loss of central contrast enhancement within the neoplasm suggested tumor necrosis. Prolonged corticosteroid therapy was necessary for symptom control. All 12 patients are currently alive (range, 7 to 63 months after diagnosis).

Chordoma and chondrosarcoma

Tumor recurrence and progression of clinical symptoms eventually occurs in most patients following conventional multimodality management of chordomas and chondrosarcomas of the skull base. In an effort to improve results, advanced cranial base microsurgical approaches and a variety of irradiation techniques have been advocated [39–41]. Although these tumors are usually considered radioresistant, some centers have reported benefit from high-dose conventional radiotherapy, brachytherapy [42], and fractionated heavy-charged-particle irradiation [43]. These techniques have been limited by tissue intolerance to high fractionated doses, by the technical difficulties associated with isotope implantation, and by the delivery of radiation to adjacent critical neurologic structures.

We used radiosurgery in the treatment of six patients with chordoma and three with chondrosarcoma [44••]. Two patients with chordoma had radiosurgery alone for clival tumors consistent with that diagnosis on CT and MR scans. All other patients had residual or recurrent tumors after prior microsurgical resection. During follow-up (mean, 21 months; range, 8 to 36 months), preradiosurgery neurologic deficits (abducens nerve palsies) improved in three patients, while the other three patients remained in stable neurologic conditions. Serial imaging studies showed that two patients had smaller tumors and four patients had no growth of the treated tumor volume.

Because the radiation dose can be delivered in a single treatment session and can spare surrounding critical brain structures, stereotactic radiosurgery has potential advantages over fractionated irradiation techniques for treating skull base chordomas and chondrosarcomas. Further follow-up with larger series of patients will be necessary to define the role of radiosurgery in contrast to other surgical techniques and methods of radiation delivery.

Other tumors

We have used radiosurgery to treat patients with other types of benign or malignant intracranial tumors. Such tumors include trigeminal and jugular foramen neurinomas ($n = 11$), solid craniopharyngiomas ($n = 5$), hemangioblastomas ($n = 6$), pineal region tumors ($n = 5$), ependymomas ($n = 6$), primitive neuroectodermal tumors ($n = 2$), malignant schwannoma ($n = 1$), locally invasive parotid adenocarcinoma ($n = 1$), and squamous cell carcinoma of the pharynx ($n = 1$) [45•].

RADIOBIOLOGIC RESEARCH FOR BRAIN TUMOR RADIOSURGERY

Efforts to improve on the results of stereotactic radiosurgery for brain tumors have consisted of advances in computer image integration and dose planning, clinical analyses of acquired experience, and modifications of dose-volume prescriptions for individual tumors. At the University of Pittsburgh, new investigations into the radiobiologic response of specific tumors have been designed.

We used a rat C6 glioma model to study the *in vivo* response of a growing malignant brain tumor to different radiosurgical doses [46••]. Our study showed that the short-term response consisted of neoplastic cell death leading to decreased tumor size. An athymic mouse subrenal capsule xenograft model for acoustic tumor radiosurgery was developed to study the response of different radiosurgical doses on tumor vasculature and cellular integrity. This study showed that radiosurgical doses of 20 and 40 Gy were sufficient to control tumor growth in the 4-month interval after radiosurgery [47••]. A similar model using an implanted human meningioma xenograft is currently being utilized. We hope these models will provide information on specific tumor dose-response relationships and on the radiobiologic mechanisms of tumor control. Currently, we are using the glioma model to study the response of radiosurgery alone versus radiosurgery in combination with whole-brain irradiation or pharmacologic radiation modifiers.

REFERENCES AND RECOMMENDED READING

Papers of particular interest, published within the annual period of review, have been highlighted as:
• Of special interest
•• Of outstanding interest

1. Leksell L: The stereotaxic method and radiosurgery of the brain. *Acta Chir Scand* 1951, 102:316–319.

2. Leksell L: Stereotactic radiosurgery. *J Neurol Neurosurg Psychiatry* 1983, 46:797–803.

3. Lunsford LD, Flickinger JC, Lindner G, *et al.*: Stereotactic radiosurgery of the brain using the first United States 201 source cobalt-60 gamma knife. *Neurosurgery* 1989, 24:152–159.

4. Columbo F, Benedetti A, Pozza F, *et al.*: External stereotactic irradiation by linear accelerator. *Neurosurgery* 1989, 16:154–160.

5. Friedman WA, Bova FJ: The University of Florida radiosurgery system. *Surg Neurol* 1989, 32:334–342.

6. Hartmann GH, Schlegel W, Sturm V: Cerebral radiation surgery using moving field irradiation at a linear accelerator facility. *Int J Radiat Oncol Biol Phys* 1985, 11:1185–1192.

7. Podgorsak EB, Olivier A, Pla M, *et al.*: Dynamic stereotactic radiosurgery. *Int J Radiat Oncol Biol Phys* 1988, 13:1553–1557.

8. Winston KR, Lutz W: Linear accelerator as a neurosurgical tool for stereotactic radiosurgery. *Neurosurgery* 1988, 22:454–464.

9. Kjellberg RN, Abe M: Stereotactic Bragg peak proton beam therapy. In *Modern Stereotactic Neurosurgery.* Edited by Lunsford LD. Boston: Martinus Nijhoff; 1988:463–470.

10. Fabrikant JI, Lyman JT, Hosobuchi Y: Stereotactic heavy-ion Bragg peak radiosurgery for intra-cranial vascular disorders: method for treatment of deep arteriovenous malformations. *Br J Radiol* 1984, 57:479–490.

11. • Kondziolka D, Lunsford LD, Flickinger JC: Stereotactic radiosurgery in children and adolescents. *Pediatr Neurosci* 1990-91, 16:219–221.
Initial experience using the gamma knife for tumors and vascular formations in children.

12. •• Kondziolka D, Dempsey P, Lunsford LD, *et al.*: A comparison between magnetic resonance imaging and computed tomography for stereotactic coordinate determination. *Neurosurgery* 1992, 30:402–407.
Accuracy of MR-determined coordinates for stereotactic surgery at 0.5 or 1.5 T in comparison to CT technique provides data for the use of MR guidance alone.

13. •• Wu A, Lindner G, Maitz AM, *et al.*: Physics of gamma knife approach on convergent beams in stereotactic radiosurgery. *Int J Radiat Oncol Biol Phys* 1990, 18:941–949.
Detailed review of radiation physics, gamma knife design, and quality assurance protocols for radiosurgery.

14. Flickinger JC: The integrated logistic formula and prediction of complications from radiosurgery. *Int J Radiat Oncol Biol Phys* 1989, 17:879–885.

15. • Lunsford LD, Flickinger J, Coffey RJ: Stereotactic gamma knife radiosurgery: initial North American experience in 207 patients. *Arch Neurol* 1990, 47:169–175.
Initial clinical experience using the gamma unit at one institution.

16. • Ebersold M, Harner S, Beatty C, *et al.*: Current results of the retrosigmoid approach to acoustic neurinoma. *J Neurosurg* 1992, 76:901–909.
Hearing preservation indications, techniques, and results for acoustic neurinoma microsurgery.

17. • Thompson BG, Coffey RJ, Flickinger JC, *et al.*: Stereotactic radiosurgery of small intracranial tumors: neuropathological correlation in three patients. *Surg Neurol* 1990, 33:96–104.
Histopathologic findings of tumors after radiosurgery.

18. •• Linskey ME, Lunsford LD, Flickinger JC, *et al.*: Stereotactic radiosurgery for acoustic tumors. *Neurosurg Clin North Am* 1992, 3:191–205.
Detailed review of tumor response and cranial nerve function preservation data for gamma knife radiosurgery in acoustic tumors (101 patients).

19. Adegbite AB, Kahn MI, Paine KWE, *et al.*: The recurrence of intracranial meningiomas after surgical treatment. *J Neurosurg* 1983, 58:51–56.

20. Simpson D: The recurrence of intracranial meningiomas after surgical treatment. *J Neurol Neurosurg Psychiatry* 1957, 20:22–39.

21. •• Kondziolka D, Lunsford LD, Coffey RJ, *et al.*: Stereotactic radiosurgery of meningiomas. *J Neurosurg* 1991, 74:552–559.
Review of the first 50 patients treated with gamma knife radiosurgery for meningiomas; up to 3-year follow-up.

22. • Flickinger JC, Lunsford LD, Wu A, *et al.*: Treatment planning for gamma knife radiosurgery with multiple isocenters. *Int J Radiat Oncol Biol Phys* 1990, 18:1495–1501.
Indications and methods for the use of multiple irradiation isocenters in radiosurgery.

23. Flickinger JC, Nelson PB, Martinez AJ, *et al.*: Radiotherapy of non-functional adenomas of the pituitary gland: results with long-term follow-up. *Cancer* 1989, 63:2409–2414.

24. Linfoot JA, Lawrence JH: Treatment of functioning pituitary tumors. In *Neurosurgery.* Edited by Wilkins RH, Rengachary SS. Toronto: McGraw-Hill; 1985:1119–1126.

25. Degerblad M, Rahn T, Bergstrand G, *et al.*: Long term results of stereotactic radiosurgery to the pituitary gland in Cushing's disease. *Acta Endocrinol* 1986, 112:310–314.

26. Rahn T, Thoren M: Radiosurgery in pituitary adenomas. In *Advances in the Biosciences.* Edited by Landolt AM, Heitz PU, Zapf J. Oxford: Pergammon; 1988:451–453.

27. • Thoren M, Rahn T, Guo WY, *et al.*: Stereotactic radio-surgery with the cobalt-60 gamma unit in the treatment of growth hormone-producing pituitary tumors. *Neuro-surgery* 1991, 29:663–668.

Further experience using the gamma unit in patients with acromegaly.

28. • Flickinger JC, Maitz AH, Kalend A, *et al.*: Treatment volume shaping with selective beam blocking using the Leksell gamma unit. *Int J Radiat Oncol Biol Phys* 1990, 19:783–789.

Indications and methods for isodose shaping using beam-blocking techniques for the gamma unit. These techniques are most useful for parasellar lesions.

29. Friedman RB, Oldfield EH, Nieman LK, *et al.*: Repeat transsphenoidal surgery for Cushing's disease. *J Neuro-surg* 1989, 71:520–527.

30. Sturm V, Kober B, Hover KH, *et al.*: Stereotactic percuta-neous single dose irradiation of brain metastases with a linear accelerator. *Int J Radiat Oncol Biol Phys* 1987, 13:279–281.

31. •• Coffey RJ, Flickinger JC, Bissonette DJ, *et al.*: Radio-surgery for brain metastases using the cobalt-60 gamma unit: methods and results in 24 patients. *Int J Radiat Oncol Biol Phys* 1991, 20:1287–1295.

Initial clinical experience in the management of solitary metastatic brain tumors, predominantly malignant melanoma.

32. •• Patchell RA, Tibbs PA, Walsh JW, *et al.*: A randomized trial of surgery in the treatment of single metastases to the brain. *N Engl J Med* 1990, 322:494–500.

This randomized prospective trial showed that surgical resec-tion plus radiotherapy provided significant increased survival compared with fractionated radiotherapy alone.

33. Lindquist C: Gamma knife surgery for recurrent solitary metastasis of a cerebral hypernephroma: case report. *Neurosurgery* 1989, 25:802–804.

34. •• Loeffler JS, Kooy HM, Wen PY, *et al.*: The treatment of recurrent brain metastases with stereotactic radio-surgery. *J Clin Oncol* 1990, 8:576–582.

Review of LINAC radiosurgery for cerebral metastases with attention to response rates, complications, and patterns of failure.

35. Bashir R, Hochberg F, Oot R: Regrowth patterns of glioblastoma multiforme related to planning of intersti-tial brachytherapy radiation fields. *Neurosurgery* 1988, 23:27–30.

36. • Bernstein M, Laperriere N, Leung P, *et al.*: Interstitial brachytherapy for malignant brain tumors: preliminary results. *Neurosurgery* 1990, 26:371–380.

Techniques and results for irradiation implants for malignant brain tumors.

37. Leibel SA, Gutin PH, Wara WM, *et al.*: Survival and qual-ity of life after interstitial implantation of removable high-activity iodine-125 sources for the treatment of patients with recurrent malignant gliomas. *Int J Radiat Oncol Biol Phys* 1989, 17:1129–1139.

38. • Dempsey P, Kondziolka D, Lunsford LD, *et al.*: The role of stereotactic radiosurgery in the treatment of glial tumors. In *Stereotactic Radiosurgery Update.* Edited by Lunsford LD. New York: Elsevier; 1992:407–410.

Preliminary experience in glioma radiosurgery; emphasizes patient selection criteria.

39. Cummings BJ, Hodson DI, Bush RS: Chordomas: the results of megavoltage radiation therapy. *Int J Radiat Oncol Biol Phys* 1983, 9:633–642.

40. Raffel C, Wright DC, Gutin PH, *et al.*: Cranial chordomas: clinical presentation and results of operative and radia-tion therapy in 26 patients. *Neurosurgery* 1985, 17:703–710.

41. Sen CN, Sekhar LN, Schramm VL, *et al.*: Chordoma and chondrosarcoma of the cranial base: an 8-year experi-ence. *Neurosurgery* 1989, 25:931–941.

42. Gutin PH, Leibel SA, Hosebuchi Y, *et al.*: Brachytherapy of recurrent tumors of the skull base and spine and iodine-125 sources. *Neurosurgery* 1987, 20:938–945.

43. Austin-Seymour M, Munzenrider J, Goitein M, *et al.*: Fractionated proton radiation therapy of chordoma and low-grade chondrosarcoma of the base of the skull. *J Neurosurg* 1989, 70:13–17.

44. •• Kondziolka D, Lunsford LD, Flickinger JC: The role of radiosurgery in the management of chordoma and chondrosarcoma of the cranial base. *Neurosurgery* 1991, 29:38–46.

Preliminary clinical experience with gamma knife radiosurgery for these tumors, with attention to dose selection and reasons for management failure.

45. • Kondziolka D, Lunsford LD: Stereotactic radiosurgery for squamous cell carcinoma of the nasopharynx. *Laryngo-scope* 1991, 101:519–522.

Defines the initial experience with extracranial radiosurgery, including its indications and limitations.

46. •• Kondziolka D, Lunsford LD, Claasen D, *et al.*: Radiobiol-ogy of radiosurgery: Part II: the rat C6 glioma model. *Neurosurgery* 1992, 31:280–288.

The first *in vivo* radiobiologic model to study the response of a malignant brain tumor to radiosurgery.

47. •• Linskey ME, Martinez AJ, Kondziolka D, *et al.*: The radio-biology of human acoustic schwannoma xenografts after stereotactic radiosurgery evaluated in the subrenal cap-sule of athymic mice. *J Neurosurg*, in press.

The first *in vivo* model to study the response of a benign tumor to radiosurgery.

Chapter 6

What's New from the Traumatic Coma Data Bank?

Lawrence F. Marshall
Sharon Bowers Marshall
Melville R. Klauber
Randall M. Chesnut

In 1979, Murray Goldstein, presently the Director of the National Institute of Neurological Disorders and Strokes but at that time Director of its Stroke and Trauma Program, initiated, with the Office of Biometry and Field Studies of that agency, requests for proposals to participate in two data banks, one for traumatic coma and one for stroke. These efforts presented a major initiative to attempt to apply modern computing technology to two serious public health problems. This chapter discusses primarily the most recent publications and observations from the Traumatic Coma Data Bank (TCDB). We would be remiss at the outset, however, if we did not mention the key figures who contributed so much to the TCDB during the 9 years in which data were being collected. Drs. William Weiss, Selma Kunitz, and Cynthia Gross from the Office of Biometry and Field Studies pioneered the design of the Data Bank and deserve enormous credit in overcoming major obstacles as they educated the neurosurgeons, neurosurgical research nurses, and local biostatisticians in the art of the possible in attempting to collect time-and event-oriented data.

Joshua Ellenberg and Mary Foulkes, at the Office of Biometry and Field Studies, shepherded the second phase of the TCDB by setting firm policies for the data analysis and publication. The principal investigators and research personnel during the Full Phase of the TCDB are listed in the Acknowledgment section [1]. It is also appropriate to recognize a few additional individuals, without whose participation the TCDB would not have fulfilled the hopes that many of us had for it. These include Dr. Donald Becker, the late Dr. Kenneth Shulman, Dr. Robert Grossman, Dr. Kamron Tabador, and Rebecca Rimel.

During the initial phase of the pilot TCDB some substantive contributions were made toward the development of rational criteria for the interpretation of computed tomography (CT) scans in head-injured patients. Toutant and colleagues [2] showed that the absence of compression of the basal cisterns was predictive of a poor outcome in these patients. Although this was not the only report on this subject (Teasdale and colleagues [3] and van Dongen and colleagues [4] reported such observations concurrently), the ability to correlate the status of the cisterns with other Data Bank elements, such as the intracranial pressure, was unique. This ability to cross-link data elements played a significant role in the development of a new classification of CT data in severe head injury. This is discussed later. Moreover, as the importance of CT scanning in predicting the patient's course of disease became increasingly clear, moves to standardize the interpretation of these scans within the TCDB resulted in a greater emphasis on the overall volume status of the intracranial contents, a major change from our previous emphasis, which rested primarily on the presence or absence of mass lesions.

Many of the publications of the Full-Phase TCDB appeared in a supplemental issue of the *Journal of Neurosurgery* in November, 1991. It is unnecessary, therefore, to review these reports in detail. Rather the focus here is to examine some of the other observations made within the TCDB and to emphasize those recently reported that may have long-term implications for patient care and research in the future. Thus, although occasional references to material previously presented are made, the emphasis is broader and yet, at the same time, focused on the future.

It is perhaps important also to note those accomplishments within the TCDB that appear to represent substantial changes from previous clinical practice or thinking so these ideas can be further modified for the better as time goes by. It should also be emphasized that the basic data format developed for the Data Bank by its founders, in a series of meetings in late 1979 and early 1980, is now being used in most head-injury centers in the world and for every major clinical trial. Therefore, at least the methodologic hopes for the

Data Bank (*ie*, the ability to collect like-data in multiple institutions throughout the United States) have been exceeded, as the TCDB data collection instruments are now being used throughout the world.

NEW DEVELOPMENTS

Therapy intensity level

During the second phase of the TCDB, when outcome comparisons between patients were made, it became increasingly clear that those who superficially appeared the same often had widely different outcomes and that one major factor that had not been incorporated into any of the analyses was the *intensity of therapy* for elevated intracranial pressure. From these observations came the development of a therapy intensity level (Table 6.1), a scale that has been significantly improved by Marmarou and colleagues [5••] at the Medical College of Virginia. It represents an alternative way of looking at intracranial pressure rather than simply looking at the levels reached during the disease course. Thus, even though two patients may have an identical intracranial pressure course, if one is receiving maximal therapy, including high doses of barbiturates, for example, that patient is viewed differently from one in whom the use of such agents (or in fact mannitol or ventricular drainage) is not required, although their intracranial pressure curves look the same. In fact, Marmarou and colleagues have graphed

Table 6.1 Scoring system for therapy intensity level scale*	
Therapy	**Score**
Barbiturates	15†
Mannitol	
>1 g/kg/h	6
≤1 g/kg/h	3
Ventricular drainage	
>4 times/h	2
≤4 times/h	1
Hyperventilation	
Intensive ($PaCO_2$ <30 mm Hg)	2
Moderate ($PaCO_2$ ≥30 mm Hg)	1
Paralysis	1
Sedation	1

*From Marmarou *et al.* [5••]; with permission.

†Maximum score is 15. Without barbiturates, the score is the sum of the other components.

the therapy intensity level scale against the intracranial pressure so one can have a visual image of the relative intensity of therapy when the intracranial pressure curves are the same. This scale is now being used in the international and domestic studies of tirilazad (Freedox, Upjohn, Kalamazoo, MI), a novel aminosteroid. Until a larger body of experience is obtained with this scale, however, a more general use of the therapy intensity level scale is probably inappropriate.

New classification of head injury

The TCDB developed a new CT classification of head injury in 1984, and its applicability is discussed in considerable detail in the TCDB supplement to the *Journal of Neurosurgery*. This classification, which is based primarily on the volume status of the brain, was an attempt to predict which patents were at risk of increased intracranial pressure and death or severe disability. Based on our experience to date with this scale, it does accomplish that end. However, the classification that is shown in Table 6.2 is far from perfect [6••]. It poorly characterizes small nonsurgical parenchymal lesions, which, if many are present, probably have an adverse impact on outcome. Further, the recent demonstration by Eisenberg and colleagues [7••] within this same cohort of patients, that subarachnoid hemorrhage is an adverse and independent risk factor in patients with severe head injury, suggests that future classifications should include subarachnoid hemorrhage within the classification scheme and not just within the data collection elements.

Extracranial complications

During the early TCDB experience, Dr. Donald Becker, now chairman of the Division of Neurological Surgery at UCLA School of Medicine, repeatedly challenged the Data Bank to determine, "why do patients die?" Most neurosurgeons have assumed that the overwhelming majority of deaths in patients with severe head injury are due to irreversible damage to the brain and that deaths due to pneumonia and other complications of coma, either short or prolonged, are responsible for the death of the patient only as a mode of exodus and not as a primary cause.

There is substantial support for the concept that many patients with severe head injury die primarily because of secondary extracranial injuries rather than from the primary impact injury itself. Greenberg and colleagues [8] demonstrated that only 20% to 25% of all patients with severe head injury who reached the hospital alive but who ultimately died had poor or absent somatosensory evoked potential responses indicative of a severe overwhelming injury. However, 80% of those admitted did not, indicating that perhaps almost half of the deaths that ultimately occur might be attributable to secondary events, some intracranial and some extracranial, given the fact that the overall mortality was 35% to 40%.

In attempting to elucidate further the influence of extracranial complications, Piek and colleagues [9••], working with the TCDB group in San Diego, began to delineate the role of extracranial complications in influencing outcome. Emphasis was placed on those

Table 6.2
Diagnostic categories of types of abnormalities visualized by computed tomography*

Category	Definition
Diffuse injury I (no visible pathology)	No visible intracranial pathology seen on computed tomography scan
Diffuse injury II	Cisterns are present with midline shift of 0–5 mm; lesion densities present; no high- or mixed-density lesion > 25 mL; may include bone fragments and foreign bodies
Diffuse injury III (swelling)	Cisterns compressed or absent with midline shift of 0–5 mm; no high- or mixed-density lesion > 25 mL
Diffuse injury IV (shift)	Midline shift > 5 mm; no high- or mixed-density lesion > 25 mL
Evacuated mass lesion	Any lesion surgically evacuated
Nonevacuated mass lesion	High- or mixed-density lesion > 25 mL; not surgically evacuated

From Marshall *et al.* [6••]; with permission.

patients in whom one would have predicted, on the basis of age and admitting Glasgow Coma Scale score, that their outcome would be a good recovery or moderate disability. Thus, the appropriate conclusion is that such patients did not suffer, at the time of impact, an overwhelming injury to the brain but rather that secondary events ultimately were responsible for their poor outcome or death.

The overall results of the study by Piek and colleagues are to be published in the *Journal of Neurosurgery* and are not completely reiterated here [9••]. The investigation demonstrated that under ideal circumstances, the mortality from acute severe head injury might be reduced by as much as 40% to 45% if the deleterious effects of shock, pneumonia, coagulopathy, and septicemia could be reversed or avoided. Shock was overwhelmingly the most important factor, pneumonia second, and the others responsible for only a modest increment in mortality and morbidity.

Chesnut and colleagues [10] carried out a detailed study on the influence of prehospital shock and hypoxia on outcome. This study demonstrated an almost doubling of mortality and morbidity in patients who had shock in the field, even though it might have been corrected at the time of hospital arrival (Table 6.3) [10]. There was almost a threefold increase in mortality (Table 6.4) in patients who remained in shock at the time of hospital arrival. Interestingly, hypoxia had surprisingly little influence when present alone, indicating that ischemia is the major insult. Unless hypoxia is combined with ischemia, however, it is very detrimental to patients with acute catastrophic injuries of the brain.

Following the impressive demonstration of the adverse consequences of prehospital shock, we carried out a rather detailed analysis of the influence of shock that occurred later in the patient's course (during the intensive care unit phase). This study demonstrated that shock under these circumstances has an equally devastating consequence, despite the fact that it occurs within the hospital setting, where it can be treated more rapidly and usually reversed.

Although this investigation is not complete, it appears that it is related to a small extent to the patient's intracranial diagnosis and primarily to patient treatment. Mannitol administration in the absence of adequate volume replacement or a philosophy that allows the cerebral perfusion pressure to fall below 70 appears to be responsible. Thus, the concept that the systolic blood pressure can fall to levels of 90 mm Hg without consequence to the patient has been shown to be incorrect.

This supports the observations of Rosner and Daughton [11••] that it is important that the cerebral perfusion pressure be maintained above 80 and that the systolic blood pressure not be allowed to drop below 100 mm Hg. Many of the patients described in this present study had very brief episodes of moderate hypotension, defined as a blood pressure less than 90 and greater than 80 systolic, and yet were irreversibly damaged by this event.

Critical levels of intracranial hypertension

Marmarou and colleagues [12••] at the Medical College of Virginia have carefully examined the rela-

Table 6.3
Outcome after secondary insult from time of injury through resuscitation at the Traumatic Coma Data Bank hospital emergency room for mutually exclusive insults*

Secondary insults	Patients, *n*	Total patients, %	Patient outcome, %		
			Good or moderate	Severe or vegetative	Dead
Total cases	717	100	43	20.2	36.8
Neither hypoxia nor hypotension	308	43	53.9	19.2	26.9
Hypoxia[†]	161	22.4	50.3	21.7	28
Hypotension[†]	82	11.4	32.9	17.1	50
Both hypoxia and hypotension	166	23.2	20.5	22.3	57.2

*From Chesnut *et al.* [10]; with permission.
[†]Hypoxia=PaO_2<60 mm Hg; Hypotension=systolic blood pressure < 90 mm Hg.

tionship between intracranial hypertension and vaso-motor instability manifested as hypotension or hyper-tension. The most striking observation from this pro-ject is the fact that the number of nursing observations in a patient in whom the intracranial pressure exceeded 20 mm Hg was a highly significant predictor in explaining outcome (Figure 6.1). In attempting to define further the role of intracranial hypertension in patients with severe head injury, other intracranial pressure cutoff points were also used by Marmarou

Table 6.4
Outcome after secondary insult at time of arrival at the Traumatic Coma Data Bank hospital emergency room for mutually exclusive insults*

Secondary insults	Patients, n	Total patients, %	Patient outcome, %		
			Good or moderate	Severe or vegetative	Dead
Total cases	699[†]	100	42.9	20.5	36.6
Neither hypoxia nor hypotension	456	65.2	51.1	21.9	27.0
Hypoxia[‡]	78	11.2	44.9	21.8	33.3
Hypotension[‡]	113	16.2	25.7	14.1	60.2
Both hypoxia and hypotension	52	7.4	5.8	19.2	75.0

*From Chesnut et al. [10]; with permission.

[†]The total number of patients is 699 instead of 717 due to missing admission data on blood pressure or arterial blood gas values in 18 patients.

[‡]Hypoxia=PaO_2<60 mm Hg; Hypotension=systolic blood pressure < 90 mm Hg.

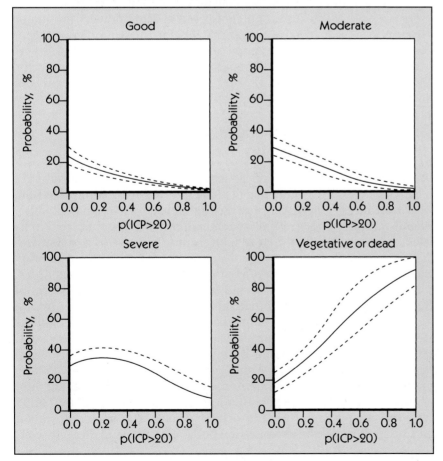

Figure 6.1

Plots of estimated outcome probability versus proportion of intracranial pressure (ICP) measurements more than 20 mm Hg (p(ICP>20)) for each outcome group. To simplify the presentation, the other mod-eled factors were fixed at the following values: age = 30 years, admission motor score = 3 (flexion), abnormal pupils = 1, and proportion of blood pressure (BP) measurements less than 80 mm Hg (p(BP<80)) = 0. Ninety-five percent asymptomatic confidence bands are plotted around each curve. (From Marmarou et al. [12••]; with permission.)

and colleagues, but none was as powerful a predictor as percent of intracranial pressure readings greater than 20 mm Hg, which strongly suggests that the detrimental effects of intracranial hypertension occur at or above this level. It is appropriate to conclude that all elevations of intracranial pressure above 20 mm Hg during the acute phase of management are of potential significance and that therapeutic intervention during the first 72 hours should be instituted at that level.

Ischemia of even a modest degree, whether due to systemic hypotension or intracranial hypertension, has much more severe adverse consequences for the severely injured brain than even previously imagined. When these observations are coupled with the observations regarding the role of subarachnoid hemorrhage in worsening head-injury outcome, one begins to have a comprehensive picture of the remarkable relationships of focal ischemia, as seen in stroke and postaneurysmal subarachnoid hemorrhage, and head injury. Head injury should be viewed not only as a process in which primary impact damage occurs at the time of injury, but also as a disease in which a series of processes are set into motion by the impact, which sensitizes the brain to even mild degrees of ischemia, or ischemia hypoxia.

Neuropsychologic and behavioral outcome

The comprehensive nature of the TCDB permitted the development of unique head injury–specific batteries of cognitive and behavioral measures that we planned to apply systematically. A major problem, however, encountered in the Data Bank and in head-injury research in general in the United States, and probably elsewhere, is our inability to have the patients routinely return for follow-up. Because most patients who suffer severe head injury are young, mobile, single men, they are frequently difficult to find during long periods of follow-up and hard to convince that returning is in their interest. Thus, attrition rates (because of poor compliance and because severe injury or death makes neuropsychologic and behavioral testing impossible) call into question the reliability of the remaining sample to predict accurately the neurocognitive outcome in the entire cohort.

Nevertheless, a remarkable number of detailed cognitive studies have been carried out within the TCDB. Levin and colleagues [13], in a select group of patients who could be adequately examined, have shown that elevated intracranial pressure appears to have little or no influence on neurocognitive recovery. This is somewhat surprising on its face but may again reflect the unique characteristics of the populations studied (ie, the ability to be examined in detail). It

may be that there is a threshold for severity of the intracranial pressure insult that must be exceeded to produce further irreversible brain damage and that the level of insult, in terms of function recovery, would be so severe that the patient cannot be tested. It should also be recalled that within the Data Bank Centers, elevations of intracranial pressure were vigorously treated with the objective of keeping to a minimum the time that the patient had an intracranial pressure above 20 mm Hg. This then is not a study of the natural history of elevated intracranial pressure on neurobehavioral outcome.

Ruff and colleagues [14] have recently shown that the 6-month neurobehavioral assessment is as strong a predictor of "return to work" as the 1-year assessment, indicating that although further changes in cognitive and behavioral function undoubtedly occur with the passage of time, a 6-month assessment, which is easier to get because of the aforementioned problems in patient compliance, can be used for long-term social and economic planning. The study also revealed the tendency for the marketplace to prefer task completion over slow but more accurate task performance. If this observation can be confirmed in a larger series, it raises some serious questions, not only with regard to the American workplace, but also on philosophies of treatment. It is not uncommon for even severely head-injured patients to recover the ability to complete a task, but the speed at which the task is completed is remarkably slowed. If a major objective in the rehabilitation phase is to ensure accurate task completion at the price of speed, this perhaps will illprepare patients for returning to society. Much more work in this area is required, but the implications are both intriguing and troubling.

Alcohol abuse and recovery from head injury

Ruff and colleagues [15] have reported on the effect of the influence of alcohol on recovery within the Data Bank. Chronic alcohol abuse was associated with a poor overall outcome in terms of mortality and morbidity (Figure 6.2), in part because of a higher frequency of CT diagnoses associated with worse prognoses, such as mass lesions, particularly subdural hematomas, and because of the systemic effects of alcohol. Intoxication at the time of impact injury, however, defined as a serum alcohol level of greater than 0.1 mg/dL, was not associated with an increased mortality in Data Bank patients or a poorer overall outcome. Within the Data Bank cohort, we were also unable to demonstrate an increase in the length of time intracranial pressure is elevated over 20 or 30 mm Hg in intoxicated patients. This latter observation calls into question both laboratory and theoretic constructs that alcohol, because of its propensity to induce free radical peroxidation within the brain or spinal cord, should be and is associated with a higher mortality and morbidity. We were unable to find evidence in this cohort of any specific deleterious effect of intoxication in patients who reached the hospital alive. Because the mortal influence of alcohol may occur primarily at the scene, it is incorrect to conclude that alcohol does not affect the mortality and morbidity from head injury in intoxicated patients. In patients arriving at the hospital alive, however, such an effect was not detected. This is an extremely important area of research, and these results should be interpreted cautiously.

IMPLICATIONS FOR THE FUTURE

The TCDB, following on the initial Multinational Data Bank of Jennett and colleagues [16], has served as the foundation for head-injury research as we approach the end of the 20th century. The data forms, and variants thereof, have been used in the recently completed nimodipine trials in head injury as well as the North American and international studies of tirilazad, a novel aminosteroid. Further, many of the concepts developed within the Data Bank are now being employed worldwide, both in head-injury management and in analyzing head-injury research data. The concept of grading complications, for example, and

determining the influence of complications, both intracranial and extracranial, has its origin within TCDB. The TCDB, following on the Multinational Data Bank, serves to add further to our understanding of severe head injury. As we approach the end of the 20th century, these studies should allow for the rational application of new treatment modalities.

The TCDB also brought together a series of interested investigators who, in turn, recruited neurosurgeons, biostatisticians, research scientists, and, perhaps most importantly, a cadre of research nurses. From this effort, major head-injury research groups have developed in many locations, not only in the United States but also throughout the world. Further, the interaction of these four centers continues 4 years after the Data Bank concluded acute data collection. The TCDB now serves as a national repository of information and provides strong evidence of the utility of computerized storage techniques for such complex medical events. The tremendous advances in microprocessing speed and power as well as the widespread distribution of such capabilities are likely to have tremendous implications for head injury research in particular and for research within the biomedical sciences in general for many years to come. Our opportunity to participate has allowed the University of California at San Diego to develop unique and important expertise both for research, and for resident training, an opportunity not likely to be duplicated for a long time to come.

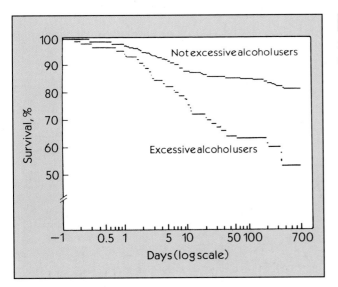

Figure 6.2

Survival rates of excessive versus not excessive alcohol users. (*From* Ruff *et al.* [15]; with permission.)

ACKNOWLEDGMENT

We would like to acknowledge the following members of the Traumatic Coma Data Bank. From the National Institute of Neurological Disorders and Stroke: Mary A. Foulkes, PhD, Project Director; Jonas H. Ellenberg, PhD, Biometry and Field Studies Branch Chief; Kathryn Chantry, Brenda Dyer, Gloria Ike, Margaret Meadows, and Alan Polis, Project Staff; Michael Walker, MD (Chairman), John Coronna, MD, Martha Denkla, PhD, Donlin Long, MD, and George W. Williams, PhD, Monitoring Committee. From the Medical College of Virginia, Richmond, VA: Harold F. Young, MD, and Anthony Marmarou, PhD, Principal Investigators; John D. Ward, PhD, Coinvestigator; Hope B. Turner, RN, MS, Nurse Coordinator; Jeff Kreutzer, PhD, Neuropsychologist; Sung Choi, PhD, Randy L. Anderson, MS, Statisticians; and Harry Lutz, PhD, James Angus, Cindy Angeil, and JoAnne Tillett, Center Personnel. From the University of California, San Diego, CA: Lawrence F. Marshall, MD, Principal Investigator; Thomas G. Luersson, MD, Coinvestigator; Sharon B. Marshall, RN, Nurse Coordinator; Ronald M. Ruff, PhD, Neuropsychologist; Melville R. Klauber, PhD, Statistician; Kathryn Hults, RN, Theresa Gautille, RN, Marjan van Berkum, RN, and Jackie Cotton, RN, Nurses; Judy Huang, MS, David Malloy, MD, Kelly Sarter, and David Young, PhD, Center Personnel. From the University of Texas Medical Branch, Galveston, TX: Howard M. Eisenberg, MD, Principal Investigator; E. Francois Aldrich, MD, Richard L. Weiner, MD, F. Guinto, MD, and G. Campbell, MD, Coinvestigators; Carol Cayard, RN, Nurse Coordinator; Harvey S. Levin, PhD, Neuropsychologist; Howard E. Gary, Jr., PhD, Statistician; Sonia Price, RN, and Barbara Turner, LVN, Nurses; and Walter M. High, Jr., PhD, Christy Saydjari, BS, Sandra Portman, PhD, Ossie Stoneham, Yolanda Santos, and Liz Zindler, Center Personnel. From the University of Virginia, Charlottesville, VA: John A. Jane, MD, PhD, Principal Investigator; T. S. Park, MD, J. A. Pershing, MD, Dennis G. Vollmer, MD, and William C. Broaddus, MD, PhD, Coinvestigators; Deborah B. Charlebois, RN, Nurse Coordinator; Jeff T. Barth, PhD, Neuropsychologist; James T. Torner, PhD, Terri Germanson, MS, MPH, and Wayne Alves, PhD, Statisticians; Nancy A. Tisdale, RN, Janice L. Hinkle, RN, MSN, and Cathy Allen, RN, Nurses; Rose Broderick, Jannine Jagger, PhD, Nancy Mays, Oswald Steward, PhD, Barbara Sadovnic, BS, and Libby Wenger, Center Personnel.

REFERENCES AND RECOMMENDED READING

Papers of particular interest, published within the annual period of review, have been highlighted as:
• Of special interest
•• Of outstanding interest

1.   Foulkes MA, Eisenberg HM, eds: National Institute of Neurological Disorders and Stroke report on the Traumatic Coma Data Bank. *J Neurosurg*, 1991, (suppl):S1–S66.

2.   Toutant SM, Klauber MR, Marshall LF, *et al.*: Absent or compressed basal cisterns on first CT scan: ominous predictors of outcome in severe head injury. *J Neurosurg* 1984, 61:691–694.

3.   Teasdale E, Cardosa E, Galbraith S, *et al.*: CT scan in severe diffuse head injury: physiological and clinical correlations. *J Neurol Neurosurg Psychiatry* 1984, 47:600–603.

4.   van Dongen KJ, Braakman R, Gelpke GJ: The prognostic value of computerized tomography in comatose head injured patients. *J Neurosurg* 1983, 59:951–957.

5.   •• Marmarou A, Anderson RL, Ward JD, *et al.*: NINDS Traumatic Coma Data Bank: intracranial pressure monitoring methodology. *J Neurosurg* 1991, 75(suppl):S21–S27.

This work from the TCDB demonstrates a methodology used to collect and analyze intracranial pressure data, and as such it serves as an important reference for workers in the field.

6.   •• Marshall SB, Klauber MR, van Berkum Clark M, *et al.*: A new classification of head injury based on computerized tomography. *J Neurosurg* 1991, 75(suppl):S14–S20.

This paper introduces the new classification of head injury that breaks down diffuse injury into four categories based on the degree of intracranial volume in the presence or absence of small, nonsurgical, hemorrhagic, or other areas.

7.   •• Eisenberg HM, Gary HE Jr, Aldrich EF, *et al.*: Initial CT findings in 753 patients with severe head injury: a report from the NIH Traumatic Coma Data Bank. *J Neurosurg* 1990, 73:688–698.

The first report on CT from the TCDB. It demonstrates the important, independent, and adverse consequence of subarachnoid hemorrhage in closed head injury when seen on the first CT scan.

8.   Greenberg RP, Newlon PG, Hyatt MS, *et al.*: Prognostic implications of early multimodality evoked potentials in severely head-injured patients: a prospective study. *J Neurosurg* 1981, 55:227–236.

9.   •• Piek J, Chesnut RM, Marshall LF, *et al.*: Extracranial complications of severe head injury. *J Neurosurg* 1992, in press.

This work highlights the extracranial complications that are responsible for a significant proportion of deaths and a remarkable increase in morbidity in patients with severe head injury.

10.   Chesnut RM, Marshall LF, Klauber MR, *et al.*: The role of secondary brain injury in determining outcome from

severe head injury: analysis of the frequency of occurrence and impact on outcome of hypotension and hypoxia and their interactions with severe multiple trauma in severely brain injured patients. *J Trauma* 1993, 34, in press.

11. •• Rosner MJ, Daughton S: Cerebral perfusion pressure management in head injury. *J Trauma* 1990, 30:933–941.

This paper supports more recent observations on the importance of maintaining the cerebral perfusion pressure certainly above 70 and perhaps above 80.

12. •• Marmarou A, Anderson RL, Ward JD, *et al.*: Impact of ICP instability and hypotension on outcome in patents with severe head trauma. *J Neurosurg* 1991, 75(suppl):S59–S66.

This work introduces in detail a concept of therapeutic intensity level and demonstrates the importance of shock when it interacts with rising intracranial pressure.

13. Levin HS, Eisenberg HM, Gary HE, *et al.*: Intracranial hypertension in relation to memory functioning during the first year after severe head injury. *Neurosurgery* 1991, 28:196–200.

14. Ruff RM, Marshall LF, Crouch JA, *et al.*: Predictors of outcome following severe head trauma: follow-up data from the Traumatic Coma Data Bank, in press.

15. Ruff RM, Marshall LF, Klauber MR, *et al.*: Alcohol abuse and neurological outcome of the severely head injured patient. *J Head Trauma Rehabil* 1990, 5:21–31.

16. Jennett B, Teasdale G, Galbraith S, *et al.*: Severe head injuries in three countries. *J Neurol Neurosurg Psychiatry* 1977, 40:291–298.

Chapter 7

Pharmacologic Advances in Cerebral Protection in Ischemia and Head Injury

Scott L. Henson
Kevin S. Lee
Jennifer B. Green
Neal F. Kassell

The high metabolic demand and limited energy storage of neurons render the brain particularly susceptible to ischemic injury. Brain injury resulting from ischemia is a common occurrence in a variety of settings, including stroke and head injury. Unfortunately, the pharmacologic agents that are now available for treating ischemic cell damage have met with only limited success (Table 7.1). The need for new neuroprotective treatments is therefore great, and intense efforts are currently underway to identify and refine viable therapeutic strategies. The following chapter examines some of the more recent approaches to this multifactorial problem, and, when appropriate, speculates about the future directions these efforts will take.

MECHANISMS AND TYPES OF ISCHEMIC DAMAGE

The identification of new therapeutic approaches has been aided by a growing understanding of the cellular mechanisms associated with ischemic damage. While a clear consensus has not been reached as to the precise sequence of molecular and cellular events responsible for ischemic pathogenesis, a general picture has emerged. As metabolic stores are reduced or depleted, the normal ionic gradients maintained by neurons become compromised. The loss of ionic homeostasis leads directly or indirectly to cellular degeneration. In the case of dense ischemia, a rapid and severe form of neuronal depolarization (ischemic depolarization) occurs, which is associated with substantial elevations of intracellular calcium, sodium, and chloride. Most neurons are irreversibly damaged when ischemic depolarization is maintained for extended periods. Cellular swelling caused by osmotically driven water entry occurs as a result of the loss of sodium and chloride gradients. In addition, a variety of normal cellular functions are disrupted or damaged by overactivation of calcium-sensitive mechanisms, lactate acidosis, and free radical generation. When allowed to continue, these events provide severe and virtually insurmountable obstacles for the therapeutic treatment of compromised neurons.

Less intense ischemia, such as occurs in the penumbra of a focal ischemic event, may present many of the same challenges; however, the opportunity for neuronal recovery is greatly enhanced. Ischemic depolarization is not usually a sustained feature of the ischemic penumbra. It is possible for mildly or moderately ischemic tissue to maintain a semblance of normal ionic balance with only intermittent and weaker disturbances of membrane polarization. Several types of pharmacologic treatments are capable of reducing cerebral infarction in the penumbra, and the development of more efficacious treatments seems likely.

It is apparent that the depth and duration of ischemia are key factors determining the outcome from cerebral ischemia. A third factor influencing this process is the intrinsic vulnerability of a given class of neuron. Certain neurons are selectively vulnerable to ischemia, perishing following ischemic events as brief as a minute or two in duration. Neurons that are highly susceptible to ischemia exhibit two general rates of degenerative response. One class of selectively vulnerable neurons exhibits a rapid form of cell death. The brevity of the ischemic events required to trigger damage (minutes) and the rapid degenerative sequence (hours or less) render these cells virtually unsalvageable unless prophylactic intervention is feasible. A second class of selectively vulnerable cells undergoes a delayed form of neuronal death requiring 2 to 4 days

for its full expression. Substantial efforts are currently underway to identify the mechanisms responsible for this slowly developing form of ischemic damage. Recent studies suggest that the therapeutic window for delayed neuronal death can range from a few hours to a day. Thus, the potential for developing successful therapeutic interventions to ameliorate delayed neuronal death is quite encouraging.

RATIONALES FOR CEREBRAL PROTECTION

Therapeutic strategies for cerebral ischemia can be divided into two broad and nonexclusive categories: 1) treatments designed to reestablish an optimal level of blood flow and 2) treatments designed to minimize cellular damage directly. In the case of cerebrovascular compromise, the first category of treatment may involve the reduction or elimination of vascular interruption via surgical intervention, the reestablishment of appropriate systemic factors (eg, restoration of adequate blood pressure, cardiac output, hematocrit), or thrombolytic therapy. Common features of this effort might include induced hypertension, hypervolemic hemodilution, and vascular dilation. The second general category of treatment targets specific cellular mechanisms participating in the initiation or expression of cellular pathology. The growing understanding of events occurring during and following ischemia has facilitated efforts to devise strategies for cerebral protection (Figures 7.1 and 7.2). The remaining sections

Table 7.1
Partial list of agents that have been or are being used for cerebral protection

Calcium channel blockers
Barbiturates
N-methyl-D-aspartate receptor blockers
Hyperosmolar agents
Free radical scavengers
Opiate agonists and antagonists
Steroids
Gangliosides
Isoflurane
Dilantin
Lidocaine
Benzodiazepines
Prostaglandin inhibitors
Iron chelators
Propranolol
Butanediol
Fluosol D-aspartate
Dimethylsulfoxide
Adenosine

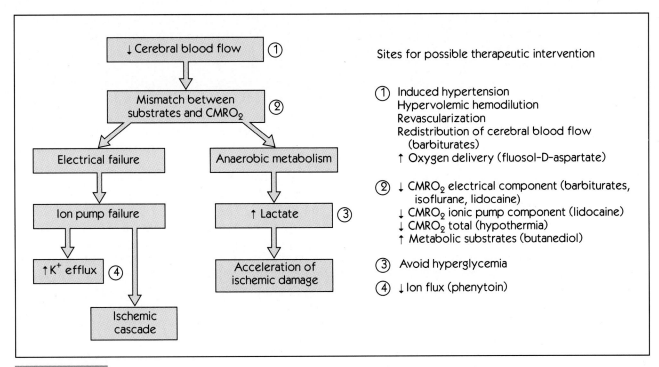

Figure 7.1

Initial steps in cerebral ischemia and sites for possible therapeutic intervention. $CMRO_2$—cerebral metabolic requirement for oxygen. (*From* Nels and Spetzler [30]; with permission.)

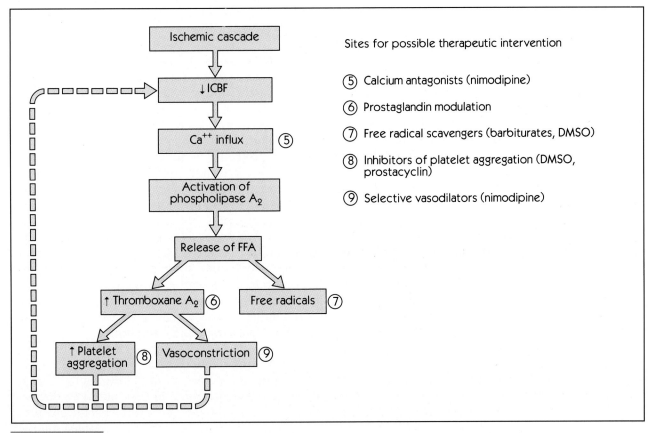

Figure 7.2

Ischemic cascade (*see* Figure 7.1) and sites for possible therapeutic intervention. Ca^{++}—calcium ion; DMSO—dimethyl sulfoxide; FFA—free fatty acid; LCBF—local cerebral blood flow. (*From* Nels and Spetzler [30]; with permission.)

of this article examine pharmacologic manipulations that modulate one or more key cellular mechanisms and analyze the utility of these manipulations for limiting ischemic damage.

CALCIUM CHANNEL BLOCKERS

Elevation of intracellular calcium ions plays a central role in the pathogenesis of ischemic cell injury. The influx of extracellular calcium and the release of intracellular stores combine to initiate a wide variety of calcium-sensitive mechanisms that when overactive can be detrimental to the cells. Because of the importance of maintaining low intracellular calcium concentrations, channel blocker therapy has received wide attention in the treatment of ischemia. Several calcium channel blockers have been investigated, including dihydropyridines (nimodipine, nifedipine, nicardipine, and nitrendipine) and diphenylalkylaminines (flunarizine, cinnarizine), each of which prevents Ca^{++} influx through voltage-sensitive channels (Table 7.2). Studies in animals indicate that these drugs may reduce delayed neuronal damage during reperfusion and increase cerebral blood flow by causing relaxation of vascular smooth muscle [1••]. Human studies using calcium channel blockers have yielded mixed results. At least four studies have shown that nimodipine reduces morbidity from vasospasm after subarachnoid hemorrhage [1••,2••]. Interestingly, these clinical trials have shown a protective effect in reducing the incidence of severe delayed ischemia deficits but have not shown a reversal of chronically spastic vessels; however, intravenous nicardipine has been shown to have a modest effect on reversal of vasospasm in a rabbit model [3•]. It has been speculated that the beneficial effects of these agents are not solely due to direct cytoprotection but may also involve the ability to dilate small resistance vessels not visible on angiography. It is noteworthy in this context that HA1077, a recently developed homopiperazine vasodilator that acts as a Ca^{++} channel blocker in vascular smooth muscle, has been shown to reverse angiographically visible, chronic cerebral vasospasm in the two-hemorrhage canine model when given intravenously [4•]. It is therefore quite important when evaluating the neuroprotective effects of calcium antagonists to distinguish between their potential effects on vascular and neuronal elements.

Clinical trials of nimodipine and nicardipine in acute ischemic stroke have yet to demonstrate clearly beneficial effects [1••, 5••,6]. The results obtained so far certainly suggest that further studies of these agents for acute cerebral infarct are justified but that treatment must be started within 6 to 12 hours to be effective. In addition, because of its hypotensive effects, treatment with nimodipine will probably be limited to therapeutic protocols using relatively low doses [1••,5••].

Clinical trials for nimodipine have also been performed in a population of 175 head-injured patients. Although ischemic neuronal damage may be the ultimate cause of cell loss after severe head injury, this trial failed to show any beneficial effect of nimodipine [7••].

The mixed results with nimodipine and nicardipine may reflect the limited actions of individual channel blockers. The elevation of intracellular calcium during ischemia results from an influx of calcium through multiple types of channels and from the release of calcium from intracellular stores. In general, calcium channel blockers are effective in blocking calcium entry at only one type of Ca^{++} channel. The activation of multiple, unblocked sources of calcium therefore places an upper limit on the utility of any agent that operates solely by blocking a single channel type. Another potential complication associated with certain calcium blockers is their hypotensive action. Although vasodilation is desirable in regions of pathologic constriction, generalized vasodilation leading to hypotension is contraindicated in the treatment of most forms of ischemia.

BARBITURATES

Barbiturates are presently the most effective pharmacologic cerebral protective agents available. They are commonly used to protect the brain against periods of ischemia during aneurysm, tumor, and arteriovenous malformation surgery. They have been shown to be neuroprotective in both focal and global ischemia but may be slightly more efficacious in focal ischemia. High-dose barbiturate therapy has been used in the treatment of severe posttraumatic brain swelling and found to have some efficacy in improving survival and outcome. Whether this is due to the effects of high-dose barbiturates on elevated intracranial pressure or to other poorly understood mechanisms is unknown. This therapy is not without complications. A study of high-dose thiopentone used in patients with severe head injuries showed a high incidence of hypotension (58%), hypokalemia (82%), respiratory complications (76%), infections (55%), hepatic dysfunction (87%), and renal dysfunction (47%) [8•].

The primary protective mechanism of the barbiturates has been attributed to their ability to decrease the cerebral metabolic rate. More specifically, it has been suggested that they selectively reduce the electrical component, or that required for synaptic transmission, while maintaining the energy required for basic cellular functions. Anesthetic agents that reduce cerebral metabolic rate to an equal level, however, do not offer the same degree of protection. It is therefore likely that barbiturates possess mechanisms of protective action in addition to the mere reduction of cerebral metabolic rate. A list of some of these possible mechanisms is given in Table 7.3.

GLUTAMATE ANTAGONISTS

The synaptic release of excitatory amino acids, in particular glutamate, is considered to be an important factor in contributing to neuronal death. Because it may be difficult to prevent the massive release of glutamate after brain injury, the most intensive efforts have been directed at blocking the action of glutamate at the receptor level. Glutamate activates at least three different types of receptors, each of which can contribute to the elevation of intracellular Ca^{++}. Perhaps the best characterized of these receptors is the N-methyl-D-aspartate (NMDA)–preferring receptor. The NMDA receptor is coupled to a channel, which allows the entry of extracellular Ca^{++}. Numerous recent studies have examined the effects of competitive and noncompetitive NMDA receptor antagonists in animal models of ischemia. In general, NMDA antagonists are ineffective or weakly effective in limiting damage following global forebrain ischemia [9••]. In contrast, these agents are effective in sparing the penumbra in models of focal cerebral ischemia.

Noncompetitive NMDA receptor antagonists can exert several additional central effects, which may mitigate against their application. One complication is a direct hypothermic effect. The noncompetitive antagonist, MK801, elicits potent and dose-dependent reductions in temperature. In addition, sedation and possible memory disturbances have been described for noncompetitive antagonists. Therefore,

there is a great interest in other agents such as dextrorphan and a new competitive glutamate antagonist, LY233053, the effects of which are less prolonged than noncompetitive antagonists. Pilot human studies are underway to evaluate the toxicity and possible applications of these drugs to several clinical situations, including acute stroke, cardiac arrest, intraoperative brain protection, and cerebral trauma [1••].

A second category of glutamate receptor is the α-amino-3-hydroxy-5-methyl-4-isoxazole (AMPA)–preferring receptor. This inotropic receptor is not directly permissive for calcium entry; however, it mediates a strong depolarizing response, which leads to the activation of voltage-dependent calcium currents. Recent animal studies examining the neuroprotective effects of an AMPA receptor antagonist (NBQX) are quite encouraging. NBQX has been shown to be neuroprotective of both global and focal ischemia in animal models [10••,11••]. Novel antagonists for AMPA receptors are currently under development, and these compounds represent a promising new avenue for treating a wide range of ischemic brain damage.

A final category of glutamate receptor is the quisqualate-preferring metabotropic receptor. These receptors can contribute to elevated intracellular calcium indirectly by increasing the second messenger IP3. The therapeutic value of targeting the metabotropic glutamate receptor is currently unknown.

FREE RADICAL SCAVENGERS

Free radicals are highly reactive chemical species whose levels increase dramatically during ischemia and following reperfusion. The reactive oxygen species generated under these conditions include the following: superoxide radical ($^{\bullet}O_2^{-}$), hydroxyl radical ($^{\bullet}OH^{-}$), hydrogen peroxide (H_2O_2), singlet oxygen ($^{1}O_2$), and nitric oxide ($^{\bullet}NO$). Substantial evidence

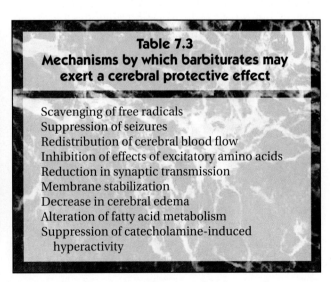

Table 7.2
Mechanisms by which calcium channel blockers may exert a cerebral protective effect

Prevention of Ca^{++} entry into cells
Prevention of Ca^{++} sequestration by mitochondria
Vasodilation
Free radical scavenging
Alteration in fatty acid metabolism
Prevention of platelet aggregation
Prevention of increases in blood viscosity

Table 7.3
Mechanisms by which barbiturates may exert a cerebral protective effect

Scavenging of free radicals
Suppression of seizures
Redistribution of cerebral blood flow
Inhibition of effects of excitatory amino acids
Reduction in synaptic transmission
Membrane stabilization
Decrease in cerebral edema
Alteration of fatty acid metabolism
Suppression of catecholamine-induced
   hyperactivity

has accumulated implicating oxygen free radicals in ischemic pathogenesis [12••]. For example, superoxide radical has been shown to increase substantially in experimental models of global and focal ischemia. The $^{\bullet}O_2^{-}$ radical can then attack proteins and polyunsaturated phospholipids in plasma membranes and other cellular constituents. This oxidative process disturbs plasma membrane function and may disrupt lysomes, mitochondria, and peroxisomes. Clearly damage to any or all of these cellular targets can have severe consequences for continued viability.

There are a number of naturally occurring enzymes that terminate the propagation of free radical cascades. Superoxide dismutase, catalase, glutathione peroxidase, α tocopherol, and ascorbic acid are all enzymes that help interrupt specific free radical actions. A primary function of these enzymes during normal cellular function is to maintain the concentrations of free radicals below a critical level, thus avoiding an autodegenerative response. Unfortunately, the effective stores of many of these enzymes are rapidly depleted during ischemia. Consequently, on reperfusion (and reoxygenation), there is a burst of unopposed free radical activity that can damage cells.

Because of the detrimental impact of excessive levels of free radicals, the potential therapeutic effects of free radical scavengers have attracted considerable attention. Laboratory studies have shown that antioxidants (eg, allopurinol and dimethylthiourea) reduce the size of cerebral infarctions following focal ischemia [10••]. Protective effects have also been reported in a model of global ischemia.

The interest in neuroprotection using antioxidant therapy has stimulated the synthesis of novel compounds that exhibit antilipolytic and free radical scavenging characteristics. A prime example of this effort is the 21-aminosteroid, tirilazad mesylate (U74006F). Tirilazad mesylate belongs to a class of compounds (lazaroids) that lacks glucocorticoid and mineralocorticoid activity but exhibits potent antilipid peroxidation activity. Tirilizad mesylate scavenges lipid peroxyl and superoxide free radicals. It also has antilipolytic properties inhibiting the release of arachidonic acid from mouse pituitary tumor cells and hypoxic pituitary tissue. Finally, a membrane-stabilizing function independent of its antioxidant and antilipolytic function has also been attributed to this compound. Tirilazad mesylate and related compounds have been tested in a variety of experimental paradigms for their protective properties against the consequences of cerebral ischemia and concussive head injury. These studies have produced mixed results, with some demonstrating substantial protective effect whereas others show little or no reduction in infarct size in ischemic animal models [13•,14•].

Clinical trials involving these agents in head injury, subarachnoid hemorrhage, and acute stroke are currently ongoing and now in phase II.

The free radical scavenger superoxide dismutase improves cerebral blood flow and reduces ischemic cerebral edema in animal models of reperfusion after stroke. It has been shown that the cytosolic free Ca^{++} in superoxide dismutase–treated animals exhibits significantly better recovery during the reperfusion period than in control animals. Additionally, the extent of focal damage is reduced in these animals [15••].

Dihydrolipoate is a biologic dithiol that has been found to have antioxidant activity. It has been tested in primary neuronal cultures and in vivo models of cerebral ischemia and found to have some protective properties. Assuming that free and sufficiently high plasma concentrations as well as good central nervous system penetration can be realized, thiols could become effective tools for the treatment of ischemia [16•].

GANGLIOSIDES

Gangliosides are naturally occurring glycosphingolipids that play a role in the promotion of developmental and regenerative processes in the central nervous system. Exogenously administered gangliosides penetrate the blood-brain barrier, actively insert into neuronal membranes, and in a variety of models of central nervous system injury may exert acute protective effects on neural tissue, presumably by preserving the functional integrity of cell membranes [17•]. Treatment with the monosialoganglioside GM_1 has been reported to limit functional deficits and cerebral edema caused by trauma. GM_1 also improves outcome and limits damage in animal models of global and focal ischemia, although one report failed to show reduction in infarct size with a focal insult [17•]. The protective effects of gangliosides in ischemia have also been demonstrated in vitro: GM_1 can attenuate glutamate-induced neurotoxicity, preserve mitochondrial structure, and preserve membrane excitability in hypoxic neural tissue [17•]. A review of nine double-blind, placebo-controlled clinical trials involving 784 patients showed a statistically significant benefit in neurologic recovery when GM_1 was administered within 48 hours after stroke. Additionally, it was concluded that treatment with GM_1 accelerated recovery from neurologic deficits during the first 2 weeks after stroke and that early administration after the stroke seems to increase the probability of a positive treatment result [18••]. In one human study of GM_1 administered to patients with subarachnoid hemorrhage, there was improved outcome as assessed by Glasgow Coma Scale scores when compared with placebo [19•].

Further study of these agents is required, however, before they can be recommended for routine clinical use in stroke and head or spinal cord injury.

STEROIDS

Laboratory investigations have yielded equivocal findings concerning the use of corticosteroids in acute ischemic injury as well as in head injury. The results of the National Acute Spinal Cord Injury Study, however, indicate that high dosages of methylprednisolone may be useful in the acute therapy of a number of cerebral insults and for prophylaxis before certain neurosurgical procedures [20••]. Methylprednisolone is thought to exert its neuroprotective action by the inhibition of lipid peroxidation. Methylprednisolone is more potent in this regard than are prednisolone, hydrocortisone, or dexamethasone. Other mechanisms such as anti-inflammatory action may also play a role. Methylprednisolone has been shown to enhance the early recovery of mice subjected to a moderately severe concussive head injury when administered at 5 minutes postinjury. Initial clinical studies of high-dose methylprednisolone in subarachnoid hemorrhage have suggested some effectiveness in the reduction of angiographically demonstrable vasospasm [20••]. Further controlled trials, however, are needed to establish this. The available experimental data argue against the use of methylprednisolone or other glucocorticoids in acute ischemic stroke [20••].

OPIATE RECEPTOR ANTAGONISTS

Opiate antagonists have been examined in central nervous system trauma and ischemia based on the hypothesis that endogenous opioids contribute to the secondary pathophysiologic response to central nervous system injury. Since 1981, a substantial body of experimental data has shown that opiate receptor antagonists can improve physiologic variables, histopathologic sequelae, and neurologic outcome following ischemic or traumatic insults. The most extensively studied opiate antagonist has been naloxone; however, the high doses required for neuroprotection suggest that either the effects are not opiate receptor mediated or that they occur through K or δ receptors, which are relatively insensitive to naloxone [21]. Current interest has centered on antagonists that exhibit greater specificity for K receptors, such as nalmefene, WIN 44,441-3, and nor-binaltorphine. In a rat model of traumatic brain injury, treatment with nalmefene significantly improved long-term neurologic outcome and was shown to improve early

changes in intracellular free magnesium concentration, ADP levels, and cytosolic phosphorylation potential [22]. Similarly, in a rabbit spinal cord ischemia model comparing nalmefene and the NMDA receptor antagonist MK-801, both drugs were comparable in improving outcome and limiting neuronal damage [21]. Results from tissue culture studies and models of forebrain ischemia show that neuroprotective effects of opiate antagonists may derive in part from an ability to attenuate NMDA receptor–mediated neurotoxicity and decrease excitatory amino acid release [21]. This should continue to be a promising area of investigation.

VOLATILE ANESTHETICS

Volatile anesthetics such as isoflurane and halothane are capable of reducing cerebral metabolic rate and producing electroencephalographic suppression in a manner similar to that of barbiturates. For these reasons, volatile anesthetics have been heavily investigated for their potential neuroprotective effects. Recent studies, however, have shown that reduction of cerebral metabolic rate is not sufficient for anesthetic-mediated brain protection. Moreover, isoflurane and halothane fail to reduce infarct size in animal ischemia models [23•]. Ongoing clinical experience still suggests that there is some neuroprotective effect with isoflurane; however, the conditions under which it is most effective and the mechanism mediating its effects remain unclear [23•,24••].

OTHER AGENTS

Several other agents deserve mention, as they may have important future roles as cerebral protectants. Dilantin applied before hypoxia in hippocampal slices slows loss of transmission during hypoxia and leads to 75% recovery of evoked potentials with reoxygenation. It appears to protect against hypoxia-induced loss of synaptic transmission and may lessen neuronal damage and cognitive dysfunction associated with stroke. Additionally, dilantin has demonstrated the ability to protect against glutamate-mediated neurotoxicity associated with ischemia in hippocampal slices [25•,26•].

Adenosine is a potent modulator in the nervous system that depresses neuronal activity by inhibiting neurotransmitter release from presynaptic nerve terminals and by altering ion conductances in postsynaptic cells. Several lines of evidence suggest that adenosine-related compounds may be useful in cerebral protection. Adenosine receptor agonists and adenosine uptake inhibitors ameliorate neuronal damage following forebrain ischemia, whereas adenosine receptor antagonists aggravate this process. Exceptions to these observations, however, have been presented [27•]. Potential obstacles for the use of adenosine-related compounds are that many of the most effective receptor agonists elicit hypothermia and exhibit limited permeability through the blood-brain barrier. The future utility of targeting the adenosine modulatory system for cerebral protection therefore depends on the development of compounds that readily cross the blood-brain barrier but have limited peripheral side effects.

The α-adrenergic antagonist idazoxan can provide protection from global cerebral ischemia. Idazoxan, however, also recognizes imidazole receptors. Oxazole rilmentidin, an agent highly selective for imidazole receptors, was examined with idazoxan in a middle cerebral artery occlusion model, and both were found to reduce focal ischemic infarction. The mechanism does not appear secondary to antagonism of α_2-adrenergic receptors or to elevation of local cerebral blood flow. Occupation of imidazole receptors, either in the ischemic zone or at remote brain sites, appears to be responsible for the neuroprotective effects of rilmentidin and idazoxan [28•].

5-Hydroxytryptamine-1A (5-HT1A) receptor agonists have been shown to reduce neuronal damage within the CA1 section of the hippocampus after 10 minutes of forebrain ischemia. This was not due to a hypothermic effect. It is postulated that the neuroprotective activity of 5-HT1A agonists is mediated by some as yet unknown inhibitory action on the neurons [29•].

Finally, it may be possible to target calcium-activated intracellular events, such as proteases and phospholipases, for cerebral protection. The elevation of intracellular calcium is believed to play a critical role in a cerebral pathology by overactivating calcium-sensitive intracellular events. Recent laboratory studies indicate that inhibitors of calcium-activated proteolysis are of benefit in limiting morphologic, biochemical, and electrophysiologic damage following ischemia. It may therefore be possible to target specific intracellular mechanisms that are activated by calcium and serve to destabilize the cells.

CONCLUSIONS

The development of a single agent that provides complete cerebral protection has been, and will likely remain, elusive. The cascade of events that is set in motion after central nervous system injury appears far too complex for a single "magic bullet." The burgeoning understanding of this cascade, however, is providing important clues for refining and extending current therapies. As the more successful of the pharmacologic approaches discussed are integrated into routine and rapid therapy, it is likely that the outcome following cerebral damage will be greatly enhanced.

REFERENCES AND RECOMMENDED READING

Papers of particular interest, published within the annual period of review, have been highlighted as:
•Of special interest
••Of outstanding interest

1. •• Grotto J: Pharmacologic modification of acute cerebral ischemia. In *Stroke: Pathophysiology, Diagnosis and Management*, 2nd ed. New York: Churchill Livingstone; 1992:943–951.
Excellent overview of the pharmacotherapy of cerebral ischemia.

2. •• Adams H: Prevention of brain ischemia after aneurysmal subarachnoid hemorrhage. *Neurol Clin* 1992, 10:251–268.
Fairly comprehensive review of the pathophysiology and treatment of ischemia related to vasospasm.

3. • Pasqualin A, Vollmer DG, Marron JA, *et al.*: The effect of nicardipine on vasospasm in rabbit basilar artery after SAH. *Neurosurgery* 1991, 29:183–188.
Modest effect of intravenous nicardipine on vasospasm in a rabbit basilar artery in subarachnoid hemorrhage model.

4. • Satoh SH, Suzuki V, Ikegaki I, *et al.*: The effects of HA1077 on cerebral circulation after SAH in dogs. *Acta Neurochir* 1991, 110:185–188.
Newly developed Ca^{++} channel blocker improves hemodynamic function in a subarachnoid hemorrhage model.

5. •• American Nimodipine Study Group: Clinical trial of nimodipine. *Stroke* 1992, 23:3–8.
Nimodipine had no overall effect when treatment was begun within 48 hours.

6. Murphy JJ, TRUST Trial Group: Randomized double-blind placebo controlled trial of nimodipine in acute stroke. *Lancet* 1990, 336:1205–1209.

7. •• Bailey I, Bell A, Gray J, *et al.*: A trial of the effect of nimodipine on outcome after head injury. *Acta Neurochir* 1991, 110:97–105.
Nimodipine failed to improve clearly the outcome from severe head injury in 175 patients.

8. • Schalen W, Messeter K, Nordstrom CH: Complications and side effects during thiopentone therapy in patients with severe head injuries. *Acta Anaesth Scand* 1992, 36:369–377.

Showed high incidence of renal, hepatic, cardiac, and respiratory infections and electrolyte disorders with high-dose thiopentone.

9. •• Siesjo BK: Pathophysiology and treatment of focal cerebral ischemia. Part I: pathophysiology. *J Neurosurg* 1992, 77:169–184.

Review article examines the pathophysiology of lesions caused by focal cerebral ischemia.

10. •• Siesjo BK: Pathophysiology and treatment of focal cerebral ischemia. Part II: mechanisms of damage and treatment. *J Neurosurg* 1992, 77:337–354.

Part II of review article that examines the mechanisms of ischemic damage and possible pharmacologic interventions.

11. •• Nellgard B, Wieloch T: Postischemic blockade of AMPA but not NMDA receptors mitigates neuronal damage in the rat brain following transient severe cerebral ischemia. *J Cereb Blood Flow Metab* 1992, 12:2–11.

α-Amino-3-hydroxy-5-methyl-4-isoxazole receptor blockade may be as important as NMDA blockade in certain types of ischemic insult.

12. •• Halliwell B: Reactive oxygen species and the central nervous system. *J Neurochem* 1992, 59:1609–1623.

Excellent review of free radicals and mechanisms of injury in the nervous system.

13. • Beck T, Beilenberg GW: The effects of two 21-aminosteroids on overt infarct size 48 hours after MCA occlusion in the rat. *Brain Res* 1991, 560:159–162.

Agents are shown to be mildly effective in reducing cortical infarct size.

14. • Lesiuk H, Sutherland G, Peeling J, *et al.*: Effect of U74006F on forebrain ischemia in rats. *Stroke* 1991, 22:896–901.

U74006F is beneficial in ameliorating ischemic neuronal injury, particularly in the neocortex.

15. •• Araki N, Greenberg J, Uematsn D, *et al.*: Effect of superoxide dismutase on intracellular calcium in stroke. *J Cereb Blood Flow Metab* 1992, 12:13–52.

The protective action of superoxide dismutase may be due to its ability to attenuate increases in intracellular calcium during the recirculation period.

16. • Prehn J, Karkonthy C, Nuglisch J, *et al.*: Dihydrolipoate reduces neuronal injury after cerebral ischemia. *J Cereb Blood Flow Metab* 1992, 12:78–87.

A biologic dithiol antioxidant has neuroprotective properties similar to those of methylthiourea.

17. • Mayer S, Pulsinelli W: Failure of GM1 ganglioside to influence outcome in experimental focal ischemia. *Stroke* 1992, 23:242–246.

GM_1 ganglioside treatment failed to reduce cerebral infarct size in permanent focal ischemia model.

18. •• Mahadik S: Gangliosides: new generation of neuroprotective agents. In *Emerging Strategies in Neuroprotection.* Edited by Marangos P. Boston: Birkhauser; 1992:196–200.

Excellent new book on the developing concepts in neuroprotection.

19. • Papo I, Benedetti A, Cartieri A, *et al.*: Monosialoganglioside in subarachnoid hemorrhage. *Stroke* 1991, 22:22–26.

GM_1 treatment produced improvement in patients with sub arachnoid hemorrhage measured by Glasgow Coma Scale scores.

20. •• Hall E: The neuroprotective pharmacology of methylprednisolone. *J Neurosurg* 1992, 76:13–22.

Outstanding and in-depth review of methylprednisolone's pharmacology and neuroprotective properties and why we should be using it more.

21. Yum S, Faden A: Comparison of the neuroprotective effects of the NMDA antagonist MK-801 and the opiate receptor antagonist nalmefene in experimental spinal cord ischemia. *Arch Neurol* 1990, 47:277–281.

22. Vink R, McIntosh T, Rhomhangi R, *et al.*: Opiate antagonist nalmefene improves intracellular free magnesium, bioenergetic state and neurologic outcome following traumatic brain injury in rats. *J Neurosci* 1990, 10:3524–3530.

23. • Warner D, Zhou J, Rasmani R, *et al.*: Reversible focal ischemia in the rat: effects of halothane, isoflurane, and methohexital anesthesia. *J Cereb Blood Flow Metab* 1991, 11:794–802.

Isoflurane fails to demonstrate as much neuroprotective ability as previously thought. Cerebral metabolic rate reduction is not sufficient criteria for anesthetic-mediated brain protection.

24. •• Todd M, Warner D: A comfortable hypothesis reevaluated: cerebral metabolic depression and brain protection during ischemia. *Anesthesiology* 1992, 76:161–164.

Insightful discussion of the role of cerebral metabolic depression in brain protection.

25. • Stanton P, Moskal J: DPH protects against hypoxia-induced impairment of hippocampal synaptic transmission. *Brain Res* 1991, 546:351–354.

Dilantin protects against hypoxia-induced loss of synaptic transmission in hippocampal slices.

26. • Potter P, Detwiler P, Thorne B, *et al.*: Diphenylhydantoin attenuates hypoxia-induced release of [3H] glutamate from rat hippocampal slices. *Brain Res* 1991, 558:127–130.

Dilantin decreased the release of glutamate in rat hippocampal slices.

27. • Mori M, Nishizaki T, Okada Y: Protective effect of adenosine on anoxic damage of hippocampal slice. *Neuroscience* 1992, 46:301–307.

Adenosine may have protective effect against anoxia or aglycemia damage of brain tissue by facilitating the resynthesis of tissue ATP during recovery phases.

28. • Maiese K, Pek L, Berger S, *et al.*: Reduction in focal cerebral ischemia by agents acting at imidazole receptors. *J Cereb Blood Flow Metab* 1992, 12:53–63.

Idazoxan blockade of imidazole receptors rather than α-adrenergic sites may be responsible for the neuroprotective actions of rilmentidin and idazoxan.

29. • Prehn J, Backharb C, Karkouthy C, *et al.*: Neuroprotective properties of 5-HT1A receptor agonists in rodent models of focal and global cerebral ischemia. *Eur J Pharmacol* 1991, 203:213–222.

5-Hydroxytryptamine-1A receptor agonists reduced damage in CA1 after 10 minutes of forebrain ischemia.

30. Nels D, Spetzler RF: Cerebral protection against ischemia. In *Cerebral Blood Flow: Physiologic and Clinical Aspects.* Edited by Wood JH. New York: McGraw-Hill; 1987:651–676.

Chapter 8

Magnetic Resonance Angiography

Robert A. Zimmerman
Thomas P. Naidich

Magnetic resonance (MR) angiography is now reaching its adolescence, a time when technological development has made considerable progress in pulse sequence design, data acquisition, postprocessing methods, and display [1•]. The next stage is the application of selected types of MR angiography to resolve specific clinical questions and to avoid diagnostic pitfalls. To these ends, MR angiography must be evaluated systematically in each disease state, compared with conventional arteriography, ultrasonography, and other established diagnostic modalities, and then correlated with pathologic findings and operative observations. The ultimate goals of MR angiography should be to improve diagnostic accuracy, to reduce patient morbidity by decreasing the need for more invasive techniques, and to add to our basic understanding of disease processes [1•].

Magnetic resonance angiography displays blood vessels by depicting the signal changes caused by blood flow. The MR angiogram is generated by one of two techniques. Time-of-flight MR angiography depends on the increase in the amplitude of the intravascular signal caused by inflow of fresh proton spins into the imaging volume. In this technique, prior application of radiofrequency pulses (called *pre-saturation pulses*) suppresses the signal from all stationary tissue in the imaging volume. Only spins that arise outside the volume and flow into the volume give MR signal, so the image displays high signal only at the site of flowing blood [2•]. Phase-contrast MR angiography is based on alterations of the phase of intravascular spins that are induced as the spins flow through a magnetic field gradient [3•]. In this technique, spins that move through a magnetic field gradient acquire a change of phase that depends on their velocity and the direction of their motion across the gradient. Stationary spins acquire no phase shift. Flowing spins do acquire a phase shift, so long as they flow across magnetic gradient lines. Spins that flow perpendicular to the gradient cross the greatest number of gradient lines and acquire the greatest phase shift. Spins that flow in the plane of the gradient, parallel to the gradient, cross no gradient lines and so acquire no phase shift. Spins that angle across the gradient acquire intermediate phase shift that is proportional to their vector component perpendicular to the gradient. Because the technique is sensitive to the velocity of the spins, estimated flow velocity must be encoded into the pulse sequences. In complex structures with differing flow rates, such as arteriovenous malformations, multiple series with different velocity encodings may be required.

In both MR angiography techniques, multiple thin sections are acquired over a period ranging from 5 to 10 minutes for time-of-flight and up to 10 to 20 minutes for phase-contrast studies. Areas of flow appear in each section as foci of high signal. Computer algorithms, such as the maximum intensity pixel projection (MIPP), are then used to identify the high-intensity pixels in each image and to connect them, slice by slice, throughout the image volume. Such "follow-the-dots" computer programs generate the MR angiographic picture. This composite image can be displayed in multiple planes, or it can be segmented into selected smaller volumes to display specific regions free from confusing superimposed vessels (Figure 8.1).

Both phase-contrast and time-of-flight MR angiography can be performed in either a three-dimensional or two-dimensional mode. Three-dimensional time-of-flight MR angiography demonstrates fast flow and consequently is good for arterial anatomy MR angiography [4•]. The major dural venous sinuses, such as the superior sagittal or transverse venous sinuses, may have flow that is fast enough to be visualized by three-dimensional time-of-flight MR angiography [4•]. Most other venous structures are not seen. Three-dimensional time-of-flight MR angiography is acquired as a thick slab of either 16, 32, 64, or 128 contiguous slices, each 0.8 to 1.5 mm in thickness. Because the data for each slice are acquired by exciting the full thickness of the slab, each slice has greater signal-to-noise ratio and shows finer vascular detail. With the three-dimensional time-of-flight technique, however, flowing spins tend to become less bright as they course distally within the imaging slab [4•]. This signal loss is due to *in-plane saturation*. As a result, the high signal intensity of inflowing blood is lost. The

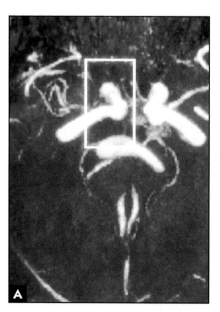

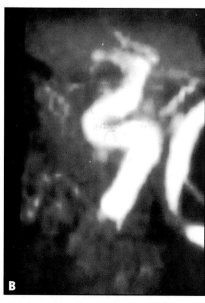

Figure 8.1

Segmentation of three-dimensional time-of-flight magnetic resonance angiography. **A,** Axial image defining the region of interest (*rectangular box*). All other data will be excluded from the reformatted image. **B,** Sagittal reformatted data shows the intrapetrous and intracavernous portions of the internal carotid artery and the adjacent basilar artery. Superimposition of the left internal carotid artery has been eliminated.

spins become saturated, and the saturated vessels fade from view (Figure 8.2). In-plane saturation affects slowly flowing spins more than rapidly flowing spins, so vessels with slow flow are poorly shown by three-dimensional time-of-flight MR angiography.

Two-dimensional time-of-flight MR angiography is a technique that demonstrates both fast and slow flow [4•]. Two-dimensional time-of-flight MR angiograms are acquired as a series of up to 64 contiguous slices. Because each slice of the two-dimensional time-of-flight series is acquired as a separate single image, each slice is an entry slice. That is, each slice displays the high signal of inflowing blood with no loss of signal from in-plane saturation. As a consequence, two-dimensional time-of-flight MR angiography is able to depict slow flow relatively well. The disadvantage of two-dimensional time-of-flight MR angiography is that patient motion between slices causes misregistration artifacts in the MIPP. These may degrade the MR angiogram or render it uninterpretable. At present, a further limitation of the two-dimensional time-of-flight technique is that the individual slices cannot be less than 2 mm in thickness. Fine detail may also be limited because the signal-to-noise ratio is limited by the thinness of the slice. However, slices can be overlapped and interpolated to provide improved vessel delineation.

The advantages of both the three-dimensional and two-dimensional techniques may be combined by performing multiple sequential three-dimensional time-of-flight MR angiograms as a series of *thin* overlapping slabs and then stacking the thin slabs just as one would the individual slices of a two-dimensional time-of-flight MR angiogram, in order to create a composite angiogram with reduced in-plane saturation, higher signal-to-noise ratio, and better edge def-

inition. This technique is designated *multiple overlapping thin-slab acquisitions* (MOTSA). MOTSA partially overcomes three MR angiography problems: 1) relatively poor spatial resolution, 2) saturation effects seen with three-dimensional time-of-flight MR angiography in smaller slow-flow vessels and in larger vessels situated at the distal end of a thick slab, and 3) signal loss from intravoxel phase dispersion resulting from turbulence [5•,6••]. Recent analysis of the value of these three different time-of-flight MR angiography techniques for evaluation of the intracranial vasculature in healthy volunteer subjects revealed that the proximal arterial circulation is best seen with a single thick volume (three-dimensional time-of-flight MR angiography) or with multiple thin-volume three-dimensional methods (MOTSA). The distal arterial branches are best appreciated by using MOTSA, and the venous circulation is best visualized by using two-dimensional time-of-flight MR angiography [7•].

Both three-dimensional and two-dimensional time-of-flight techniques are limited by the turbulence of flow that occurs where vessels bifurcate, where vessels change direction, and where vessels are narrowed by atherosclerotic disease [2•]. Turbulence produces dephasing of the moving protons within the blood vessel. This dephasing causes loss of signal from flowing spins. Even where blood flow is present, signal loss from dephasing mimics, and may be misinterpreted as, absence of signal from vascular stenosis or from a filling defect within the vessel. Such dephasing can be minimized by using a higher matrix size (smaller voxel), by decreasing the echo time, and by the injection of an intravascular paramagnetic contrast agent, such as gadopentetate dimeglumine (Magnevist; Berlex Laboratories, Cedar Knolls, NJ) to shorten relation times.

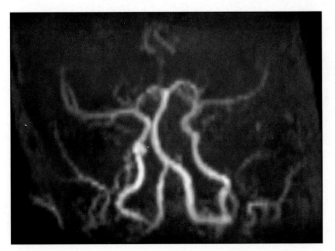

Figure 8.2

In-plane saturation effects. Coronally reformatted three-dimensional time-of-flight magnetic resonance angiogram obtained with 128 partitions from a single slab shows progressive loss of signal in the distal middle cerebral artery branches due to saturation effects.

Use of a relaxation agent such as gadopentetate dimeglumine may substantially improve the image quality of MR angiography by increasing the conspicuity of peripheral small vessels and by eliminating or reducing areas of signal loss from turbulence (Figure 8.3). These relaxing agents increase the contrast of vessels versus the background by selectively shortening the T_1 value of blood more than the T_1 value of stationary tissues [8]. This advantage is lost whenever the perivascular "background" tissue also shows enhancement. Thus, a relative contraindication to the use of contrast-enhanced MR angiography is the presence of an adjacent perivascular lesion, such as a subacute infarct or a brain tumor. In such cases, contrast enhancement within the perivascular lesion produces high MR signal that is detected and displayed by the MIPP algorithm, obscuring the vascular anatomy. Another potential disadvantage of using contrast enhancement for MR angiography is that venous structures that were not seen on routine noncontrast three-dimensional time-of-flight MR angiography may now become visible and may be superimposed on the arterial anatomy.

Magnetic resonance angiography images may be improved by using appropriate imaging coils. Small peripheral intracranial vessels are consistently imaged better by using a surface coil than by using a head coil, provided that the small field of view is kept constant. More centrally located vessels are visualized as well or better when a standard head coil is used [9].

Improvements in MR resolution may also be achieved by a technique called *magnetization transfer suppression*. This technique takes advantage of the fact that blood has a lower concentration of macromolecules than does the stationary perivascular brain tissue. The protons within macromolecules are relatively immobile, have shorter T_2 relaxation times, and resonate over a broader frequency range than do the more mobile protons that exist in the free water. Application of a low-power radiofrequency pulse (called the magnetization transfer suppression pulse) at a frequency that is slightly off the resonant proton frequency successfully saturates the immobile, more broadly responsive protons in the macromolecules but leaves the protons within free water relatively unaffected [10••]. Because stationary perivascular brain tissue has a significantly higher concentration of macromolecules than does intravascular blood, magnetization transfer suppression saturation of these macromolecules suppresses the background signal far more than the blood signal. This increases the relative contrast of blood to background and provides sharper definition of the blood vessels.

Magnetic resonance angiography techniques can also be used to measure actual flow velocities within blood vessels, not just to display vascular anatomy. By use of a modified MR angiography sequence [11••], the flow velocities have been measured in the middle cerebral arteries in six volunteers under differing conditions of "static" and "active" cerebral function. Mea-

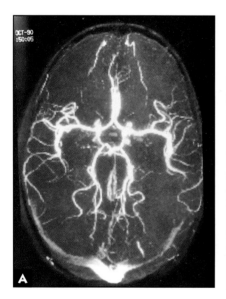 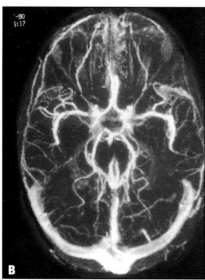

Figure 8.3

Normal three-dimensional time-of-flight magnetic resonance angiogram with and without gadopentetate dimeglumine. **A,** Precontrast angiogram. **B,** Postcontrast angiogram. Note that the postcontrast examination shows greater conspicuity of small vessels but also shows well the dural venous sinuses and the internal cerebral vein.

surements of the average values for mean maximal middle cerebral artery flow velocities were 69.8 cm/s before brain activation by finger movement, 77.2 cm/s during brain activation, and 69.6 cm/s afterward (Table 8.1). This MR flow technique compares well with transcranial Doppler: the increase in flow velocity with brain activation was 11% as measured by MR angiography and 11.3% as measured by transcranial Doppler sonography.

Future technical developments in MR angiography are likely to be helpful to the operating neurosurgeon. These include stereoscopic MR angiography [12] as well as MR angiography for planning stereotactic procedures. Ehricke and colleagues [13•] have shown that computer algorithms can be used to combine MR imaging and MR angiography data sets to produce a three-dimensional surface reconstruction that reveals both the gyral surface and the vascular anatomy. The three-dimensional image (Figure 8.4) may then be shaved and peeled to display the precise relationships of the vessels to the brain surface. The information derived has practical implications for planning stereotactic biopsy or implantation procedures.

Table 8.1
Maximal velocities measured with magnetic resonance imaging in the middle cerebral artery before, during, and after finger movement*

	Maximal velocities, *cm/s*	
	Mean ± SD	Range
At rest before finger movement	69.8 ± 9.1	53–84
During finger movement	77.2 ± 8.6	58–92
At rest after finger movement	69.6 ± 9.3	56–86
Difference between velocities measured before and during finger movement	7.1 ± 2.9	1–12
Difference between velocities measured during and after finger movement	7.2 ± 4.0	2–13

*From** Mattle *et al.* [11••]; with permission

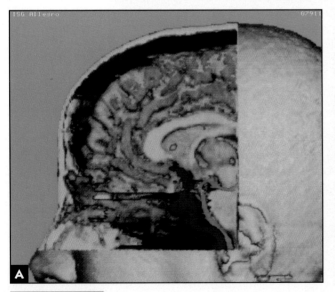 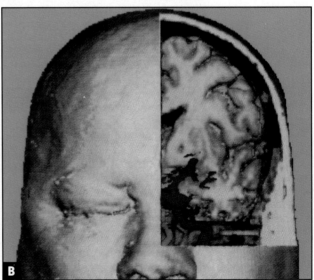

Figure 8.4

Sagittal (**A**) and coronal (**B**) views of the anatomic relationship of the left internal carotid artery to the brain and surface anatomy. There is a distal left internal carotid artery aneurysm.

CLINICAL APPLICATIONS

Table 8.2 lists the present indications for MR angiography.

Aneurysms

It is appealing to consider using MR angiography as a screening test for the diagnosis of unruptured aneurysms (Figure 8.5). If MR angiography is highly accurate, there is the opportunity to deal with these aneurysms before rupture to reduce the associated morbidity and mortality. Aneurysms as small as 3 to 4 mm have been detected with three-dimensional time-of-flight MR angiography with a spatial resolution of 0.9 mm [14]. In one series of 19 patients with 21 aneurysms confirmed by angiography, there was an incremental increase in sensitivity from 67% with MR angiography images alone to 86% when the MR angiogram was evaluated together with the individual axial slices of the original three-dimensional data set and the conventional MR image [14]. Other authors have found that with three-dimensional time-of-flight MR angiography they could demonstrate the morphology of aneurysms and their relationships to the vessels of origin more accurately with smaller aneurysms than they could with larger aneurysms (> 0.8 to 1 cm in diameter) [14,15]. Larger aneurysms can reduce the inflow and washout of fresh (unsaturated) spins within the lumen of the aneurysm, so MR angiography displays an artifactual reduction in the signal intensity within the aneurysm [15]. In the setting of a relatively recent (subacute) hematoma, the high signal intensity of methemoglobin on MIPP MR angiography images may obscure an adjacent aneurysm or the vessel that is suspected of harboring an aneurysm. This occurs because the signal of methemoglobin is high enough to be incorporated with the high signal of intravascular flow when the MIPP algorithm is reconstructed. With an older subacute thrombus that contains methemoglobin of only moderately increased signal intensity in the periphery of the aneurysm, the signal intensity of this site may be somewhat reduced on the MIPP MR angiogram, whereas the patent lumen is more intense [15]. In the

Table 8.2
Indications for magnetic resonance angiography in adult and pediatric patients*

Vascular occlusion
(*eg*, from emboli, thrombosis, vasculitis, atherosclerosis, focal compression, or increased intracranial pressure)

Diminished flow within a vessel leading to decrease in size of the vessel
(*eg*, congenital hypoplasia of a blood vessel, diminished flow and diminished vessel size due to either more proximal stenosis or to diminished distal runoff from vascular occlusion or increased intracranial pressure)

Focal narrowing of a blood vessel wall by a disease process within the wall
(*eg*, vasculitis, atherosclerosis, dissection)

Filling defect within the vascular lumen
(*eg*, embolus, thrombus)

Increased flow within a vessel resulting in an increase in size of the vessel lumen
(*eg*, arteriovenous malformation)

Increase in number of vessels
(*eg*, nidus in an arteriovenous malformation, hypervascular tumor)

Collateral blood flow
(*eg*, around the site of vascular occlusion, luxury perfusion, Moyamoya disease)

Vascular encasement (*eg*, meningioma, cranial base rhabdomyosarcoma) and vascular displacement
(*eg*, craniopharyngioma, acoustic schwannoma)

Anomalous vascular position
(*eg*, internal carotid artery passing through the middle ear, congenital tortuosity of common or internal carotid arteries, and anomalous vessels such as persistent trigeminal artery, otic artery, or hypoglossal artery)

Intracerebral bleeds
(*eg*, rule-in vascular causes, such as arteriovenous malformation, aneurysm, embolus, venous thrombosis)

Pre- and postprocedure evaluation
(*eg*, interventional neuroradiology, neurosurgery, extracorporeal membrane oxygenation)

From Zimmerman and Bilaniuk [4•]; with permission.

setting of an acute or chronic thrombus, the periphery of the aneurysm may not be visible at all [16].

Houston and colleagues [17••] studied 12 patients with 14 aneurysms with three-dimensional time-of-flight and three-dimensional phase-contrast MR angiography and compared these findings with those of conventional angiography. They found that the three-dimensional phase-contrast method was better for showing the patent aneurysm lumen, especially in aneurysms larger than 15 mm in size. Three-dimensional time-of-flight MR angiography was necessary to show the presence or absence of subacute thrombus and was equal to three-dimensional phase-contrast MR angiography for aneurysms that were 3 to 15 mm in size. Blatter and colleagues [6••] used the MOTSA technique in 13 patients with 19 aneurysms. In the 14 aneurysms that were demonstrated by conventional angiography, one aneurysm 1.8 mm in diameter arising at the origin of the anterior choroidal artery was not seen on MR angiography. Tsuruda and colleagues [18] evaluated five patients with cerebral aneurysms treated by endovascular balloon occlusion. These postoperative aneurysm patients are ideal for evaluation by MR imaging or MR angiography because the balloons are essentially free of the metallic artifact that is found with even the nonferromagnetic aneurysm clips. Both patients treated with occlusion of the proximal internal carotid artery showed lack of flow on MR angiography. In the three patients with partially treated aneurysms with residual flow on conventional angiography, three-dimensional time-of-flight MR angiography detected residual flow in two but failed to show flow in one. This failure resulted from the presence of methemoglobin,

which produced a signal intensity similar to blood flow, and from progressive saturation of the slow flow within the residual aneurysmal lumen, so signal was not produced.

Postoperative complications may also be shown by MR angiography. In a series of nine patients with fusiform dilatation of the internal carotid artery following childhood surgery for craniopharyngioma, the aneurysms were demonstrated in all seven patients examined with three-dimensional time-of-flight MR angiography [19]. MR angiography may thus prove to be valuable in the postoperative assessment of these and other patients at risk.

Other concerns presently limit the broad application of MR angiography to aneurysm work-up, including the well-appreciated facts that conventional MR imaging may not detect acute subarachnoid hemorrhage [20]; that uncooperative patients may move during the study, precluding the possibility of integrating the individual images into an MR angiogram [4•]; and that vascular spasm can reduce the degree of flow into the aneurysm, thereby reducing the ability of MR angiography to display its lumen [16].

Arteriovenous malformations

The cerebral arteriogram remains the gold standard for the diagnosis of arteriovenous malformations. However, MR angiography has been found to be valuable in the initial screening, whether or not there has been an intracerebral bleed [4•]. When suspicion of possible arteriovenous malformation is raised by the presence of an increased number of or tortuosity of flow voids on MR imaging, MR angiography has been

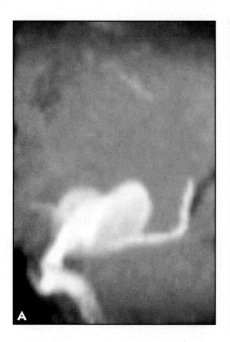
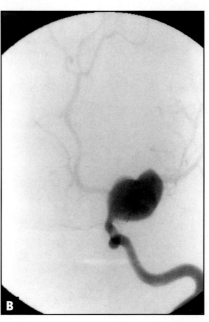

Figure 8.5

Distal internal carotid artery aneurysm. **A,** Coronal oblique reformatted three-dimensional time-of-flight magnetic resonance angiogram of a distal internal carotid artery aneurysm. No neck is identified. **B,** Oblique anteroposterior projection of the internal carotid arteriogram shows the same aneurysm, and again, no neck is identified. The aneurysm appears to share a common wall with the internal carotid artery where it extends into the proximal middle cerebral artery.

useful in differentiating among an arteriovenous malformation (Figure 8.6), prominent normal vessels, and collateral blood flow related to more proximal vascular occlusions. When the intracerebral hematoma is hyperacute (oxyhemoglobin) and does not yet show high signal intensity on T_1-weighted images, three-dimensional time-of-flight and three-dimensional phase-contrast MR angiography are both satisfactory imaging techniques [4•]. When the hematoma has progressed to the stage of methemoglobin and does exhibit high signal intensity on T_1-weighted images, three-dimensional phase-contrast MR angiography is necessary to eliminate the high signal intensity of methemoglobin from the background [4•].

In a series of 10 patients with arteriovenous malformations studied by three-dimensional phase-contrast MR angiography, Nussel and colleagues [21] found that successful MR angiography display of key diagnostic information regarding the blood supply to the arteriovenous malformation, the size of the nidus, and the nature of the draining veins depended on lesion size. Three-dimensional phase-contrast MR angiography provided complete diagnostic information in all six large arteriovenous malformations (3 to 7 cm in size) but in only one of four small arteriovenous malformations (< 2 cm in size). In the three patients with small arteriovenous malformations, MR angiography failed to provide complete information. Less optimistic results were reported by Houston and colleagues [17••] using three-dimensional time-of-flight and three-dimensional phase-contrast MR angiography in a series of 17 patients with vascular anomalies: 11 arteriovenous malformations, one arteriovenous fistula in the brain, one dural fistula, one venous angioma, one slow-flow arteriovenous malformation, one cavernous angioma of the thalamus, and one cryptic arteriovenous malformation. The slow-flow arteriovenous malformation and the thalamic cavernous angioma were not seen on MR angiography but were seen on gadopentetate-enhanced MR imaging. The authors found that the number of feeders to the arteriovenous malformations demonstrated

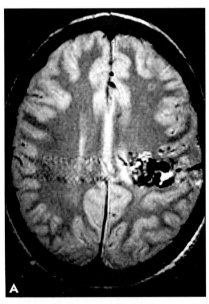

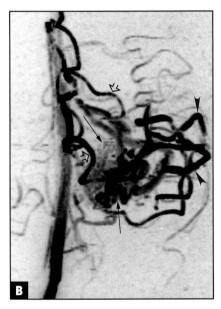

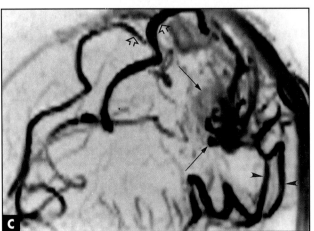

Figure 8.6

Arteriovenous malformation. **A,** Axial long repetition time, short echo time magnetic resonance (MR) image shows areas of mixed low and increased signal intensity in the left parietal lobe. Phase-encoding artifacts are generated across the image in a horizontal band due to the pulsation of the blood vessels. Serpiginous hypointensities represent vessels in the nidus of an arteriovenous malformation. **B,** Axial three-dimensional time-of-flight MR angiogram shows enlarged feeding branches of the middle cerebral artery (*arrowheads*), the nidus of the arteriovenous malformation (*arrows*), and enlarged branches of the anterior cerebral artery (*open arrows*). **C,** Sagittal oblique reformatted MR angiogram shows the enlarged feeding branches of the anterior cerebral artery (*open arrows*), the nidus of the arteriovenous malformation (*arrows*), and feeding branches of the middle cerebral artery (*arrowheads*).

by MR angiography was quite variable and that in only one patient did they identify the same feeders by MR angiography as by the conventional angiogram [17••]. These authors point out that with three-dimensional phase-contrast MR angiography the velocity encoding is a key technical factor, so multiple series performed at differing velocity encodings may be necessary to display all of the venous and arterial structures. With three-dimensional phase-contrast MR angiography and a velocity encoding of 10 to 20 cm/s, slow-and medium-velocity venous structures are identified. With three-dimensional phase-contrast MR angiography and a velocity encoding of 60 cm/s, the feeding arteries, nidus, and high-velocity draining veins are identified.

Blatter and colleagues [6••] used MOTSA MR angiography in 26 patients with arteriovenous anomalies, 12 of which were brain arteriovenous malformations, and found a good correlation between conventional angiography and MR angiography in those arteriovenous malformations fed by a single pedicle. In complex cases with multiple feeders or draining veins, the correlation was difficult.

A significant current limitation of MR angiography is the inability to demonstrate the temporal sequence of filling of vessels passing into and out of the arteriovenous malformation. To image selectively the individual circulations (ie, left internal carotid, right internal carotid, or vertebrobasilar territories) passing into the arteriovenous malformation, one must selectively presaturate the other parent vessels to suppress signal from them [4•,22]. MR angiography and MR imaging remain superior methods for demonstrating the location and relationships of the arteriovenous malformation nidus to the brain tissue [17••].

Acquired cerebrovascular disease

Stroke from acquired cerebrovascular disease continues to be the most common life-threatening and disabling neurologic disease of adult life [23]. MR angiography of the extracranial and intracranial circulation holds out the promise that an accurate noninvasive method of evaluating the cerebral vasculature may be at hand. Together with MR imaging of the brain, MR angiography has the potential to give the most comprehensive picture possible of the anatomic structures involved in cerebrovascular disease. A number of recent studies have tried to address the issues of the accuracy of MR angiography when compared with either conventional angiography or carotid ultrasonography [24•]. Unfortunately, differences in technique and choice of categories of stenosis make it difficult to compare these studies directly.

Extracranial cerebrovascular disease

In one series of three-dimensional time-of-flight studies of 12 patients, 22 carotid arteries were evaluated for the bifurcation. Lesions were graded on a five-point scale (normal—0%, mild—1% to 30%, moderate—30% to 70%, severe—70% to 99%, occlusion—100%). In this series the authors found good agreement between MR angiography and conventional angiography in all but one case of severe stenosis that was graded indeterminate by MR angiography. In cases of severe stenosis, however, the MR angiogram tended to overestimate the degree of distal stenosis [25].

After refining their MR angiography technique by using three-dimensional time-of-flight MR angiography with a shorter echo time (7 ms) than in the prior study (13 ms), the same investigators [26•] evaluated a further series of 65 carotid arteries in 38 patients. Correlation coefficients between digital subtraction arteriograms and MR angiography for left-sided vessels was 0.97 and for right-sided vessels 0.95 with this improved MR technique.

Anderson and colleagues [27] compared two-dimensional time-of-flight and three-dimensional time-of-flight MR angiography, ultrasonography, and x-ray angiography. Thirty-one of 61 patients had all three examinations. A five-point scale of stenoses was used, ranging from normal to occlusion. Spearman rank correlations for internal carotid artery origins were 0.94 (MR angiography and x-ray arteriography), 0.85 (MR angiography and ultrasonography), and 0.82 (x-ray angiography and ultrasonography). Of 16 possible ulcers detected by x-ray angiography, 11 were noted by MR angiography, none by ultrasonography.

Other investigators [28•] used two-dimensional time-of-flight MR angiography to evaluate 94 carotid arteries. Two independent readers evaluated the studies using a five-point scale (normal—0% to 15%, mild—16% to 49%, moderate—50% to 79%, severe—80% to 99%, occlusion—100%). One observer reported a 70% agreement between MR angiography and conventional angiography, whereas the other found only a 56% agreement. The best correlation was in the severely stenotic category. The worst was in the occluded category [28•].

Two-dimensional time-of-flight MR angiography was also evaluated by Heiserman and colleagues [29] in 73 carotid arteries. Four readers independently evaluated the MR angiograms and the conventional angiograms using a five-point stenosis score similar to, but not identical to, the two scores just presented. Overall agreement between MR angiography and conventional angiography was found to be 79%. Severe stenosis was characterized by signal void (flow gap) at the level of the stenosis and within the poststenotic segment of the artery; signal was recovered and flow reappeared within the distal segment of the vessel.

Polak and colleagues [30•] used three independent readers to compare two-dimensional time-of-flight MR angiography, color Doppler sonography, and digital subtraction angiography studies in 42 carotid bifurcations in 23 patients (Figure 8.7). Overall, 85% of MR angiography studies were in agreement with digital subtraction angiography. The narrowing of the vessel (percent lumen diameter) seen on digital subtraction angiography was correlated with the length of the zone of signal loss on MR angiography. Greater than 50% stenosis on digital subtraction angiography correlated with a flow gap on MR angiography with a correlation coefficient of 0.69.

Pavone and colleagues [31] proved that two-dimensional time-of-flight MR angiography could be performed on a 0.2-T permanent magnet. Correlation was made between digital subtraction angiography and MR angiography in 54 carotid arteries of 31 patients. Good correlation was found in five normal and 18 mild stenoses. In eight cases of intermediate-grade stenosis on digital subtraction angiography, MR angiography overestimated the degree of stenoses. In one case of severe stenosis on digital subtraction angiography, MR angiography underestimated the degree.

Applegate and colleagues [32•] used two-dimensional phase-contrast MR angiography to evaluate the patency of 35 carotid and vertebral arteries. In this examination, large anatomic regions were studied by a single slice 20 to 60 mm thick. Slice acquisition time is relatively rapid (3.5 minutes). Methemoglobin does not present a problem because only the moving protons in blood contribute to the image signal. No postprocessing MIPP reconstruction is required. This technique showed promise, but the report did not systematically evaluate the accuracy of the method relative to other techniques or to the degree of vascular stenoses.

It should be noted in assessing the worth of these comparative studies that even conventional intra-arterial angiography may misdiagnose the presence or absence of mural ulceration (present in up to one third of carotid arteries) [33,34]. Therefore, MR angiography is similarly likely to misdiagnose ulceration [23]. All authors have shown that the degree of vascular stenosis can be overestimated when turbulence-induced dephasing occurs beyond the stenotic segment (Figure 8.8). Although overestimation of stenosis may be preferred to underestimation in a screening test, problems are still present [23]. The North American Symptomatic Carotid Endarterectomy Trial [35] has demonstrated efficacy of endarterectomy in patients with 70% stenosis. The efficacy increases, however, with increasing degrees of stenosis. MR angiography may not be able to differentiate the 70% from 80% from 90% stenosis [36•] and may fail to identify those patients most suitable for surgery.

The distinction between severe stenosis and complete occlusion is also critical (Figure 8.9). In this distinction, MR angiography has not yet proved itself [28•,36•]. At present, as Ackerman and Candia [36•] suggest, MR angiography studies are best used to rule in an x-ray arteriogram, rather than to rule one out. X-ray arteriography is the gold standard for lumen size, intraluminal thrombus, tandem lesions, and adequacy of collateral flow. It is likely, however, that improvements in vessel visibility and, as a result, the detection of clinically significant disease will be forthcoming with further technical improvements in generating MR angiography [24•].

Other extracranial manifestations of cerebrovascular disease have also been studied by MR angiography. These include subclavian steal, thoracic outlet

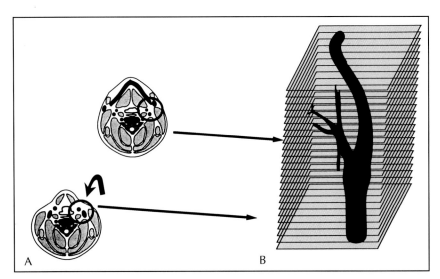

Figure 8.7

The two main steps in obtaining and displaying magnetic resonance projection angiograms of the carotid bifurcations. A series of transaxial gradient refocused images (**A**) is first acquired over an 8-cm-long segment of the neck centered on the carotid bifurcation. A small region of interest is defined on these images (*curved arrow*). Images are then used to create projection angiograms (**B**) with the maximum intensity pixel projection algorithm. (*From* Polak *et al.* [30•]; with permission.)

A   B

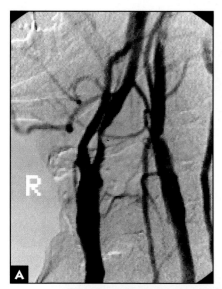

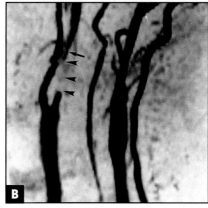

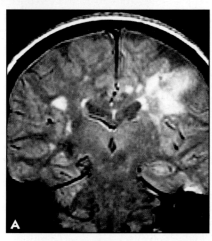

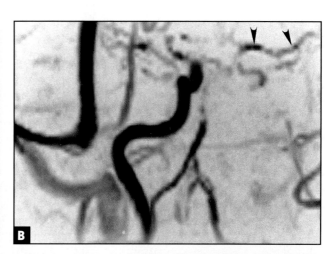

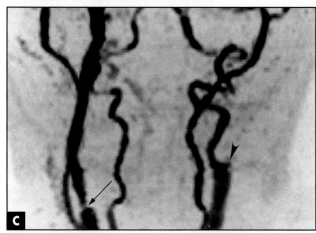

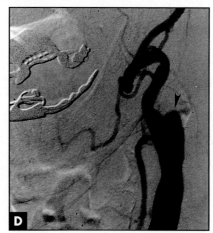

Figure 8.9

Cerebral infarction with occlusion of the left internal carotid artery. **A,** Coronal long repetition time, short echo time magnetic resonance (MR) image shows increased signal intensity at the site of a posterior left frontal infarct. **B,** Oblique coronal reformatted three-dimensional time-of-flight MR angiogram shows absence of the left internal carotid artery with evidence of flow in the left middle cerebral artery (*arrowheads*).

C, Coronal reformatted two-dimensional time-of-flight MR angiogram of neck vessels shows partial stenosis at the origin of the right internal carotid artery (*arrow*) and absence of flow in the left internal carotid artery (*arrowhead*) starting from its origin and continuing distally. **D,** Anteroposterior left common carotid arteriogram shows complete occlusion of the left internal carotid artery at the site of origin (*arrowhead*).

syndrome, Takayasu's arteritis, and fibromuscular disease. Turjman and colleagues [37] demonstrated the presence of subclavian steal by MR angiography in three patients. They used presaturation pulses on cephalad flow to the brain and then on caudad flow from the brain, so as to demonstrate a reversal of flow in the brachiocephalic vessels involved in the steal. Ohkawa and colleagues [38] demonstrated stenosis of the subclavian artery with the patient's arm abducted in comparison with the normal appearance when the arm was not abducted. Oneson and colleagues [39] used three-dimensional time-of-flight MR angiography to demonstrate narrowing of the brachiocephalic vessels at sites of involvement by Takayasu's arteritis. Heiserman and colleagues [40] and Brant-Zawadski and Gillan [23] have found that artifacts associated with MR angiography can produce images that mimic the angiographic findings of fibromuscular dysplasia, decreasing the sensitivity and specificity of MR angiography for detection of fibromuscular dysplasia. Conventional angiography remains the gold standard for the diagnosis of fibromuscular dysplasia.

Venous thrombosis

Magnetic resonance imaging already constitutes an excellent modality with which to demonstrate the presence of clot in cortical veins, in deep venous structures (internal cerebral veins, vein of Galen, straight sinus), or in the more superficial dural venous sinuses (sagittal and transverse) (Figure 8.10A) [41]. MR angiography performed with presaturation of arterial inflow has proven to be an informative additional step in demonstrating venous thrombosis [42]. Two-dimensional time-of-flight MR angiography is used when there is no evidence of methemoglobin on MR imaging, and three-dimensional phase-contrast

MR angiography is used when methemoglobin is present (Figure 8.10B). Chaudhuri and colleagues [43] showed in three cases of calvarial metastases that MR angiography was valuable in identifying sinus thrombosis missed by computed tomography.

Occlusive intracranial cerebrovascular disease

There is still little literature comparing the value of MR angiography and digital subtraction angiography for intracranial vascular occlusive disease. This reflects the problems encountered in evaluating adults in whom the cerebral blood flow is adversely affected by poor cardiac output or proximal extracranial carotid stenosis, both of which further decrease the rate of flow in both proximal and distal intracranial vessels. The single-slab three-dimensional time-of-flight technique suffers from in-plane saturation effects, so vessels much beyond the circle of Willis are poorly visualized. However, this technique best correlates with conventional angiography in demonstrating vascular narrowing of proximal intracranial vessels [44]. Using three-dimensional phase-contrast MR angiography, Warach and colleagues [45••] demonstrated occlusions or severe stenoses of major intracranial vessels in 16 of 24 patients with infarcts greater than 2 cm in diameter. The inability to demonstrate smaller areas of branch occlusion was thought to be related to insufficient spatial resolution. Three-dimensional phase-contrast MR angiography correlated well with occlusion of the proximal middle cerebral artery branch and could be used to assess collateral flow patterns [44].

The MOTSA technique has been used in evaluating intracranial cerebrovascular disease in 58 patients and correlated to x-ray angiography in 20 [6••]. Proximal stenoses of the anterior circulation shown by x-

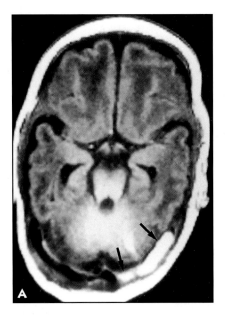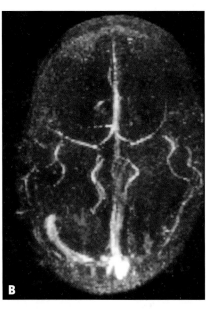

Figure 8.10

Transverse venous sinus thrombosis. **A,** Axial short repetition time, short echo time magnetic resonance (MR) image shows hyperintense methemoglobin clot in the left transverse venous sinus (*arrows*). **B,** Axial three-dimensional phase-contrast MR angiogram shows absence of flow in the left transverse venous sinus.

ray angiography correlated with MR angiography findings of segmental narrowing or nonvisible vessels and with decreased distal vessel signal intensity. In seven patients suspected of having cerebrovascular emboli, four with normal x-ray angiography had normal MR angiography, whereas three with emboli on x-ray angiography had MR angiography evidence of cutoff vessels, nonvisualization of a vessel segment, or decreased signal in the vessel distally.

Magnetic resonance angiography is particularly useful in patients with symptoms of vertebrobasilar insufficiency (Figure 8.11). Of 10 patients in the series of Blatter and colleagues [6••], five were normal by both studies. Basilar stenoses or occlusions were correctly demonstrated by x-ray angiography and MR angiography in three patients, and occlusions of the posterior cerebral artery were shown in two patients. In the pediatric population, MR angiography has been successful in evaluating sickle cell patients for potential large-vessel occlusive disease [46], in evaluating the intracranial and extracranial collateral circulation in infants treated with extracorporeal membrane oxygenation [47,48], in evaluating children with spontaneous onset of acute hemiplegia (Figure 8.12) [49], in those suffering traumatic vascular injuries [50], and in those with Moyamoya disease (Figure 8.13) [49,51].

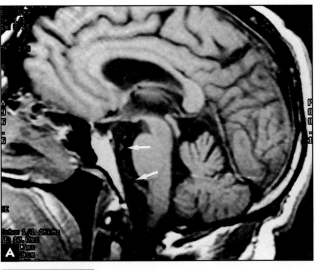

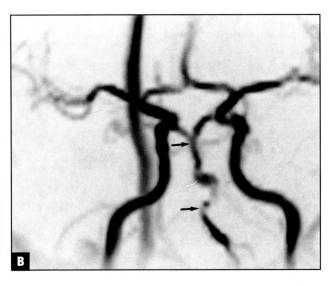

Figure 8.11

Basilar artery stenosis. **A,** Sagittal short repetition time, short echo time magnetic resonance (MR) image shows marked irregular narrowing of the flow void in the basilar artery (*arrows*). **B,** Coronal reformatted MR angiogram shows irregular narrowing of the stenotic basilar artery (*arrows*).

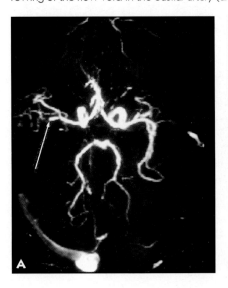

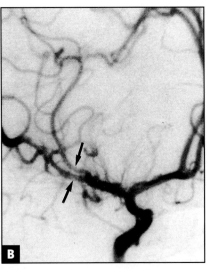

Figure 8.12

Embolus or thrombus in the proximal middle cerebral artery branches. **A,** Axial three-dimensional time-of-flight magnetic resonance angiogram shows a complete cutoff of the proximal left middle cerebral artery at its point of bifurcation (*arrow*). **B,** Right internal carotid arteriogram. Oblique anteroposterior projection shows filling defects (*arrows*) in two branches of the middle cerebral artery arising at the point of bifurcation.

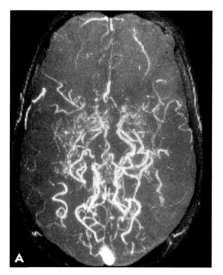
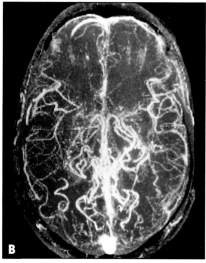

REFERENCES AND RECOMMENDED READING

Papers of particular interest, published within the annual period of review, have been highlighted as:
• Of special interest
•• Of outstanding interest

1. • Litt AW: MR angiography. *AJNR* 1991, 12:1141–1142.
A worthwhile commentary on the maturity or lack thereof of MR angiography. Refers to the paper by Lewin and Laub (*AJNR* 1992, 12:1133–1139).

2. • Keller PJ: Time-of-flight magnetic resonance angiography. *Neuroimaging Clin North Am* 1992, 2:639–656.
Basic concepts of time-of-flight angiography are explained in an understandable fashion.

3. • Dumoulin CL: Phase-contrast magnetic resonance angiography. *Neuroimaging Clin North Am* 1992, 2:657–676.
Phase-contrast MR angiography is explained by its developer and advocate.

4. • Zimmerman RA, Bilaniuk LT: Pediatric brain, head and neck, and spine magnetic resonance angiography. *Magn Reson Q* 1992, 8:264–290.
A comprehensive review of the central nervous system applications in pediatrics.

5. • Parker DL, Blatter DD: Multiple thin slab magnetic resonance angiography. *Neuroimaging Clin North Am* 1992, 2:677.
Multiple overlapping thin-slab acquisition MR angiography is explained by the developer.

6. •• Blatter DD, Parker DL, Ahn SS, *et al.*: Cerebral MR angiography with multiple overlapping thin slab acquisition. Part II: early clinical experience. *Radiology* 1992, 183:379–389.
Multiple overlapping thin-slab acquisition MR angiography systematically applied in 164 patients in a multi-institutional study produces excellent image quality in 90% and good diagnostic results.

7. • Lewin JS, Laub G: Intracranial MR angiography: a direct comparison of three time-of-flight techniques. *AJNR* 1992, 12:1133–1139.
An example of how MR angiography investigation should be carried out. Looks at choices between three pulse sequences in evaluating different parts of the vascular anatomy in normal volunteers.

8. Marchal G, Michiels J, Bosmans H, *et al.*: Contrast-enhanced MRA of the brain. *J Comput Assist Tomogr* 1992, 16:25–29.

9. Hendrix LE, Strandt JA, Daniels DL, *et al.*: Three-dimensional time-of-flight MR angiography with a surface coil: evaluation in 12 subjects. *AJR Am J Roentgenol* 1992, 159:103–106.

10. •• Edelman RR, Ahn SS, Chien D, *et al.*: Improved time-of-flight MR angiography of the brain with magnetization transfer contrast. *Radiology* 1992, 184:395–399.
Discusses improved MR angiography with magnetization transfer contrast.

11. •• Mattle H, Edelman RR, Wentz KU, *et al.*: Middle cerebral artery: determination of flow velocities with MR angiography. *Radiology* 1991, 181:527–530.
New physiologic application with modified MR angiography pulse sequence measures flow velocities in intracranial vessels. Changes demonstrated with activation corresponded to that of transcranial Doppler sonography.

12. Wentz KR, Mattle HP, Edelman RR, *et al.*: Stereoscopic display of MR angiograms. *Neuroradiology* 1991, 33:123–125.

13. • Ehricke HH, Schad LR, Gademann G, *et al.*: Use of MR angiography for stereotactic planning. *J Comput Assist Tomogr* 1992, 16:35–40.

Surface display of skin underlying the brain with superimposed vessels.

14. Ross JS, Masaryk TJ, Modic MT, *et al.*: Intracranial aneurysms: evaluation by MR angiography. *AJNR* 1990, 11:449–456.

15. Sevick RJ, Tsuruda JS, Schmalbrock P: Three-dimensional time-of-flight MR angiography in the evaluation of cerebral aneurysms. *J Comput Assist Tomogr* 1990, 14:874–881.

16. Ruggieri PM, Masaryk TJ, Ross JS, *et al.*: Intracranial magnetic resonance angiography. *Cardiovasc Intervent Radiol* 1992, 15:71–81.

17. •• Houston J, Rufenacht DA, Ehman RL, *et al.*: Intracranial aneurysms and vascular malformations: comparison of time-of-flight and phase-contrast MR angiography. *Radiology* 1991, 181:721–730.
Evaluation of intracranial vascular anomalies by phase-contrast MR angiography and time-of-flight MR angiography yields results suggesting that the former may be more important.

18. Tsuruda JS, Sevick RJ, Halbach VV: Three-dimensional time-of-flight MR angiography in the evaluation of intracranial aneurysms treated by endovascular balloon occlusion. *AJNR* 1992, 13:1129–1136.

19. Sutton LN, Gusnard D, Bruce DA, *et al.*: Fusiform dilatations of the carotid artery following radical surgery of childhood craniopharyngiomas. *J Neurosurg* 1991, 74:695–700.

20. Bradley WG, Schmidt PG: Effect of methemoglobin formation on the MR appearance of subarachnoid hemorrhage. *Radiology* 1985, 156:99–104.

21. Nussel F, Wegmuller H, Huber P: Comparison of magnetic resonance angiography, magnetic resonance imaging and conventional angiography in cerebral arteriovenous malformation. *Neuroradiology* 1991, 33:56–61.

22. Mattle HP, Wentz KU: Selective magnetic resonance angiography of the head. *Cardiovasc Intervent Radiol* 1992, 15:65–70.

23. Brant-Zawadski M, Gillan G: Extracranial carotid magnetic resonance angiography. *Cardiovasc Intervent Radiol* 1992, 15:82–90.

24. • Heiserman JE: The role of magnetic resonance angiography in the evaluation of cerebrovascular ischemic disease. *Neuroimaging Clin North Am* 1992, 2:753–767.
Good review of the role of MR angiography in the evaluation of extracranial vascular disease.

25. Masaryk TJ, Modic MT, Ruggieri PM, *et al.*: Three dimensional (volume) gradient echo imaging of the carotid artery bifurcation: preliminary clinical experience. *Radiology* 1989, 171:801–806.

26. • Masaryk AM, Ross JS, Di Cello MC, *et al.*: 3DFT MR angiography of the carotid bifurcation: potential and limitations as a screening examination. *Radiology* 1991, 179:797–804.
Progress in MR angiography studies of extracranial vascular disease with good correlation between MR angiography and digital subtraction angiography.

27. Anderson CM, Saloner D, Lee RE, *et al.*: Assessment of carotid artery stenosis by MR angiography: comparison with x-ray angiography and color-coded Doppler ultrasound. *AJNR* 1992, 13:989–1003.

28. • Litt AW, Eidelman EM, Pinto RS, *et al.*: Diagnosis of carotid artery stenosis: comparison of 2DFT time-of-flight MR angiography with contrast angiography in 50 patients. *AJNR* 1991, 12:149–154.
Looks at extracranial vascular disease with MR angiography in comparison with conventional angiography, exploring intraobserver variability.

29. Heiserman JE, Drayer BP, Fram EK, *et al.*: Carotid artery stenosis: clinical efficacy of two dimensional time of flight MR angiography. *Radiology* 1992, 182:761–768.

30. • Polak JF, Bajakian RL, O'Leary DH, *et al.*: Detection of internal carotid artery stenosis: comparison of MR angiography, color Doppler sonography, and arteriography. *Radiology* 1992, 182:35–40.
Compares two-dimensional time-of-flight MR angiography with color Doppler sonography and conventional arteriography. Looks at the relationship between degree of stenosis and length of zone of signal loss distal to stenosis.

31. Pavone P, Marsili L, Catalano C, *et al.*: Carotid arteries: evaluation with low-field-strength MR angiography. *Radiology* 1992, 184:401–404.

32. • Applegate GR, Talagala SL, Applegate LJ: MR angiography of the head and neck: value of two-dimensional phase-contrast projection technique. *AJR Am J Roentgenol* 1992, 159:369–374.
Two-dimensional phase-contrast MR angiography is a technique with real promise that has largely been ignored. Application yields good results in 84 patients with mixed diseases.

33. Edwards JH, Kricheff I, Riles T, *et al.*: Angiographically undetected ulceration of the carotid bifurcation as a cause of embolic stroke. *Radiology* 1979, 132:369–373.

34. Eikelboom B, Riles T, Mintzer R, *et al.*: Inaccuracy of angiography in the diagnosis of carotid ulceration. *Stroke* 1983, 14:882–885.

35. Barnett HJM, and the North American Symptomatic Carotid Endarterectomy Trial Collaborators: Beneficial effects of carotid endarterectomy in symptomatic patients with high-grade carotid stenosis. *N Engl J Med* 1991, 325:445–453.

36. • Ackerman RH, Candia MR: Assessment of carotid artery stenosis by MR angiography. *AJNR* 1992, 13:1005–1008.
A well thought out commentary on the weakness of MR angiography in the assessment of carotid extracranial atherosclerotic disease.

37. Turjman F, Tournut P, Baldy-Porcher C, *et al.*: Demonstration of subclavian steal by MR angiography. *J Comput Assist Tomogr* 1992, 16:756–759.

38. Ohkawa Y, Isoda H, Hasegawa S, *et al.*: MR angiography of thoracic outlet syndrome. *J Comput Assist Tomogr* 1992, 16:475–477.

39. Oneson SR, Lewin SJ, Smith AS: MR angiography of Takayasu arteritis. *J Comput Assist Tomogr* 1992, 16:478–480.

40. Heiserman JE, Drayer BP, Fram EK, *et al.*: MR angiography of cervical fibromuscular dysplasia. *AJNR* 1992, 13:1454–1457.

41. Barron TF, Gusnard DA, Zimmerman RA, *et al.*: Cerebral

venous thrombosis in neonates and children. *Pediatr Neurol* 1992, 8:112–116.

42. Padayachee TS, Bingham JB, Graves MJ, *et al.*: Dural sinus thrombosis: diagnosis and follow-up by magnetic resonance angiography and imaging. *Neuroradiology* 1991, 33:165–167.

43. Chaudhuri R, Tarnawski M, Graves MJ, *et al.*: Dural sinus occlusion due to calvarial metastases blind spot. *J Comput Assist Tomogr* 1992, 16:30–34.

44. Pernicone JR, Thorp KE, Ouimette MV, *et al.*: Magnetic resonance angiography in intracranial vascular disease. *Semin Ultrasound CT MRI* 1992, 13:256–273.

45. •• Warach S, Li W, Ronthal M, Edelman RR: Acute cerebral ischemia evaluation with dynamic contrast-enhanced MR imaging and MR angiography. *Radiology* 1992, 182:41–47.
Correlation of size of infarct to MR angiography demonstration of intracranial vascular abnormalities.

46. Wang Z, Bogdan AR, Zimmerman RA, *et al.*: Evaluation of stroke in sickle cell disease by 1H nuclear magnetic resonance spectroscopy. *Neuroradiology*, 1992, 35:57–65.

47. Lago P, Rebsamen S, Clancy RR, *et al.*: Magnetic resonance imaging and angiography abnormalities following neonatal ECMO (extracorporeal membrane oxygenation) therapy. 1: focal parenchymal brain lesions and cerebrovascular response to carotid artery and jugular vein ligation. Submitted, *Ann Neurol.*

48. Wiznitzer M, Masaryk TJ, Lewin J, *et al.*: Parenchymal and vascular magnetic resonance imaging of the brain after extracorporeal membrane oxygenation. *Am J Dis Child* 1990, 144:1323–1326.

49. Zimmerman RA, Bogdan AR, Gusnard DA: Pediatric magnetic resonance angiography: assessment of stroke. *Cardiovasc Intervent Radiol* 1992, 15:60–64.

50. Zimmerman RA: Vascular injuries of the head and neck. *Neuroimaging Clin North Am* 1991, 1:443–459.

51. Yamada I, Matsushima Y, Suzuki S: Moyamoya disease: diagnosis with three-dimensional time-of-flight MR angiography. *Radiology* 1992, 184:773–778.

Chapter 9

Endovascular Occlusion of Cerebral Aneurysms

Lee R. Guterman
Arvind Ahuja
Leo N. Hopkins

Endovascular neurosurgery is an alternative treatment for cerebrovascular disease. Rather than use open surgical techniques, microcatheters are used to enter the cerebral circulation after percutaneous femoral access. During the past 10 years, astonishing engineering advances in microcatheter technology have permitted access to distal branches of the cerebral circulation. The superselective placement of microcatheters into distal branches of the anterior, middle, and posterior cerebral circulation has enabled endovascular surgeons to treat lesions that had been deemed inoperable by conventional methods. Catheters can be placed into aneurysms in any position in the cerebral circulation, yet not all cerebral aneurysms are amenable to endovascular treatment.

Microcatheters serve as a pathway for the delivery of thrombogenic devices into or around an aneurysm. The introduction of thrombogenic devices into cerebral aneurysms has revolutionized their treatment. Platinum coils, silicone and latex balloons, polymers, stents, and other materials are being used to treat intracranial aneurysms.

This chapter reviews basic techniques for the endovascular treatment of cerebral aneurysms, with the results of treatment presented in a historical fashion. Methods of device preparation and catheter placement are described. The rationale of patient selection is discussed. Perioperative management, including the philosophy of intensive care management, is reviewed and presented.

BALLOONS

Microcatheters are used to deliver inflatable silicone or latex balloons into the aneurysm cavity in order to induce thrombosis (Figure 9.1). Inflatable balloons are secured onto the tips of microcatheters and directed into the body of the aneurysm. Ideally, the balloon conforms to the dimensions of the aneurysm cavity after inflation (Figure 9.2). The aneurysm cavity thromboses. If successful, the neck of the aneurysm is completely obliterated, and endothelial cells cover the orifice of the aneurysm. Subsequent reendothelialization results in permanent exclusion of the aneurysm cavity from the lumen of its parent vessel.

The first description of a catheter-based treatment of a cerebral aneurysm was published in 1964 by Luessenhop and Velasquez [1]. They reported an unsuccessful attempt to induce aneurysm thrombosis by placing a silicone balloon into an aneurysm of the supraclinoid carotid artery. Over the next 25 years, anecdotal case reports grew into large patient series. Two groups dominated the contribution of patients to the international database. In the USSR, neurosurgeons in Kiev and Moscow, and in the United States, interventional neuroradiologists at The University of California at San Francisco, defined our present knowledge concerning the treatment of cerebral aneurysms with latex and silicone balloons, respectively.

In 1973, Serbinenko [2] performed the first successful treatment of a saccular aneurysm with a detachable latex balloon. The aneurysm cavity thrombosed while patency of the lumen of the parent artery was maintained. One year later, Serbinenko [2] reported on 300 cases of balloon catheter occlusion of major cerebral vessels. Catheter placement was achieved by direct puncture of the internal carotid artery. Only three of 300 reported cases involved successful treatment of cerebral aneurysms (one basilar artery and two supraclinoid carotid artery aneurysms) with detachable balloons. Serbinenko described his technique but did not report patient follow-up. Before these successful cases, two deaths were reported during the treatment of basilar artery aneurysms.

In 1981, Hieshima and colleagues [3] described a technique for therapeutic transcatheter occlusions. An inflatable and detachable Silastic (Dow Corning, Midland, MI) balloon was secured to a coaxial catheter system by a miter valve. In the same year, Debrun and colleagues [4] reported on nine patients with giant unclippable aneurysms treated with detachable balloons. Four patients had a superficial temporal artery to middle cerebral artery bypass before sacrifice of the parent vessel by detachable balloon occlusion. One patient had an arterial ligation without bypass. The authors concluded that sacrifice of the parent artery appeared safer than direct aneurysm obliteration.

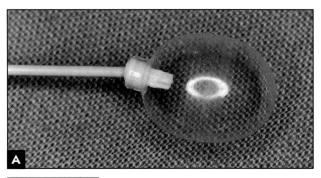
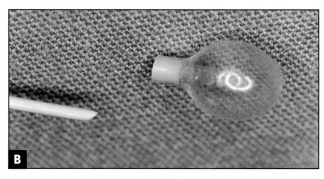

Figure 9.1

Detachable silicone balloon (Interventional Therapeutics Corporation, South San Francisco, CA). **A,** The balloon is attached to the delivery catheter by inserting the distal catheter tip through the miter valve at the proximal end of the balloon. **B,** Once the balloon is positioned in the aneurysm cavity, it can be detached. The balloon can be inflated with contrast material to allow fluoroscopic image analysis during placement. After placement, the contrast can be exchanged for 2-hydroxy-ethyl-methacrylate (HEMA). The solidified polymer prevents balloon deflation after detachment.

In 1982 Romodanov and Shcheglov [5] reported on 137 intravascular occlusions of saccular aneurysms of the cerebral arteries using a detachable balloon catheter. Between 1974 and 1980, 119 patients were treated. Follow-up varied between 1 month and 6 years but details were not provided. Fifteen patients had the parent vessel obliterated. Only two patients were treated following subarachnoid hemorrhage. One hundred four patients presented in "satisfactory" neurologic condition before embolization. Complete obliteration of the aneurysm cavity without compromise of the parent vessel was achieved in 93 patients. Only three of 119 patients experienced recanalization of the aneurysm lumen. Four deaths were reported, three from thrombosis of the internal carotid artery and one from pneumonia.

In 1984 Berenstein and colleagues [6] reported on 14 patients with giant aneurysms of the cavernous carotid and vertebral arteries. The lumen of the parent vessel was sacrificed in all cases. In one case, an attempt was made to treat the aneurysm cavity, but this resulted in recanalization, and the parent artery was subsequently sacrificed.

In 1986, Hieshima and colleagues [7] placed two detachable silicone balloons into a left carotid oph-

thalmic artery aneurysm. After 8 months, complete angiographic obliteration of the aneurysm was maintained. In that same year, Hieshima and colleagues [8] reported balloon occlusion of a distal basilar artery aneurysm with proximal basilar artery stenosis. Balloon angioplasty was employed to widen the proximal basilar artery and facilitate placement of the silicone balloons. The patient developed slight dysmetria. Angiography revealed bilateral narrowing of the proximal posterior cerebral arteries.

In 1987 Higashida and colleagues [9] reported on a patient who was asymptomatic 1 year after balloon embolization of a giant cavernous carotid artery aneurysm. No follow-up angiogram was obtained. In the same year, Fox and colleagues [10] published a series of 68 patients with unclippable aneurysms. Thirty-five patients had an extracranial-intracranial arterial bypass (EIAB) before balloon occlusion of the parent artery. Balloon placement was either distal to or proximal and distal to the aneurysm orifice. Direct treatment of the aneurysm cavity was not attempted. Later that year, Hieshima and colleagues [11] reported balloon occlusion of a midbasilar artery aneurysm that had bled repeatedly. After placement of two balloons, the patient developed a subtle right hemiparesis and was placed on sodium warfarin. Follow-up angiography 3 months later demonstrated obliteration of the aneurysm cavity with preservation of the lumen of the parent vessel.

In 1988 Higashida and colleagues [12] reported 80% occlusion of a carotid ophthalmic artery aneurysm after balloon embolization. Attempted EIAB, clipping, and wrapping had failed. In the same year, Goto and colleagues [13] used a polymer (2-hydroxy-ethyl-methacrylate, HEMA) that when injected into a silicone balloon within an aneurysm cavity resulted in permanent solidification of the inflated balloon shape. Initiating the polymerization reaction was simple, reproducible, and facilitated at physiologic temperatures. Later that year, Higashida and colleagues [14] reported complete obliteration of a cavernous carotid artery aneurysm with a silicone balloon filled with HEMA. The aneurysm remained occluded 1 year later.

In 1989 Higashida and colleagues [15] published a series of 25 patients with 26 aneurysms of the posterior circulation. Fifteen patients had previous subarachnoid hemorrhage. Ten patients had mass effect. In 17 cases, the lumen of the parent artery was preserved. Nine cases required total occlusion of the parent artery. There were five deaths, three strokes, and three transient ischemic attacks. Patients were heparinized during the procedure. Protamine was used to normalize the coagulation process after the procedure. Sixty percent of the

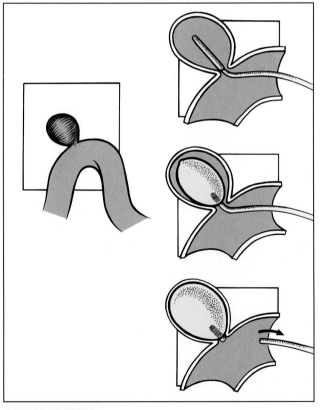

Figure 9.2

The placement of a detachable balloon into an aneurysm cavity. In this representation, the balloon fills the aneurysm cavity after placement. This is not usually the case.

patients were neurologically intact and stable 2 to 43 months after the procedure.

In a 1990 review article, Hieshima and colleagues [16] cited 4% morbidity and 6% stroke rates in more than 200 patients with intracranial vascular abnormalities treated by balloon embolization. Angiography after balloon placement revealed a decreased mass effect. Preliminary data indicated that if an aneurysm remained occluded after 6 months, the risk of rebleeding decreased. Only one patient was reported to have had subarachnoid hemorrhage 6 months after balloon occlusion of an aneurysm.

In 1990, Higashida and colleagues [17] reported on a series of 84 patients with intracranial aneurysms treated with detachable silicone balloons, 59 in the anterior circulation and 25 in the posterior circulation. Thirty-one patients presented with acute subarachnoid hemorrhage. The time interval between initial bleed and balloon embolization was not reported. Treatment was restricted to patients who either failed surgical clipping or could not tolerate general anesthesia, or to those with anatomically inaccessible aneurysms (cavernous carotid artery, midbasilar region). Balloon embolization was felt to be the sole alternative for intervention in this group. Fifteen deaths were reported, 10 of which resulted from growth and rupture of the aneurysm cavity after balloon placement. There were nine strokes after balloon placement. Most were caused by the release of fresh thrombus within the aneurysm cavity during placement of the detachable balloon. In one case, the HEMA was liberated from a ruptured balloon. The polymer migrated distally into the cerebral circulation resulting in thrombotic stroke. Nineteen of the 84 aneurysms treated were larger than 3 cm in diameter. Sixty-five of the 84 aneurysms were totally occluded by placement of one or more balloons. Nineteen were subtotally treated—only 85% of the aneurysm cavity was occluded.

In 1990 Shcheglov [18] presented the results of the Kiev experience at the Stonwin lectures. During a 14-year period, 725 treatments of intracerebral aneurysms were performed using latex balloons. In each case, the balloon shape was tailored to the angiographic appearance of the aneurysm. In 91% of cases, the aneurysm was treated without compromise of the lumen of the parent vessel. Seventeen of the 725 cases were performed less than 3 weeks after subarachnoid hemorrhage. Aneurysms larger than 5 cm in diameter were treated with multiple balloons followed by surgical clipping. In 617 patients, the outcome was reported as good in 80% and fair in 20%. The definitions of good and fair are not provided in the report. Thirty-three patients died, a mortality of 5.4%. At the same conference, Serbinenko presented the Moscow experience [19] of 267 patients treated during a 19-year period. Most procedures involved inoperable aneurysms. In 67% of cases, the aneurysm was occluded from the parent vessel with good results. Thirty-seven patients had EIAB before endovascular therapy. Thromboembolism of cerebral vessels occurred in 7.9% of cases. Postoperative mortality was 7.5%.

Methods for balloon placement into cerebral aneurysms

The placement of detachable silicone balloons into the distal cerebral circulation requires the introduction of a rigid 9-French guide catheter into the proximal carotid or vertebral artery. Interventional Therapeutics Corporation (ITC, South San Francisco, CA) developed a coaxial delivery catheter system that can be placed over a guidewire (Figure 9.3). The inner catheter is longer and more flexible than the outer catheter, and once the coaxial system is positioned the wire is removed. The outer catheter is advanced as the inner catheter is withdrawn. This coaxial design permits the placement of a large internal diameter catheter while minimizing vessel lumen trauma. Silicone balloons contain a miter valve that permits the introduction of a catheter for inflation. The valve is included within the balloon so that most of its surface is not exposed to blood as a potential source of thrombus. On withdrawal, the valve closes, maintaining the inflation pressure and desired size and shape of the balloon.

The balloon delivery system is also coaxial (Figure 9.4). The inner catheter is placed through the miter valve in the balloon. The outer catheter acts as a ballast for detachment. Once the catheter system is assembled, contrast (isosmotic metrizamide) is used to inflate the balloon and purge the system of air. Inflation of the balloon with contrast enables visualization during fluoroscopy. Silicone balloons are made of a semipermeable membrane; therefore, mixture of the metrizamide solution should produce an isosmotic solution to prevent swelling of the balloon after intravascular inflation. By holding the outer catheter stationary and pulling the inner catheter back, the balloon can be detached.

Placement of the balloon into the aneurysm cavity can be challenging. Tortuous vessels with areas of stenosis proximal to the aneurysm orifice can block access to the body of the aneurysm. The ITC coaxial balloon catheter system does not accept a guidewire. Placement of the balloon relies on blood flow. If the aneurysm orifice is small, maneuvering the balloon into the aneurysm cavity can be difficult. At times, a second balloon catheter can be used to push the balloon into the aneurysm cavity (Figure 9.5). Use of the ITC system is limited by the skill of the intervention-

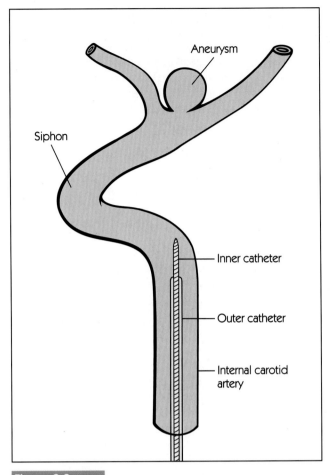

Figure 9.3

This coaxial balloon delivery system can be placed over a guidewire. Once the coaxial system is positioned, the wire is removed.

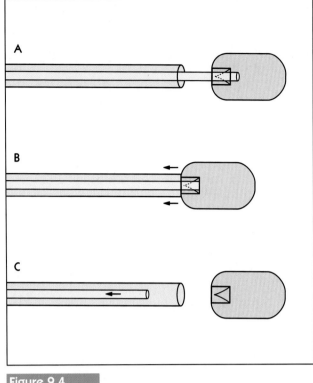

Figure 9.4

Coaxial balloon delivery system. **A,** The balloon is attached to the inner catheter. **B,** The inner catheter is then pulled back so that the balloon miter valve abutts the outer catheter. **C,** The inner catheter is then pulled out of the miter valve and the balloon is released.

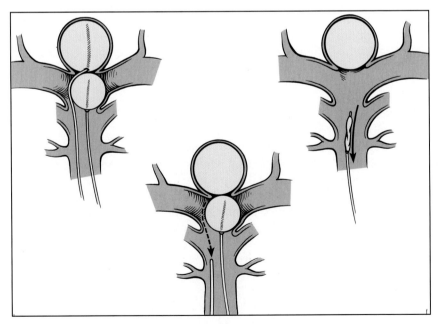

Figure 9.5

Basilar artery aneurysm. Two balloon catheters are being used—one to deliver a balloon directly into the aneurysm cavity, and the nondetachable balloon catheter to help position the detachable balloon in the aneurysm cavity.

ist. Nelson [20] reported on the use of a Tracker 18 catheter (Target Therapeutics, Freemont, CA) with a latex balloon. Using a Tracker catheter to deliver the detachable balloon enables the use of an 0.018-in wire to position the balloon.

Once the balloon has been placed into the aneurysm cavity, it is inflated according to its volumetric specifications. After detachment, balloons filled with isosmotic metrizamide have been reported to deflate. If this occurs before aneurysm thrombosis, the potential for distal embolization of balloon debris could result in infarction. To prevent deflation and rupture, Goto and colleagues [13] used a permanent inflation system with a hydrophilic polymer. When the balloon had been inflated within the aneurysm cavity, metrizamide was exchanged with a mixture of HEMA, initiator, and catalyst. A polymerization reaction turning methacrylate monomers into polymethyl methacrylate occurred in the balloon cavity, forming a solid cast of the balloon. Thus, premature deflation was avoided.

Giant aneurysms require multiple balloons to induce thrombosis. Motion of the balloon within the aneurysm cavity can result in aneurysm rupture. A ball valve effect can result if a balloon allows entry of blood into the aneurysm cavity during systole but blocks outflow of blood during diastole. The resulting expansion of the aneurysm cavity ends in rupture. Kwan and colleagues [21] reported on two patients with basilar artery aneurysms treated by intraaneurysmal balloon occlusion. In one case, follow-up angiography demonstrated aneurysmal enlargement of a subtotally treated aneurysm neck. In the second case, a HEMA-filled balloon migrated distally into the sac of a midbasilar artery aneurysm. This patient rebled and later died. In some cases, migration of the HEMA-filled balloon has been documented within an organized thrombus.

The endovascular treatment of patients in the acute phase after subarachnoid hemorrhage is a controversial topic. The Kiev experience reported on 17 patients who were treated with balloon embolization after acute subarachnoid hemorrhage [5,18]. Soaking the latex in thrombin before embolization facilitated clotting in the aneurysm cavity. If the aneurysm was angiographically obliterated, patients were considered protected from rebleeding. In the San Francisco series of posterior circulation aneurysms treated with silicone balloons, more than 50% of procedures were performed on patients after subarachnoid hemorrhage [15]. The time interval after the hemorrhage was not reported. Ten of 15 deaths were from rebleeding after balloon embolization.

In 1990 George and colleagues at the Lariboisière [22] reported on 92 cases of intracranial aneurysms treated by detachable latex balloon occlusions. Forty-eight parent artery occlusions and 44 selective aneurysm occlusions were performed. Thirty of the patients undergoing selective occlusion had experienced recent subarachnoid hemorrhage prior to treatment. In this group, there were five deaths—three aneurysm ruptures before balloon placement and two vascular occlusions. Two patients in this group experienced subarachnoid hemorrhage during or after treatment. There were 10 cases of balloon deflation. Forty-three percent of these patients had good results.

In the parent artery occlusion group, 85% of patients had good results. There were two deaths—one balloon embolized in the middle cerebral artery (MCA) and one patient experienced total occlusion of the basilar trunk. There were four ischemic complications and one subarachnoid hemorrhage.

In 1991 Forsting and colleagues [23] reported on the treatment of a giant aneurysm at the junction of the vertebral and basilar arteries with a detachable balloon. Temporary occlusion of both vertebrals was performed without neurologic deficit. Electrophysiologic monitoring revealed no changes during occlusion. With the patient under general anesthesia, permanent occlusion was performed. Death occurred secondary to ischemic infarction of the pons and medulla. At autopsy, the left anterior-inferior cerebellar artery and three pontine branches that arose from the dome of the aneurysm were totally occluded.

Hodes and colleagues [24•] reported 16 cases of parent artery occlusions of unclippable aneurysms using detachable balloons. Follow-up varied between 1 and 8 years. Twelve patients had an excellent outcome. There were four deaths—two were procedure-related, one from rupture of another aneurysm, and one from thrombosis of the MCA. Four patients demonstrated recanalization of the parent vessel and one developed an aneurysm on a different location of the same vessel.

In 1988, Target Therapeutics marketed a series of platinum coils designed to induce thrombosis after delivery into an aneurysm cavity using the Tracker catheter system. Our experience demonstrated that these coils were easily placed within the body of the aneurysm. Unfortunately, the thrombogenic potential of the platinum varied. Coil migration out of the aneurysm cavity into the distal cerebral circulation was reported [25,26].

In 1990, Graves and colleagues [27••] reported on the treatment with platinum coils of 21 experimental lateral wall aneurysms in a canine model. Simple or complex curves in the platinum wire did not induce thrombosis and lacked spatial stability after placement into the aneurysm cavity. Coils with configurations similar to flower petals that were augmented with silk fibers were more thrombogenic and did not migrate out of the aneurysm cavity. These coils resulted in total thrombosis of the aneurysm cavity in only 40% of the treated aneurysms. Partial thrombosis of the parent vessel was present in 50% of treated aneurysms, although thrombus dissolved within 21 days of coil placement.

Target Therapeutics improved the thrombogenicity of the coils by incorporating polyethylene terephthalate (Dacron, Dupont, Wilmington, DE) threads into the tertiary coil structure (Figure 9.6). Although the thrombogenicity improved and the amount of migration after placement decreased, control during coil placement was limited. Once the coil was ejected from the catheter tip, its final position was flow-directed (Figure 9.7). No mechanism for retrieval was available.

In 1990 Dowd and colleagues [28] reported on the placement of platinum coils into three cerebral aneurysms. One patient with a left posterior inferior cerebellar artery aneurysm was left with a partially treated residual neck. Two patients were discharged in good neurologic condition with thrombosed aneurysms.

In 1991 Arnaud and colleagues [29•] reported on the preoperative embolization of a ruptured MCA aneurysm. The patient had subarachnoid hemor-

rhage with a large temporal lobe hematoma producing a mass effect. The aneurysm was partially thrombosed with platinum coils, and the hematoma was evacuated by craniotomy. The rationale was that partial thrombosis of the aneurysm would decrease the risk of intraoperative hemorrhage. Lane and Marks [30•] reported on a case of recent subarachnoid hemorrhage (Hunt and Hess grade IV) with an anterior communicating artery aneurysm. Angiography revealed extravasation of contrast through the dome of the aneurysm. Balloon occlusion of the aneurysm failed, and two platinum coils were placed. Ten months after treatment, the aneurysm remained completely occluded. Higashida and colleagues [31] reported on the treatment of a vertebrobasilar artery aneurysm by platinum microcoils coated with Dacron threads. Four months after treatment, the aneurysm remained completely occluded.

During the 1991 Congress of the World Federation of Interventional Therapeutic Neuroradiology, more than 50 patients with intracranial aneurysms treated by thrombogenic microcoils were reported. Pruvo and colleagues [26] reported 16 aneurysms treated with platinum microcoils. Eleven aneurysms were angiographically obliterated; four were partially treated. In three patients, coils migrated out of the aneurysm after placement, resulting in complete motor paralysis. Lemme-Plaghos and colleagues [32] reported on 11 aneurysms treated with Flower coils (Target Therapeutics). Six treated aneurysms were

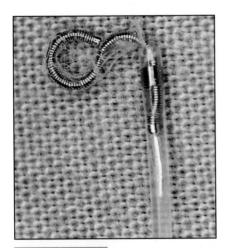

Figure 9.6

Coated platinum microcoil and Tracker catheter delivery system (Target Therapeutics, Freemont, CA). A gold-tipped wire is used to push the coils through the microcatheter into the aneurysm cavity. There is very little control over the final position of the coils in the aneurysm cavity.

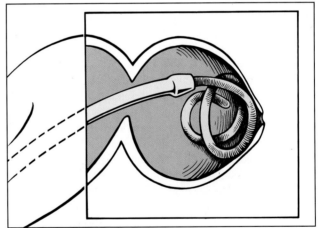

Figure 9.7

A coil being delivered into an aneurysm cavity.

intracavernous: three were subtotally occluded, two were angiographically obliterated, and one hemorrhaged, resulting in death shortly after treatment. One patient had a fatal bleed shortly after treatment. Fox and colleagues [33] reported on the treatment of five patients with Flower coils. Four procedures were performed in the acute phase of subarachnoid hemorrhage. After treatment, all aneurysms had residual necks. Casasco and colleagues [34] reported on 16 patients treated with microcoils. Five were asymptomatic and 11 had experienced previous subarachnoid hemorrhage. In 12 patients, more than 90% of the aneurysm was angiographically occluded. After 1 year, they reported no rebleeds.

Method for placement of coils into cerebral aneurysms

Platinum coils are placed through a Tracker catheter system. In our facility, a gentle curve is steamed into a 6-French Royal Flush catheter (Cook, Bloomington, IN). This catheter is soft and easily placed into the proximal internal carotid or vertebral artery. The Tracker system represents a milestone in technologic advancement in catheter design and atraumatic guidewire production. The catheter's unibody extrusion and torquability facilitated easy access to distal branches of the cerebral circulation. The Tracker catheter is advanced through the guide catheter, and the tip of the Tracker is placed within the aneurysm cavity (Figure 9.8). Potential exists to push the catheter or the guidewire through the dome of the aneurysm cavity. A radiolucent guidewire with a gold tip is used to advance the coil through the catheter. In this way, the catheter tip can be distinguished from the coil during fluoroscopy. As the coil is advanced through the catheter, the Tracker catheter tip can move forward into the aneurysm cavity. Visualization of the Tracker catheter tip at the moment of delivery of the coil will help prevent rupture of the dome of the aneurysm.

The final position of coils after delivery is directed by blood flow. If the final position partially occludes the parent vessel, coils cannot easily be repositioned. Target Therapeutics recently developed a snare catheter used for the emergent retrieval of coils that threaten to occlude the lumen of the parent vessel (Graves *et al.* Paper published at the American Society of Neuroradiology Meeting; 1992; St Louis, MO.)

Numerous small series have been reported in abstracts and case reports over the past 2 years, but no large patient series have been reported. Four cases of distal embolization of coils after release within the aneurysm cavity have been reported [25,26]. The small size of these coils and lack of control severely limit their usefulness.

Guglielmi detachable coils

Guglielmi and colleagues [35••], in conjunction with engineers at Target Therapeutics, began the development of an electrically detachable coil system in 1990 (Guglielmi Detachable Coil, GDC) that would overcome the aforementioned problems. Coils were attached to a stainless steel guidewire by a solder junction (Figure 9.9). The coils are malleable and are available in lengths ranging from 2 to 40 cm. Once delivered, they assume a helical structure with a diameter between 2 and 20 mm. Detachment is achieved by electrolysis of the steel core of a portion of the guidewire close to the solder junction that secures the coil to the guidewire. The proximal end of the guidewire is attached to a battery. A ground is placed in the patient's groin. As current is run from cathode to anode in a conducting solution, the stainless steel degrades, resulting in detachment of the coil from the guidewire. For electrolysis to occur, the

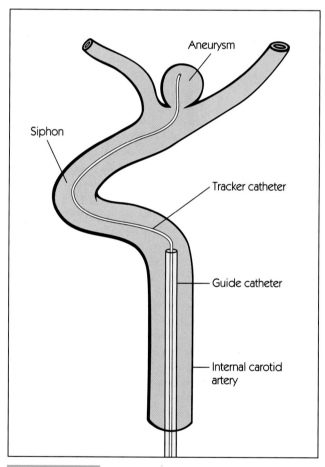

Figure 9.8

Method for placement of coil into a cerebral aneurysm. The Tracker catheter (Target Therapeutics, Freemont, CA) is advanced through the guide catheter, and the tip of the Tracker is placed within the aneurysm cavity.

stainless steel junction must be outside the delivery catheter. This ensures exposure of the surface to an ionic environment required for electrolysis.

The coil system permits the delivery of a large mass of coils into the body of the aneurysm and decreases the chance of migration of detached coils out of the aneurysm. The coil's tertiary structure is compliant, assuming the shape of the aneurysm into which it is delivered. Multiple coils of various sizes can be delivered into an aneurysm in an attempt to completely thrombose the aneurysm cavity. If loops of coil bulge into the lumen of the parent vessel during delivery or delivery threatens rupture of the aneurysm cavity, coils can be retrieved before detachment.

In 1991 Guglielmi and colleagues [35••,36•] reported on the treatment in 15 patients, 21 to 69 years of age. Eight patients had experienced recent subarachnoid hemorrhage. Electrothrombotic coils were placed to occlude 70% to 100% of the aneurysm cavity. One parent artery harboring an aneurysm was thrombosed. No patients experienced permanent neurologic deficit. Aneurysms of the posterior circula-tion were subtotally occluded, while aneurysms of the anterior circulation were radiographically obliterated.

In 1992, Guglielmi and colleagues [37] reported the combined results of the GDC investigators in North America. The results for 43 aneurysms of the posterior fossa were presented. A 70% to 98% thrombosis rate of the aneurysm neck was achieved in 22 of 26 wide-necked aneurysms and in three of 16 small-necked aneurysms. Complete aneurysm occlusion was obtained in 13 of 16 aneurysms with small necks and in four of 26 with wide necks.

Method of detachable coil placement

As with other coil techniques, a 6-French guide catheter is placed into the proximal carotid or verte-bral artery. For the delivery of detachable coils, the Tracker catheter has been modified to include a prox-imal and distal mark at the catheter tip (Figure 9.10). Overlap of these marks with radiopaque marks on the guidewire ensure that the junction between coil and guidewire is outside the catheter before current is

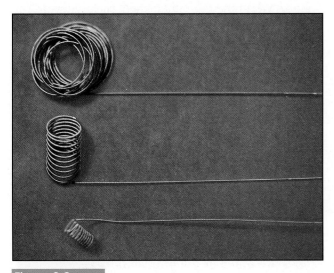

Figure 9.9

Electrically detachable coils.

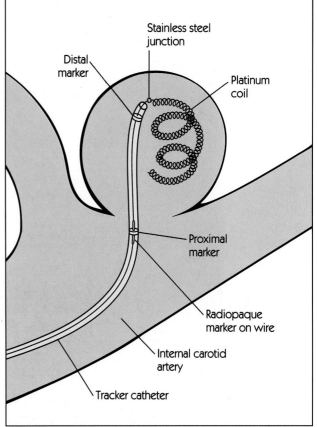

Figure 9.10

Guglielmi Detachable Coil (GDC) system (Target Therapeutics, Freemont, CA). Note proximal and distal catheter markers, and the marker on the coil and stainless steel junction.

applied. This junction must be surrounded by an ionic environment in order for electrolysis of the stainless steel to occur.

The position of the Tracker catheter within the aneurysm cavity is crucial. Coils should be loaded into the aneurysm cavity from the dome downward. The first coil chosen should be the largest size that can be accommodated by the aneurysm cavity. Coils placed subsequently will push the larger mass down toward the orifice (Figure 9.11). Building the coil mass from the dome downward prevents the release of smaller coils out of the aneurysm and into the distal cerebral circulation.

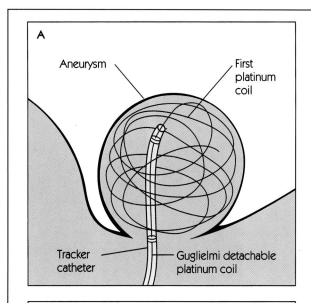

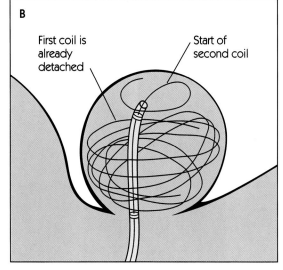

Figure 9.11

The position of the Tracker catheter (Target Therapeutics, Freemont, CA) within the aneurysm cavity is crucial. Coils placed subsequent to the first will push the larger mass down toward the orifice.

Determination of the aneurysm size is crucial in the selection of the appropriate coils for delivery. We routinely place 1-cm washers on the anterior and lateral aspect of the forehead during digital angiography (Hieshima G, personal communication, 1990). These act as standards of measurement for approximating the size of the aneurysm. The diameter of the aneurysm at its widest point is used to determine the appropriate coil size.

The delivery of coils is performed using fluoroscopy to ensure proper placement. The coils should flow out of the catheter without resistance and assume a tertiary structure that conforms to the shape of the aneurysm body. Once the coil has been delivered and the solder junction between coil and guidewire is outside the catheter tip, current can be applied. The current generator operates in a current clamp mode maintaining 0.5 mA by varying the voltage applied between anode and cathode. As the stainless steel junction begins to degrade, a higher voltage is automatically applied between anode and cathode to maintain the 0.5-mA level. The progress of detachment can be monitored by viewing the increase in voltage. When the coil is detached, the guidewire can be removed and an angiogram performed. After placement of the first coil, the angiographic appearance of the aneurysm cavity determines the size of the next coil to be placed. The endpoint for coil delivery is reached when the maximum number of coils has been placed without causing occlusion of the vessel harboring the aneurysm.

Coils are available in two wire gauges. Both 0.018-in and 0.010-in coils are available in an array of tertiary diameters and lengths. Coils made from 0.010-in wire are softer and more malleable. As a result they are less traumatic to the aneurysm cavity. Unfortunately these properties make the 0.010-in coils more vulnerable to remodeling by blood flow. Recanalization secondary to coil remodeling or migration has been reported (Paper presented at the Interventional Neuroradiology Morbidity and Mortality Conference; August, 1992; Jackson Hole, WY; Figures 9.12 and 9.13).

PATIENT SELECTION

Many devices for the treatment of intracranial aneurysms are experimental. Food and Drug Administration approval is pending. As a result, investigators must be participating in an approved protocol before devices are distributed. These studies require specific application of the technology to a well-defined patient population.

In our facility, each patient harboring a cerebral circulation aneurysm is evaluated by a panel of cere-

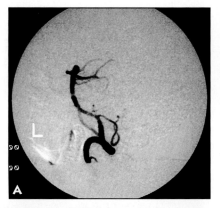

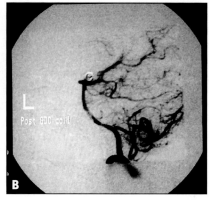

Figure 9.12

A 38-year-old woman, Hunt and Hess grade 1. **A,** Left vertebral artery injection demonstrating a basilar artery aneurysm. **B,** One day after treatment with electrically detachable coils, the aneurysm cavity that was initially occluded is now patent. **C,** Patient was taken to surgery. When the clip was applied, coils broke through the aneurysm dome.

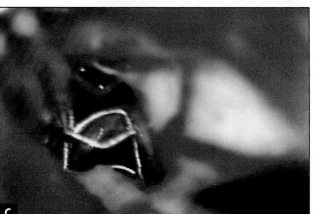

Figure 9.13

A, Left common carotid artery injection demonstrating an anterior communicating artery aneurysm. **B,** The aneurysm after completion of treatment with electrically detachable coils. **C,** Thirteen months after initial treatment with electrically detachable coils. **D,** Retreatment with electrically detachable coils.

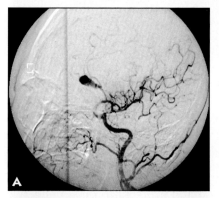

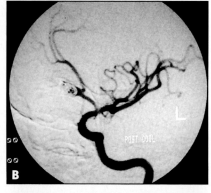

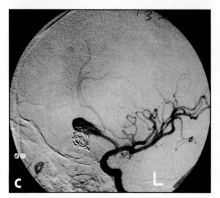

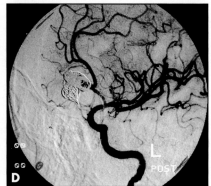

brovascular neurosurgeons. The neurologic status on presentation, Hunt and Hess grade, and medical condition are carefully reviewed. Patients with giant posterior circulation or intracavernous carotid artery aneurysms are strongly considered for endovascular occlusion. If the aneurysm has a wide neck, placement of coils or balloons into the aneurysm cavity is difficult. Turbulent flow after device placement can cause the device to dislodge and embolize into the cerebral circulation. The result can be permanent occlusion of a distal vessel and irreversible neurologic deficit.

Patients who will not tolerate general anesthesia secondary to recent myocardial infarction, poor pulmonary function, lung disease, or acute subarachnoid hemorrhage with a poor Hunt and Hess grade will be considered for endovascular occlusion even if the aneurysm is surgically accessible. Calcification of the aneurysm neck may complicate placement of a clip across the neck of the aneurysm during surgery. In these cases, endovascular occlusion is strongly considered.

Aneurysms with small necks have been permanently thrombosed with coils and balloons. Traditionally, these lesions have been adequately treated with open surgical techniques. Documented surgical morbidity and mortality set a high standard against which all other procedures must be judged. Justifying a change in the routine for treatment of small-neck anterior circulation aneurysms is difficult. Subjecting a patient population to an unproved treatment method that may have a high morbidity and mortality violates a code of ethics all physicians are sworn to uphold. Yet the neurosurgical community must apply scrutiny equally to both existing and nonestablished treatment methods. Biased scrutiny of competing technologies will result in a protectionist policy. This stance will be misconstrued by the public as mercenary in origin. Presently, public opinion will not tolerate the slightest innuendo of protectionism at the public expense.

All studies performed to date have included patients who were deemed unsuited for open surgical techniques. These studies have demonstrated that balloons or coils represent a treatment with an acceptable level of morbidity and mortality compared with the natural history of the disease. As the technology matures, the morbidity and mortality will surpass that achieved by open surgery.

PERIOPERATIVE MANAGEMENT

Recent subarachnoid hemorrhage

Patients who have sustained recent subarachnoid hemorrhage present complex management problems. The basic tenets of treatment established during the past 20 years apply whether the treatment is endovascular or open surgery. Protection from rebleeding is accomplished with sedation and induced hypotension. All patients are started on nimodipine and intravenous steroids. If possible, 24 hours of dexamethasone and nimodipine are completed before endovascular therapy.

Most endovascular procedures can be performed in an awake yet sedated patient. The ability to avoid general endotracheal anesthesia decreases the risk of morbidity and mortality for patients with cardiovascular or pulmonary disease. Recent subarachnoid hemorrhage complicates the treatment plan. Successful completion of endovascular treatment of aneurysms requires that the patient remain still throughout the procedure. Patients with subarachnoid hemorrhage are usually confused and the degree of cooperation varies depending on their perioperative Hunt and Hess grade. In our institution, uncooperative patients who have not been intubated have required an excessive degree of intravenous sedation to complete the procedure. As a result, the ability to perform a neurologic assessment during the procedure was lost. The decision to perform an endovascular procedure using intravenous sedation compromises control of the patient's blood pressure, ventilation, oxygen delivery, and fluid status. The control of these parameters is a powerful tool for prevention of sudden changes in transmural pressure across the aneurysm wall that result in rebleeding in patients with recurrent subarachnoid hemorrhage.

The decision to use general endotracheal anesthesia is a difficult one. Our service has experienced two intraoperative fatal subarachnoid hemorrhages secondary to inadequate control during the procedure. As a result, all endovascular treatments of aneurysms on patients with recent subarachnoid hemorrhage are done with the patient under general endotracheal anesthesia employing the techniques of hypotension and barbiturate cerebral protection proven effective in open surgery.

Unruptured aneurysms

The elective treatment of unruptured, asymptomatic aneurysms has always presented a less complex problem than the treatment of freshly ruptured aneurysms. Elective endovascular procedures can be performed using intravenous sedation. With proper preoperative counseling, patients are cooperative and will remain still during the procedure. If painful portions of the procedure are anticipated and analgesia is administered, excessive motion can be avoided.

Patients are started on nimodipine and dexamethasone 24 hours before the procedure. Routine preoperative laboratory tests are obtained. Bleeding time is obtained and platelet function tests are used when indicated. An electrocardiogram and chest radiograph are obtained. Heparin traps are placed into both arms and intravenous hydration is begun 12 hours before treatment. A Foley catheter (C. R. Bard, Cleveland Heights, OH) is placed in the patient prior to arrival in the angiography suite. The groin is shaved and an intramuscular injection of atropine, midazolam hydrochloride (Versed, Hoffmann-LaRoche, Nutley, NJ), and meperidine hydrochloride (Demerol, Sanofi-Winthrop, New York) is administered. On arrival at the angiography suite, the patient is monitored for cardiac rhythm, oxygen saturation, and blood pressure. Oxygen is administered through nasal cannulae.

Intensive care management

The philosophy of intensive care management after the endovascular occlusion of cerebral aneurysms depends on whether postoperative patients are considered to be protected from rebleeding. Fresh thrombus is a dynamic entity. Thrombus can be lysed before enzymatic crosslinking, resulting in recanalization. Does a complete angiographic obliteration of the aneurysm cavity at the completion of the procedure guarantee permanent occlusion? If the aneurysm cavity harbors thrombus before endovascular device delivery, patients may be at risk for aneurysm rupture, even if angiography displays total obliteration of the aneurysm after the completion of device delivery. Statistically significant evidence has not yet been compiled, although protocols are in place to answer this question.

After the treatment of cerebral aneurysms with coils, patients should be placed on standard subarachnoid hemorrhage precautions if bleeding preceded treatment. Hypotension may be induced to reduce fluctuations in blood pressure. Patients may be subjected to judicious volume expansion if vasospasm develops, but hypertensive therapy should be avoided. A lower threshold for cerebral angioplasty should be employed. In patients with unruptured aneurysms, more liberal postoperative precautions may be used. Unfortunately there is still no guarantee that this patient population is protected from rebleeding. Some centers have suggested that aneurysms be treated with electrically detachable coils in a staged fashion rather than attempting complete endovascular occlusion in one procedure. If this philosophy is employed, are these patients considered protected from rebleeding before the final treatment? Some suggest that isolation of the aneurysm dome from the hemodynamic forces produced during systole provides protection from rebleeding [29•]. Suzuki and Ohara [38] demonstrated that most aneurysms (85%) rupture at the dome. Forces generated by systole can result in a dissection from the aneurysm neck to the dome [39]. This may explain the findings of Suzuki and Ohara.

Our endovascular service bases all clinical intensive care management decisions on the principles of neurosurgical intensive care. Cerebral blood flow and rheology are optimized. Nimodipine is continued to prevent cerebral ischemia at the cellular level. Dexamethasone is continued to combat mass effect of treated aneurysms. Transcranial Doppler is used in patients with recent subarachnoid hemorrhage to follow flow velocity and help establish the need for emergent angiography and treatment. Routine angiography is performed at 1 week, 6 months, and 1 year after treatment.

CONCLUSIONS

Endovascular neurosurgery presently provides an alternative treatment for cerebral aneurysms that are not amenable to surgical intervention. The morbidity and mortality associated with endovascular treatments exceeds that reported for open surgery. As new devices and catheter delivery systems are developed, the present complication rates will decrease. Although electrically detachable coils represent a significant advancement for endovascular treatment of aneurysms, this technique will not replace open surgery. The neurosurgical community must recognize the potential benefits of catheter-based treatments of cerebrovascular disease and help shape future developments in this field.

The perioperative care of patients for endovascular therapy must assume that treated patients are protected from hemorrhage. Patients presenting after subarachnoid hemorrhage introduce a particular treatment dilemma. Little data exist concerning the endovascular treatment of acutely ruptured aneurysms. Standard intensive care management must be modified to allow time for the aneurysm to become irreversibly thrombosed. After endovascular therapy of cerebral aneurysms, normotension and normovolemia may help to ensure aneurysm thrombosis. Vigilant angiographic follow-up of patients treated with coils over 5 or 10 years will provide the data necessary to define their role in the treatment of cerebral aneurysms.

Endovascular neurosurgery presents an opportunity to revolutionize the treatment of cerebrovascular disease. The development of new treatments and algorithms for perioperative patient care must come from the neurosurgical community, since the ultimate responsibility for patient care rests on our shoulders.

REFERENCES AND RECOMMENDED READING

Papers of particular interest, published within the annual period of review, have been highlighted as:
• Of special interest
•• Of outstanding interest

1. Luessenhop AJ, Velasquez AC: Observations on the tolerance of intracranial arteries to catheterization. *J Neurosurg* 1964, 21:85–91.

2. Serbinenko FA: Balloon catheterization and occlusion of major cerebral vessels. *J Neurosurg* 1974, 41:125–145.

3. Hieshima GB, Grinnell V, Mehringer CM: A detachable balloon for therapeutic transcatheter occlusions. *Radiology* 1981, 138:227–228.

4. Debrun GM, Fox AJ, Drake C, *et al.*: Giant unclippable aneurysms: treatment with balloons. *AJNR* 1981, 2:167–173.

5. Romodanov AP, Shcheglov VI: Intravascular occlusion of saccular aneurysms of the cerebral arteries by means of a detachable balloon catheter. In *Advances and Technical Standards in Neurosurgery*, vol. 2. Edited by Krayenbühl H, Sweet WH. New York: Springer-Verlag; 1982:25–49.

6. Berenstein A, Ransohoff J, Kupersmith M, *et al.*: Transvascular treatment of giant aneurysms of the cavernous carotid and vertebral arteries: functional investigation and embolization. *Surg Neurol* 1984, 21:3–12.

7. Hieshima GB, Higashida RT, Halbach VV, *et al.*: Intravascular balloon embolization of carotid-ophthalmic artery aneurysm with preservation of the parent vessel. *AJNR* 1986, 7:916–918.

8. Hieshima GB, Higashida RT, Wapenski J, *et al.*: Balloon embolization of a large distal basilar artery aneurysm: case report. *J Neurosurg* 1986, 65:413–416.

9. Higashida RT, Halbach VV, Mehringer CM, *et al.*: Giant cavernous aneurysm associated with trigeminal artery: treatment by detachable balloon. *AJNR* 1987, 8:757–758.

10. Fox AJ, Viñuela F, Pelz DM, *et al.*: Use of detachable balloons for proximal artery occlusion in the treatment of unclippable cerebral aneurysms. *J Neurosurg* 1987, 66:40–46.

11. Hieshima GB, Higashida RT, Wapenski J, *et al.*: Intravascular balloon embolization of a large mid-basilar artery aneurysm: case report. *J Neurosurg* 1987, 66:124–127.

12. Higashida RT, Halbach VV, Hieshima GB, *et al.*: Treatment of a giant carotid ophthalmic artery aneurysm by intravascular balloon embolization therapy. *Surg Neurol* 1988, 30:382–386.

13. Goto K, Halbach VV, Hardin CW, *et al.*: Permanent inflation of detachable balloons with a low-viscosity hydrophilic polymerizing system. *Radiology* 1988, 169:787–790.

14. Higashida RT, Halbach VV, Hieshima GB, *et al.*: Cavernous carotid artery aneurysm associated with Marfan's syndrome: treatment by balloon embolization therapy. *Neurosurgery* 1988, 22:297–300.

15. Higashida RT, Halbach VV, Cahan LD, *et al.*: Detachable balloon embolization therapy of posterior circulation intracranial aneurysms. *J Neurosurg* 1989, 71:512–519.

16. Hieshima GB, Higashida RT, Halbach, VV: Intravascular treatment of aneurysms. *Clin Neurosurg* 1990, 38:338–343.

17. Higashida RT, Halbach VV, Barnwell SL, *et al.*: Treatment of intracranial aneurysms with preservation of the parent vessel: results of percutaneous balloon embolization in 84 patients. *AJNR* 1990, 11:633–640.

18. Shcheglov VI: Endosaccular detachable balloon catheter treatment of cerebral saccular aneurysms. *AJNR* 1990, 11:224–225.

19. Konovalov AN, Serbinenko FA, Filatov JM, *et al.*: Endovascular treatment of arterial aneurysms. *AJNR* 1990, 11:225.

20. Nelson M: A versatile, steerable, flow-guided catheter for delivery of detachable balloons. *AJNR* 1990, 11:657–658.

21. Kwan ESK, Heilman CB, Shucart WA, *et al.*: Enlargement of basilar artery aneurysms following balloon occlusion: "water-hammer" effect. *J Neurosurg* 1991, 75:963–968.

22. George B, Aymard A, Gobin P, *et al.*: Traitment endovasculaire des anévrysmes intracrâniens: intérêt et perspecitve d'aprés une série de 92 cas. *Neurochirurgie* 1990, 36:273–278.

23. Forsting M, Resch KM, von Kummer R, et al.: Balloon occlusion of a giant lower basilar aneurysm: death due to thrombosis of the aneurysm. *AJNR* 1991, 12:1063–1066.

24. • Hodes JE, Aymard A, Gobin YP, *et al.*: Endovascular occlusion of intranial vessels for curative treatment of unclippable aneurysms: report of 16 cases. *J Neurosurg* 1991, 75:694–701.
Report of 16 parent artery occlusions for the treatment of unclippable aneurysms that resulted in death in four patients and recanalization of the parent vessel in an additional four patients.

25. Kohne D, Nahser HC: Staged endovascular treatment of cerebral aneurysms with coils. *Neuroradiology* 1991, 33:S145.

26. Pruvo JP, LeClerc X, Soto Ares G, *et al.*: Endovascular treatment of 16 intracranial aneurysms with microcoils. *Neuroradiology* 1991, 33:S144.

27. •• Graves, VB, Strother CM, Partington, CR, *et al.*: Flow dynamics of lateral carotid artery aneurysms and their effect on coils and balloons: an experimental study in dogs. *AJNR* 1992, 13:189–196.
Report of treatment with platinum coils of 21 experimental aneurysms in a canine model. Only 40% of the aneurysms treated by polyethylene terephthalate (Dacron)–coated coils

(DuPont, Wilmington, DE) with complex curves thrombosed completely. Partial thrombosis of the parent vessel was seen in 50% of treated aneurysms.

28. Dowd CF, Halbach VV, Higashida RT, *et al.*: Endovascular coil embolization of unusual posterior inferior cerebellar artery aneurysms. *Neurosurgery* 1990, 27:954–961.

29. • Arnaud O, Gobin YP, Mourier K, *et al.*: Embolisation préopératoire en urgence par coils d'un anévrysme sylvien rompu: a propos d'un cas. *Neurochirurgie* 1991, 37:196–199, 1991.

Preoperative embolization of an MCA aneurysm after acute subarachnoid hemorrhage. Coils were placed to protect against rebleeding during evacuation of a hematoma.

30. • Lane B, Marks MP: Coil embolization of an acutely ruptured saccular aneurysm. *AJNR* 1991, 12:1067–1069.

Patient with an anterior communication artery aneurysm after acute subarachnoid hemorrhage. An aneurysm treated with two coils remained totally occluded 10 months later.

31. Higashida RT, Halbach VV, Dowd CF, *et al.*: Interventional neurovascular treatment of a giant intracranial aneurysm using platinum microcoils. *Surg Neurol* 1991, 35:64–68.

32. Lemme-Plaghos LA, Schonholz CJ, Ceciliano AL: Transarterial platinum coil embolization of aneurysms. *Neuroradiology* 1991, 33:S144.

33. Fox AJ, Lownie SP, Drake CG: Endovascular therapy of aneurysms with platinum coils following subarachnoid hemorrhage. *Neuroradiology* 1991, 33:S145.

34. Casasco A, Rogopoulos A, Aymard A, *et al.*: Endovascular treatment of surgical and nonsurgical intracerebral aneurysms with metallic coils. *Neuroradiology* 1991, 33:S145.

35. •• Guglielmi G, Viñuela F, Sepetka I, *et al.*: Electrothrombosis of saccular aneurysm via endovascular approach. Part 1: electrochemical basis, technique, and experimental results. *J Neurosurg* 1991, 75:1–7.

First description of electrically detachable coils and experimental results in a swine aneurysm model.

36. • Guglielmi G, Viñuela F, Dion J, *et al.*: Electrothrombosis of saccular aneurysms via endovascular approach. Part 2: preliminary clinical experience. *J Neurosurg* 1991, 75:8–14.

Treatment of 15 patients with cerebral aneurysms using electrically detachable coils. In most cases, a residual neck was left untreated. All aneurysms were considered inoperable before coil treatment.

37. Guglielmi G, Viñuela F, Duckwiler G, *et al.*: Endovascular treatment of posterior circulation aneurysms by electrothrombosis using electrically detachable coils. *J Neurosurg* 1992, 77:515–524.

38. Suzuki J, Ohara H: Clinicopathological study of cerebral aneurysms: origin, rupture, repair, and growth. *J Neurosurg* 1978, 48:505–514.

39. Strother CM, Graves VB, Rappe A: Aneurysm hemodynamics: an experimental study. *AJNR* 1992, 13:1089–1095.

Chapter 10

The Poor-Grade Aneurysm Patient

Peter D. le Roux
H. Richard Winn

Every year 30,000 people suffer subarachnoid hemorrhage (SAH) in the United States. Two thirds of these individuals die or are disabled. Although many factors determine outcome (Tables 10.1 and 10.2), the level of consciousness at admission is the strongest predictor of outcome (Table 10.2). Generally patients who are alert at presentation do well, whereas those who have altered consciousness, particularly coma, do poorly.

Several large studies strongly suggest that surgery improves on the natural history of aneurysmal SAH [1,2]. Most series, however, included patients in good neurologic condition only; poor-grade (unconscious) patients invariably were excluded or died. In the past decade, there have been significant advances in understanding the pathogenesis, pathophysiology, and management of SAH, which have led to a greater enthusiasm for treating poor-grade patients. The approach to these poor-grade patients and the results of such treatment are reviewed in this chapter.

EPIDEMIOLOGY AND GRADING

Even in this technological era, crucial decisions about patient care depend on an accurate assessment of the clinical condition. To better define surgical risk and prognosis, patients with SAH have been graded. Over 40 such systems have been developed, the Hunt and Hess scale being the most popular [3]. More recently, the World Federation of Neurologic Surgeons Scale, incorporating the Glasgow Coma Scale, has become popular [4]. Although variability can occur in interpreting a patient's grade (most commonly intermediate or grade III), it is clear from numerous studies that coma (*ie*, grades IV and V) is a poor prognostic factor [1–3,5,6•,7••,8•,9•].

In addition to coma, the time from hemorrhage to hospitalization has a strong influence on outcome. Alvord and colleagues [5], in an attempt to define natural history, created probability tables based on the time from SAH and admission grade using the data from Pakarinen's population-based study [10]. On the day of hemorrhage, grade IV patients have a 35% chance of surviving, whereas grade V patients have a 5% chance of surviving. Approximately 30% of SAH patients suffer grade IV or V hemorrhage. Until recently, these patients were excluded from treatment, but they are now being treated as the pathophysiology of SAH is better understood.

PATHOLOGY

The clinical grade correlates both with mortality and morbidity as well as the severity of cerebral pathophysiology. In autopsy studies of patients dying from ruptured cerebral aneurysms, SAH, intracranial hematoma, intraventricular hemorrhage, infarction, and cerebral edema (often in combination) are found. In poor-grade patients, intracranial findings are marked and associated with increased intracranial pressure, often as a result of intracranial hematoma (Figure 10.1). These findings further differentiate poor-grade from good-grade patients [11–13].

Table 10.1
Factors predicting outcome of subarachnoid hemorrhage at presentation

Age
Preexisting medical condition
Admission Glasgow Coma Scale score (level of consciousness)
Admission subarachnoid hemorrhage grade, *eg*, Hunt and Hess grade
Amount of subarachnoid hemorrhage visible on computed tomography
Intraventricular hemorrhage
Intracerebral hemorrhage
± Site and size of aneurysm

Table 10.2
Consciousness level at admission determines outcome in the International Cooperative Study on the timing of aneurysm surgery[*†]

Consciousness level	Good recovery, %	Moderately disabled, %	Severely disabled, %	Vegetative survival, %	Dead, %	Total, *n*
Alert	74.3	7.5	4.1	1.0	13.1	1722
Drowsy	53.5	11.0	6.3	1.7	27.6	1136
Stuporous	30.2	13.8	8.0	4.3	43.7	348
Comatose	11.1	5.4	7.9	3.5	72.1	315
Total	57.6	9.1	5.5	1.8	26.0	3521

[*]*From* Kassel *et al.* [65]; with permission.
[†]Relationship between admission level of consciousness and outcome: chi-square=720.5; $P<0.001$.

Intracranial hematoma complicates about 30% of SAH, being most prevalent in poor-grade patients, and it usually results from ruptured aneurysms surrounded by brain parenchyma, such as middle cerebral artery aneurysms (Figure 10.2) [14••,15–17]. Level of consciousness is often correlated with the size of the clot; those greater than 50 mL in volume invariably cause coma. Intracranial hematoma adversely affects outcome in all grades, particularly if midline shift is observed on head computed tomographic (CT) scan [7••,9•,11,14••,15,16,18]. Intraventricular hemorrhage occurs in nearly three quarters of poor-grade patients and is usually associated with intracranial hematoma. Hydrocephalus and increased intracranial pressure result, particularly if blood fills the entire ventricular system. Ependymal and subependymal cells and arachnoid villi can be damaged, which may lead to chronic hydrocephalus [2,7••,19,20, 21••,22,23•,24].

Aneurysms rarely rupture into the subdural space (<0.5%). Kamiya and colleagues [25•] reviewed 484 patients with SAH; 15 had subdural hematoma, 10 of which were grade IV or V. The associated SAH was usually small. Seven patients underwent prompt surgical evacuation of the subdural hematoma, and a good outcome occurred in five of these patients. None of the eight patients treated conservatively survived.

Cerebral infarction is common in poor-grade patients, particularly those who survive more than 1 day [26,27]. Infarction can result from vasospasm. Indeed, the amount of subarachnoid blood, but not its clearance, correlates with infarction [28]. Furthermore, the presence of hypotension and intracranial hematoma increases the risk of infarction threefold [26,27,29]. Lastly, intracranial hematoma and resultant brain herniation (especially with middle cerebral artery aneurysms) can lead to strangulation of the posterior cerebral artery and consequent occipital infarction. Without question, many poor-grade patients have suffered severe damage, but the prompt evacuation of mass and relief of intracranial hypertension can improve outlook.

PATHOPHYSIOLOGY

Intracranial pressure

Experimental and clinical studies demonstrate a rapid rise in intracranial pressure after aneurysmal rupture. In good-grade patients, the intracranial pressure rapidly returns to normal, but it remains elevated in poor-grade patients. B waves are common, indicating poor compliance. Intracranial pressure, size of hemorrhage, and clinical grade correlate (grade I/II, <15 mm Hg; grade III, 15 to 40 mm Hg; grade IV, 30 to 75 mm Hg; and grade V, >75 mm Hg) [11–13,30,31]. Systemic hypertension may accompany SAH, and although this may be a homeostatic attempt to overcome increased intracranial pressure, Brinker and colleagues [32•] suggest that this may be deleterious and aggravate intracranial hypertension because of impaired autoregulation.

Cerebral blood flow

Cerebral blood flow is 30% to 40% of normal following SAH; after the initial ictus, there is a rapid return to normal in good-grade patients but not in poor-grade patients. Although increased intracranial pressure can contribute to a low cerebral blood flow, knowledge of systemic arterial blood pressure and intracranial pressure alone may be insufficient to calculate cerebral blood flow. Several investigators have evaluated cere-

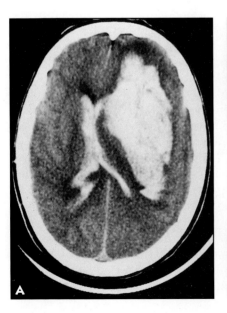 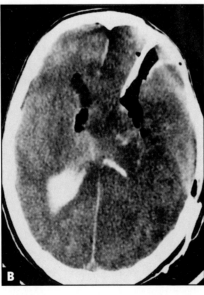

Figure 10.1

A, Intracerebral and intraventricular hemorrhage leading to cerebral swelling and intracranial hypertension are frequently present in poor-grade patients. **B,** Extensive decompression and ventriculostomy are often necessary at the time of aneurysm obliteration.

bral blood flow after SAH. For example, Fazl and colleagues [33••] studied 58 SAH patients and 49 controls with xenon-133. Cerebral blood flow correlated with both the Miller-Fisher [34] and Hunt and Hess [3] grades, and ranged between 48.6±12.3 mL/100 g/min in grade I and 37.3±9.6 in grade V patients. Similar results were obtained by Mountz and colleagues [35•], who used a portable xenon-133 unit. Cerebral blood flow was decreased, particularly in poor-grade patients. Following surgery, cerebral blood flow improved immediately in good-grade patients and slowly in poor-grade patients. Attempts have been made to correlate electrophysiologic findings with ischemia. Whereas somatosensory evoked potential (SSEP) central conduction time is often prolonged, particularly in poor-grade patients, cerebral blood flow and central conduction time only correlate when cerebral blood flow is less than 30 mL/100 g/min. Thus marginal ischemia may not be identified [33••].

Many variables contribute to diminished cerebral blood flow, such as intracranial hematoma, intraventricular hemorrhage, hydrocephalus, edema, vasospasm, sedation, and metabolic rate. Evaluation of cerebral metabolism may help determine the cause. For example, Carpenter and colleagues [36••] studied 11 patients following SAH with positron emission tomography. Before the development of vasospasm, there was a 25% reduction in the cerebral metabolic rate of oxygen ($CMRO_2$) but no change in oxygen extraction fraction, suggesting that depressed $CMRO_2$ may contribute to decreased cerebral blood flow. Following the development of vasospasm, oxygen extraction fraction increased, suggesting that the decreased $CMRO_2$ was then secondary to low cerebral blood flow. In contrast to cerebral blood flow, cerebral blood volume is often increased [37]. This probably reflects vasodilatation of the distal microcirculation in an attempt to compensate for either low cerebral blood flow or spasm in proximal or basal vessels. This vasodilation, however, contributes to decreased compliance and autoregulation.

Autoregulation and carbon dioxide reactivity

Under normal circumstances, the cerebral circulation can autoregulate itself in response to changes in systemic arterial blood pressure and respond to changes in $PaCO_2$. Autoregulation keeps cerebral blood flow constant despite variations in cerebral perfusion pressure. In SAH, however, especially in poor-grade patients, both autoregulation and carbon dioxide reactivity (CO_2R) are impaired [38–40]. The autoregulatory curve is shifted to the right, so even a small fall in systemic arterial blood pressure can lead to a passive decrease in cerebral blood flow and contribute to

cerebral ischemia. This in turn may lead to edema, an increase in intracranial pressure, and further impairment of cerebral blood flow.

Hyperventilation is one method of treating raised intracranial pressure. To be of benefit, CO_2R should be intact. This is not always the case in poor-grade patients. Using transcranial Doppler, Klingelhöfer and colleagues [41•] studied CO_2R in 20 volunteers (3.7% ± 0.5%) and 40 patients with SAH (2% ± 1.1%). Poor-grade patients demonstrated a very small response (0.8% ± 0.3%). Hyperventilation may therefore be effective in reducing intracranial pressure in good-grade patients, but not poor-grade patients. In view of this, the determination of CO_2R may be helpful in directing appropriate treatment in critically ill individuals.

Acetazolamide, a carbonic anhydrase inhibitor and cerebral vasodilator, can be used to assess circulatory reserve. If the cerebral microcirculation is maximally dilated, no cerebral blood flow increase is observed after acetazolamide is administered. Shinoda and colleagues [42•] studied 42 SAH patients with single-photon emission CT (SPECT) after acetazolamide administration and found that the vasodilatory response was reduced, particularly in poor-grade patients and those with intracranial hematoma or vasospasm. This lack of vascular reactivity, however, provides a means of alleviating vasospasm through the use of hypervolemic, hypertensive therapy. If autoregulation is impaired, then an increase in the systemic arterial blood pressure may result in an increase in cerebral blood flow and collateral flow, so avoiding the ischemic threshold. Excessive elevation of systemic arterial blood pressure beyond the reset autoregulatory curve may contribute to edema or even hemorrhage; therefore, knowledge of the time course of impaired autoregulation is important. Immediately after experimental SAH in primates, autoregulation is impaired at both the lower and upper ends but only at the upper end of the autoregulatory curve 1 week later [43•]. Myonecrosis induced by the SAH and vasospasm probably prevent the vessels from constricting when blood pressure increases.

Although basal vessels may constrict, distal parenchymal vessels tend to dilate after SAH. For example, Vollmer and colleagues [44••] studied rabbit basilar and parenchymal arteries *in vitro* after SAH. Although vascular reactivity was impaired in the basilar artery, microcirculatory vessels retained their vasoreactivity. The mechanism of this is not known. As subarachnoid blood does not often extend into the Virchow-Robin spaces, distal vessels are usually unaffected by red blood cell breakdown products. Alternatively, atrial natriuretic factor, released when intracranial pressure is elevated, may dilate pial vessels. The release of atrial natriuretic factor may also contribute to hypoperfusion, as Nakao and colleagues [45•] observed when measuring cortical blood flow with a laser Doppler. This finding, however, may reflect edema in the surrounding parenchyma rather than a direct effect on the vessels.

There are many clinical implications of impaired autoregulation, the most important being meticulous control of systemic arterial blood pressure and volume and the prevention of hypovolemia and hypotension [46].

Volume and electrolytes

Patients with SAH, particularly those in poor grades, have decreased systemic intravascular volume [47••,48]. Paradoxically, sodium is also decreased. The cause of these changes is unclear, but the presence of these abnormalities is important to recognize because cerebral ischemia may be aggravated [49]. Previously, hyponatremia was attributed to the syndrome of inappropriate antidiuretic hormone (SIADH), but it is now apparent that cerebral salt wasting and natriuresis that result from release of atrial natriuretic factor may play a role. The mechanism for this is not known, although recent clinical studies have demonstrated that high levels of atrial natriuretic factor are related to intraventricular hemorrhage, suprasellar SAH, or vasospasm [50•,51••]. Hyponatremia may have numerous deleterious effects; among them attenuated autoregulation or CO_2R has been observed [52•]. These findings emphasize the importance of maintaining euvolemia despite hyponatremia. Dehydration and fluid restriction are contraindicated in poor-grade aneurysm patients, and diuretics should be used with caution [49]. Other electrolyte abnormalities such as hypokalemia and hypocalcemia are common and can contribute to cardiac arrhythmias and cardiac dysfunction.

Cardiorespiratory function

Abnormalities in cardiac rhythm and function are common in poor-grade patients [53,54••,55]. The electrocardiographic changes may resemble those observed in myocardial infarction. Prolonged QT waves are common and may predispose to ventricular tachycardia. Therefore, care is necessary when hemodynamic monitoring lines are inserted. In some patients, subendocardial hemorrhage and necrosis may occur. Electrocardiographic changes, however, that correlated to this are inconstantly observed; instead cardiac dysfunction is more closely related to the severity of neurologic injury. Occasional evaluation of cardiac enzymes and echocardiography may be necessary to rule out myocardial infarction. Surgery, however, should not be delayed on the basis of electrocardiographic changes only.

The poor-grade patient is at high risk for pulmonary complications. A depressed level of consciousness attenuates laryngeal reflexes; cough and the ability to take deep breaths so predisposing to the development of atelectasis and pneumonia. Patients with severe SAH may occasionally develop neurogenic pulmonary edema, impaired lung compliance, and decreased functional residual capacity [56]. This condition may prove refractory to oxygen therapy alone and require positive end-expiratory pressure (PEEP). Although PEEP can increase intracranial pressure, such an increase is unusual, unless PEEP is greater than 15 cm H_2O. PEEP, however, can decrease cardiac output, which may pose a significant risk to the patient.

In summary, care of poor-grade aneurysm patients requires intensive efforts: intubation, mechanical ventilation, and meticulous control of cardiovascular and intracranial dynamics. Also required is continuous invasive monitoring: electrocardiography, arterial pressure, pulmonary artery pressure, cardiac output, intracranial pressure, transcranial Doppler, and frequent CT scans to mention a few. In addition, efficient organization of paramedical services ensures early implementation of this policy.

CLINICAL MANIFESTATIONS AND DIAGNOSIS

A significant depression in consciousness is the sentinel neurologic feature of poor-grade aneurysm. Other neurologic findings may include a dilated pupil and asymmetric motor and reflex responses. In the comatose patient, the diagnosis may often not be readily apparent because a history is not obtainable. Altered consciousness as a presenting sign in SAH was recently reviewed in a retrospective review of 286 cases of all grades by Adams and colleagues [57••], who found that consciousness was altered in 68%, in most cases transiently, but only 43 patients remained unconscious at admission. The most consistent clinical observation in these patients was neck stiffness. Respiratory irregularity or arrest is common in comatose patients and may exacerbate SAH by contributing to anoxic cerebral edema. For example, in a defined SAH population, Ramirez-Lassepas and Ahmed [58•] found that 14% of the patients suffered cardiorespiratory arrest. This represented 4.9% of all cardiorespiratory arrest patients who were successfully resuscitated before arrival at the emergency department. All were grade V at admission. Cardiorespiratory arrest was more common in women and those with intraventricular hemorrhage and intracranial hematoma. Consistent with these observations are forensic studies that suggest that 5% of unexpected deaths may be attributed to aneurysm rupture, frequently in association with intraventricular hemorrhage and intracranial hematoma. The diagnosis of SAH should be suspected in nontraumatic coma patients, particularly in women in their fourth and fifth decades. An immediate CT scan should be obtained to confirm the diagnosis. Lumbar puncture is contraindicated in the poor-grade patient because most have increased intracranial pressure, and many harbor space-occupying lesions.

To identify the location of the aneurysm requires angiography. Angiography, however, requires a significant amount of time (at least 30 to 60 minutes). Thus, a dilemma is created in patients with intracranial hematoma who need immediate surgery. CT scanning can be used to diagnose SAH, intraventricular hemorrhage, and intracranial hematoma, but there is overlap between the CT characteristics of aneurysmal and nonaneurysmal intracranial hematoma. Furthermore, no CT feature can definitively exclude aneurysm rupture. By contrast, infusion CT scanning is useful in these patients to determine the cause of an intracranial hematoma [59]. Infusion CT requires about 10 to 15 minutes to perform and is able to detect 97% of aneurysms greater than 3 to 5 mm in size. This technique is particularly useful in the deteriorating grade V patient with evidence of brainstem compression. In these patients even the time required for single-vessel angiography (30 to 60 minutes) can be life-threatening. By contrast, with the use of CT infusion studies, the patient can be taken quickly to the operating room knowing that an aneurysm is present. In addition, sufficient anatomic information is provided to perform both hematoma evacuation and aneurysm clipping (Figure 10.2). In the patient who is neurologically stable and in whom urgent intracranial hematoma evacuation is planned, limited angiography, tailored by the infusion scan, may be useful (Figure 10.3). A middle cerebral artery aneurysm requires only an ipsilateral carotid injection, whereas anterior communicating artery aneurysms need bilateral carotid studies. Four-vessel angiograms should be performed in all other patients not going directly to the operating room.

SURGERY

Timing

Apart from the effect of the initial hemorrhage, vasospasm and rebleeding are the leading causes of mortality and morbidity after SAH. Several recent prospective studies have demonstrated that the risk of rebleeding is highest in the first 24 to 48 hours after SAH and not later as previously thought [60,61]. Rebleeding is twofold to threefold more common in poor-grade patients [23•,62–64]. Only definitive surgical obliteration can prevent rebleeding.

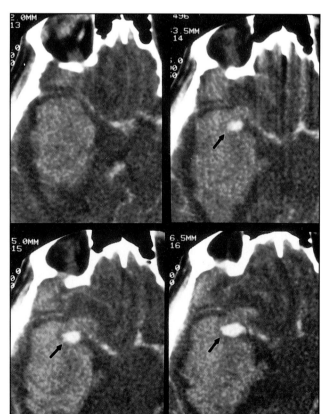

Figure 10.2

Computed tomographic infusion scans demonstrating the M_1 segment and middle cerebral artery aneurysm (*arrows*) responsible for the intracerebral hemorrhage.

Until recently, surgeons were reluctant to operate early after aneurysmal rupture, fearing a swollen brain and consequent technical difficulties. Although this sentiment may have been appropriate 20 years ago, several large-scale studies culminating in the International Cooperative Study have demonstrated that technical difficulties are no more likely with early surgery than delayed surgery. Furthermore, overall management results for early or late surgery are similar [65]. A significant advantage for good-grade patients undergoing early surgery was found when North American Centers involved in this study [66••] were separately analyzed. Vasospasm was the leading cause of unfavorable outcome. These results may reflect the period in which the patients were evaluated—before the widespread use of hypervolemia, calcium channel blockers, and angioplasty, all of which are effective, to differing degrees, in managing vasospasm. Aneurysm obliteration before the use of hypervolemia and angioplasty is advisable because these modalities may increase the risk of rupture of an unsecured aneurysm.

Early surgery has also been thought to exacerbate vasospasm. Recently, Findlay and colleagues [67••] tested this hypothesis in a primate model of SAH, and demonstrated that mechanical manipulation of vasospastic vessels did not exacerbate vasospasm. It is possible, therefore, that other factors, such as hypovolemia or hypotension, contributed to the poor outcome that surgeons previously observed after early surgery. A distinct benefit may be provided by early surgery, as it allows more aggressive treatment of vasospasm. For example, Solomon and colleagues [8•] evaluated 145 SAH patients and found that the incidence of delayed ischemic neurologic deficit was lower in patients undergoing early surgery. Further-

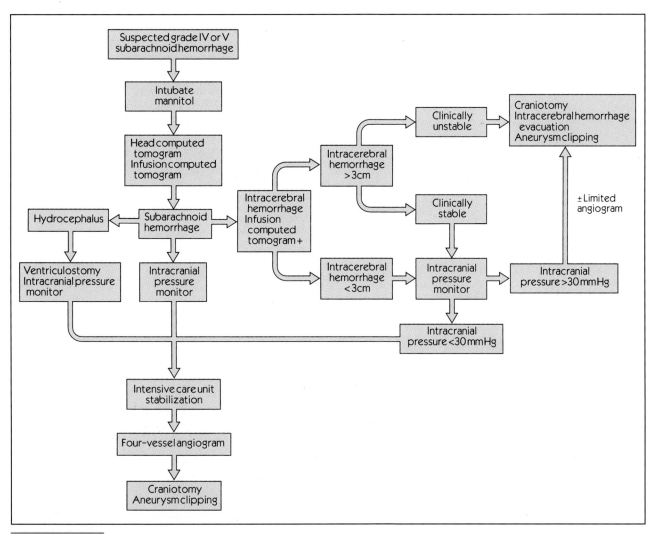

Figure 10.3

Algorithm illustrating preoperative assessment and care of poor-grade aneurysm patients.

more, the timing of surgery did not aggravate vasospasm, provided that an intensive policy to prevent vasospasm was implemented. Further evidence for the role of early surgery and aggressive vasospasm management is provided by Säveland and colleagues [7••]. After evaluating 276 SAH patients they found that 81% of good-grade patients were able to return to work. By contrast 58% of good clinical grade (I or II) patients admitted to the Cooperative Study were able to return to their premorbid state [65]. The use of early surgery, hypervolemia, and calcium channel blockers was thought to contribute to this difference. Almost all researchers have found that vasospasm is more likely to develop in poor-grade patients. Thus, early surgery may allow more effective management of vasospasm, once the aneurysm is secure.

A third potential advantage of early surgery is the relief of intracranial pressure. Most poor-grade patients have increased intracranial pressure from intracranial hematoma, hydrocephalus, or edema. Bailes and colleagues [11] studied 54 grade IV or V SAH patients; mean intracranial pressure was 40.2 mm Hg. Nineteen patients were not operated on; all died from intracranial hypertension. A total of 27 patients died, 19 of whom had intracranial hematoma. Delaying surgery can lead to deleterious ischemia and infarction. Early operation has been considered dangerous, but when considering overall management outcome, maybe advantageous. For example, Winn and colleagues [18] demonstrated that outcome was substantially improved when poor-grade patients were treated aggressively with early surgery. In addition, neither early surgery nor the patient's neurologic condition was correlated with operative morbidity. The ability to perform early surgery in these poor-grade patients is related, to a significant extent, to advances in neuroanesthesiology.

Anesthetic considerations

Together with the development of the operating microscope and the refinement of microinstruments and technique, advancements in neuroanesthesia have improved the safety of early surgery. This has not come about through the development of a single pharmacologic agent, but rather through an understanding of the pathophysiology of SAH and the effect of anesthetic agents on cerebral hemodynamics. The maintenance of cerebral perfusion, cerebral protection, brain relaxation, and prevention of aneurysm rupture are central to the successful treatment of the poor-grade patient. Thus, invasive monitoring is an important component of neuroanesthesia management. All poor-grade patients should have arterial blood pressure and Swan-Ganz catheters placed. Electrocardiography, pulse oximetry, end-tidal carbon dioxide, retrograde jugular catheterisation, Foley catheterisation, esophageal temperature monitoring, and frequent blood sampling are also required in these patients. Intubation is necessary if the level of consciousness is depressed and should preferably be instituted before the patient's arrival in the operating room. Induction should not be started until vascular hemodynamics can be closely and continuously monitored.

The goal of induction is to lower the risk of rupture by minimizing transmural pressure of the aneurysm wall. This can be achieved by lowering blood pressure but at the risk of exacerbating cerebral ischemia. Poor-grade patients have raised intracranial pressure, which may theoretically protect against rerupture. Therefore, attempts to maintain cerebral perfusion pressure without sudden changes in either systemic arterial blood pressure or intracranial pressure are preferable. A variety of anesthetic agents can achieve this. In general, intravenous agents are better than inhalational agents, as the latter tend to have a greater effect on cerebral blood flow. A combination of fentanyl and thiopental is our preferred anesthetic. Provided there are no motor deficits, paralysis can be achieved by administering succinylcholine. Its tendency to increase intracranial pressure can be prevented by deep anesthesia [68]. Alternatively, nondepolarizing agents, such as vecuronium, can be used. Pancuronium tends to increase systemic arterial blood pressure and should be used cautiously.

There are no data on the influence of different anesthetic agents on outcome for aneurysm surgery. Rather than rely on a specific anesthetic agent, successful treatment of poor-grade aneurysm patients depends on the ability of the surgical and anesthesia teams to act in unison, with management tailored to the individual patient. Maintenance of anesthesia requires the provision of a relaxed brain and cardiac and cerebral hemodynamic stability. Short-acting narcotics, such as fentanyl or sufentanil, combined with isoflurane provide satisfactory conditions. In addition, isoflurane in low doses can decrease $CMRO_2$ without influencing cerebral blood flow. By contrast, when high doses are used, systemic arterial blood pressure may decrease. Nitrous oxide is a cerebral vasodilator and may attenuate brain relaxation. This effect can be lessened by combining it with intravenous agents. Poor-grade aneurysm patients are usually left intubated at the end of the procedure. This facilitates the use of intravenous-based anesthesia, but dosage must be tapered to allow clinical assessment.

If on opening the dura the brain remains tight, a continuous infusion of thiopental may prove useful. Further adjuncts to brain relaxation include cerebrospinal fluid drainage, osmotic diuresis, and hyperventilation. Lumbar drains can be inserted in poor-grade aneurysm patients provided that no mass lesion is present. If a lumbar drain is going to be placed, it is best to do so after institution of anesthesia to prevent increases in blood pressure. Alternatively, a ventriculostomy can be used. This requires transgression of brain tissue but has the advantage of providing decompression in the postoperative period. Sudden loss of cerebrospinal fluid must be avoided. Mannitol coupled with furosemide should be given to all patients at induction provided fluid status is carefully and continuously monitored, because mannitol can acutely decrease peripheral vascular resistance and systemic arterial blood pressure. Thereafter cardiac output may increase. Thus in patients with marginal cardiac function, failure can be precipitated. Similarly, there may be a transient rise in cerebral blood flow and intracranial pressure before intracranial pressure is lowered [69,70].

Within the physiologic range, cerebral blood flow and $PaCO_2$ demonstrate a linear relationship. In poor-grade patients, however, CO_2R is impaired; therefore operating conditions must be continuously assessed to optimize carbon dioxide to minimize intracranial pressure [39,71]. In addition, excessive hyperventilation can exacerbate ischemia. Calculation of the optimal $PaCO_2$ to maintain adequate cerebral blood flow may be achieved through continuous monitoring of venous oxygen saturation with a retrograde jugular catheter. Needless to say, positioning is crucial to ensuring brain relaxation. Furthermore, care must be taken not to impede venous return in the neck by restrictive dressings or encircling tape or ties. Fluid status must be carefully controlled to maintain normovolemia before and hypervolemia after the aneurysm is clipped. Normal saline is the most physi-ologic solution; both Ringer's lactate, which is hyposmolar, and glucose may aggravate the effects of ischemia.

Technical considerations

Although aneurysms can be easily clipped through small craniotomies, in poor-grade patients large bone flaps are preferable to prevent brain herniation and strangulation (Figure 10.4). If possible, the sphenoid should be extensively taken down, during the pterional approach, to minimize brain retraction. In cases with a large intracranial hematoma and elevated intracranial pressure, removal of the skull base may not be possible and therefore partial clot removal, distant from the aneurysm, may be necessary for decompression.

Uncontrollable cerebral swelling and premature aneurysm rupture are the feared complications of early surgery. Prudent anesthetic management may prevent the former and attenuate the effects of the latter. Traditionally, systemic hypotension has been used during aneurysm dissection to prevent rupture. Poor-grade patients, however, have deficient autoregulation. Systemic hypotension, therefore, decreases global cerebral blood flow and potentially worsens ischemia and swelling. For example, Giannotti and colleagues [72••] reviewed 41 aneurysm ruptures that occurred during 276 operations. The use of hypotension did not decrease the risk of rupture. Furthermore, hypotension was deleterious to outcome if rupture occurred—only 38% of patients had a good outcome, whereas 89% did well when systemic arterial blood pressure was normal. Rather than globally decrease cerebral blood flow, temporary clips have been advo-

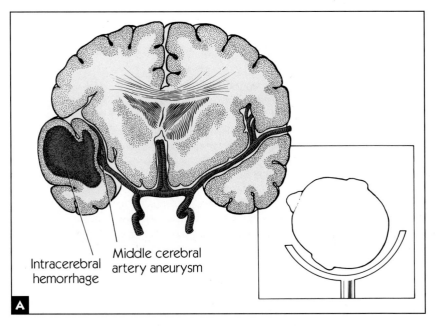

A

Intracerebral hemorrhage

Middle cerebral artery aneurysm

Figure 10.4

The operative technique for the poor-grade aneurysm patient with a large intracerebral hemorrhage (ICH). **A,** Coronal schematic of a right middle cerebral artery aneurysm and temporal lobe ICH. **Inset,** Head position: the head is rotated more toward the midline than for a standard aneurysm approach.

(Continued on next page)

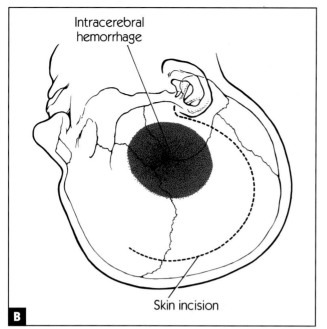

Intracerebral hemorrhage

Skin incision

B

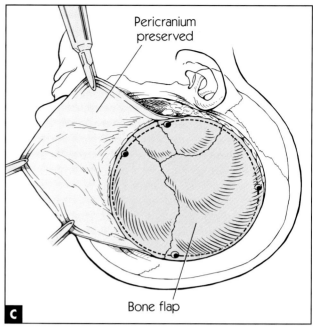

Pericranium preserved

Bone flap

C

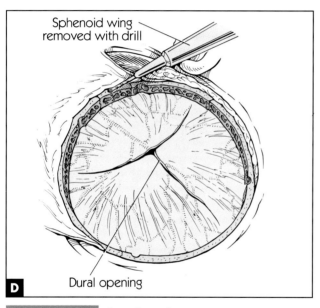

Sphenoid wing removed with drill

Dural opening

D

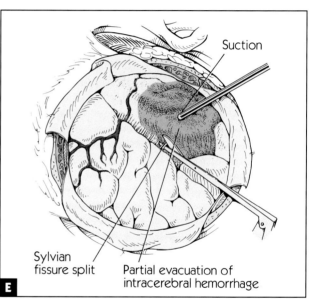

Suction

Sylvian fissure split

Partial evacuation of intracerebral hemorrhage

E

Figure 10.4 *(continued)*

B, Outline of the skin incision. **C,** A large free bone flap is prefer-able to prevent brain strangulation. The pericranium is preserved for dural augmentation if needed at closure. **D,** Judicious brain relaxation allows part of the lesser sphenoid wing to be removed using the air drill. **E,** After the dura is opened, part of the ICH, distant from the aneurysm, can be removed to improve exposure and brain relaxation. Standard microvascular techniques are used to open the sylvian fissure. **F,** The frontal lobe is carefully retracted to expose the internal carotid artery and establish proximal con-trol as needed. The deeper arachnoid is opened with Yasargil microscissors. **G,** Microdissection is continued to expose the aneurysm neck and its parent vessel. Hematoma over the aneurysm

dome is left undisturbed. It is unwise to approach the aneurysm through the ICH. Following application of the clip, aneurysm obliteration is confirmed by puncturing the aneurysm dome. **H,** The remaining ICH is removed after confirming occlusion of the aneurysm. If cerebral swelling persists a lobectomy may be nec-essary. **I,** To prevent postoperative intracranial hypertension, dural augmentation with pericranium and closure without replacing the bone flap is useful in some patients exhibiting cerebral swelling. *Arrows* indicate where edge of pericranium is tacked to dura. **J,** A ventricular catheter, particularly if there is intraventricular hemorrhage, and an intracranial pressure monitor are placed.

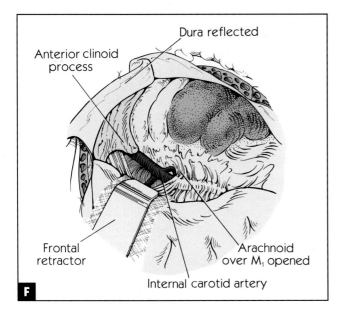

F Anterior clinoid process · Dura reflected · Frontal retractor · Arachnoid over M₁ opened · Internal carotid artery

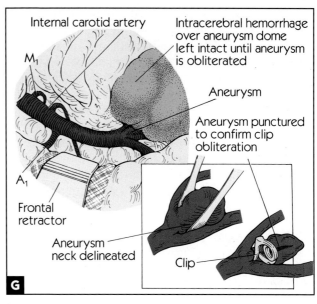

G Internal carotid artery · M₁ · A₁ · Frontal retractor · Aneurysm neck delineated · Intracerebral hemorrhage over aneurysm dome left intact until aneurysm is obliterated · Aneurysm · Aneurysm punctured to confirm clip obliteration · Clip

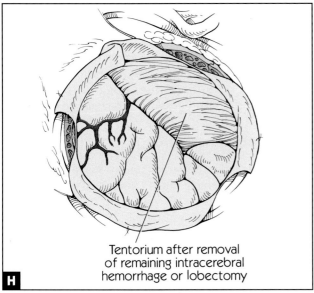

H Tentorium after removal of remaining intracerebral hemorrhage or lobectomy

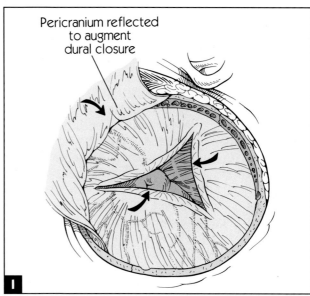

I Pericranium reflected to augment dural closure

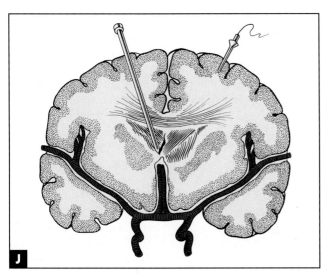

J

cated to diminish local transmural pressure in the aneurysm. Improvements in clip design have reduced the risk of vessel damage. Alternatively, endovascular techniques such as balloon occlusion can be used, particularly for vertebrobasilar or paraclinoid carotid aneurysms [73•]. Care must be taken not to overinflate the balloon and damage the endothelium. Heparinized saline should be infused locally to prevent distal emboli. An added advantage of endovascular occlusion is that intraoperative angiography can confirm aneurysm occlusion and vessel patency. The latter may also be measured by microvascular Doppler.

Cerebral protection can be useful when temporary clips are applied. Cerebral protection may be provided in a number of ways. For example, free radical scavengers (mannitol) or pharmacologic suppression of $CMRO_2$ using barbiturates, etomidate, and isoflurane have been used. In addition, recent experimental evidence suggests that mild brain hypothermia (33°C to 35°C) may also provide protection whereas hyperthermia (>38°C) can be harmful [74,75]. Temperature should therefore be carefully controlled. No randomized studies exist to guide the choice of cerebral protectant, but clinical experience dictates that their effect on both cerebral and cardiac function must be closely monitored. Isoflurane and barbiturates can both lower blood pressure, particularly when used in large doses [76•]. In addition to using cerebral protectants, efforts should be made to improve collateral flow, rheology, and blood pressure when temporary clips are applied. Etomidate has become popular as a cerebral protectant because there are few reported cardiovascular side effects. In a rat model of incomplete forebrain ischemia, however, Watson and colleagues [77••] found that etomidate only provided protection where moderate rather than severe reduction in cerebral blood flow occurred. This insult was usually insufficient to abolish an electrophysiologic response.

When temporary clips are used, it is difficult, however, to predict the duration of tolerable occlusion time. Electrophysiologic monitoring (electroencephalography [EEG], brainstem auditory evoked potentials [BAEP], and SSEP) can be used to detect ischemia. Monitoring must be tailored to that region of the brain that most likely will be affected by ischemia to improve sensitivity and specificity of the test [78••,79•]. For example, Mizoi and Yoshimoto [79•] used SSEP monitoring (median nerve) in 17 poor-grade patients. The N_{20} peak (cortex) was attenuated after 75% of middle cerebral artery occlusions, usually within 8 minutes. By contrast, N_{20} attenuation occurred after only 7% of internal carotid artery occlusions. No changes were observed after anterior cerebral artery occlusion even when the posterior tibial nerve was stimulated. The N_{20} peak disappeared when cerebral blood flow (measured with cortical thermal diffusion) was less than 40% of the preocclusion flow. Therefore, SSEP monitoring may be useful in detecting middle cerebral artery ischemia, but not after internal carotid artery or anterior cerebral artery occlusion. Poor sensitivity after vertebrobasilar occlusion has similarly been found. EEG indicates global ischemia, but is best used to determine the optimal dose of a cerebral protectant. There is no benefit to increasing the dose beyond electrocerebral silence [77••]. Transcranial Doppler assessment of blood flow velocity and retrograde assessment of jugular oxygen saturation may prove useful in the future to determine the effect of cerebral protectants.

Although many factors may lead to ischemia during temporary vascular occlusion, attention should be paid to technique to prevent vessel injury or delayed ischemia. In addition, Ogawa and colleagues [80•] recently observed that internal carotid artery occlusion, trapping, and prolonged occlusion, even if residual circulation is relatively well maintained, can lead to neurologic deficits in good-grade patients. Temporary clips should therefore be intermittently released every 6 to 8 minutes. Others suggest that slightly longer periods (8 to 20 minutes) may not be harmful.

Intracerebral hemorrhage

The presence of intracranial hematoma after aneurysmal rupture adversely affects outcome, particularly if the hematoma is greater than 3 cm in diameter and associated with shift and coma [7••,9•,14••,15,16,18]. A single prospective study, evaluating the management of intracranial hematoma in all grade aneurysm patients, exists [15]. Mortality was 80% in the nonoperative group and 27% after surgical treatment. It is important to occlude the aneurysm at the same time as hematoma evacuation, as removal of the intracranial hematoma alone is associated with nearly a threefold increase in mortality [17]. Angiography is thus necessary before surgery; however, the delay can be life-threatening in patients with evidence of brainstem compression. Most studies have advised against treating these grade V patients who harbor massive intracranial hematoma, reporting mortalities of nearly 100%. Based on plain CT findings, empiric exploration of the sylvian fissure has been reported in two case reports with limited success. CT characteristics, however, are not always definite. To overcome this, we have used CT infusion scanning in 25 patients with aneurysmal intracranial hematoma and evidence of brainstem compression, and proceeded directly to surgery without the delay incurred in obtaining angiography (Figure 10.3). Without surgery, all would have died, but with aggressive management half survived. Furthermore, 32% were independent and living at home with only mild disability. We did not find any preoperative factor that predicted outcome and believe that surgery should not be withheld from poor-grade patients with intracranial hematoma. Prognosis becomes readily apparent in the postoperative period—12 of the 13 patients who died did so within 4 days, whereas all eight patients who were independent at 6-month follow-up were able to follow commands within 72 hours.

We believe, however, that the successful management of poor-grade aneurysm patients, with intracranial hematoma, requires intensive efforts beginning with an efficient paramedic service. Cerebral swelling and intracranial hypertension are frequently present; therefore, mannitol must be given immediately on diagnosis to temporarily improve cerebral dynamics. Alternatively, a ventriculostomy can be placed, but rapid or excessive cerebrospinal fluid drainage must be avoided. The operative technique is illustrated in Figure 10.4. A large craniotomy is necessary to prevent brain strangulation and provide the easiest and safest access to the intracranial hematoma. With judicious brain relaxation and careful bony decompression of the sphenoid wing, proximal control should first be obtained and aneurysm clipping attempted before hematoma evacuation. Occasionally, partial hematoma evacuation, away from the aneurysm, is necessary. We use standard microvascular principles when clipping the aneurysm. After definitive aneurysm obliteration, the remaining intracranial hematoma can be safely evacuated. To approach the aneurysm through the clot, or evacuate the entire intracranial hematoma before aneurysm occlusion invites disaster. If cerebral swelling remains, lobectomy, ventriculostomy, or preferably duraplasty without bone replacement can be used. Postoperatively angiography should be performed to confirm aneurysm obliteration. Hypervolemic therapy is then instituted and intracranial pressure carefully monitored. We have found that in grade V patients with intracerebral hemorrhage, an extensive decompression prevents intracranial hypertension. Patients who do not survive usually declare themselves within 48 to 72 hours, failing to respond to management of intracranial pressure.

Hydrocephalus and intraventricular hemorrhage

The incidence of acute hydrocephalus varies depending on the criteria used for diagnosis. It is clear, however, that the presence of intraventricular hemorrhage and poor clinical grade are the strongest predictors of hydrocephalus. Vasospasm may often accompany hydrocephalus [2,7••,19,20,21••,24].

Intraventricular hemorrhage is also associated with intracranial hemorrhage and poor outcome. In addition, intraventricular hemorrhage may stimulate release of atrial natriuretic factor, leading to hyponatremia and decreased intravascular volume [50•]. Although acute hydrocephalus is well recognized, there is no consensus on its management because ventricular drainage may be associated with rebleeding [81•]. Whether ventriculostomy alters the natural history (ie, increases the rate of rebleeding or improves survival) is presently unclear. With this caveat in mind, review of the literature indicates that rebleeding after ventriculostomy is not usually immediate but occurs 24 hours later [23•]. Moreover, the same authors observed that catheter drainage of intraventricular hemorrhage resulted in clinical improvement in 13 of 29 grade IV/V patients. More than half had good outcome. Bailes and colleagues [11] have had similar success with careful, controlled cerebrospinal fluid drainage (to 15 cm H_2O). Occasionally, insertion of the ventricular catheter is difficult because of shift or ventricular effacement. Similarly, drainage may be poor, particularly with extensive intraventricular hemorrhage. In the acute stage, ventricular drainage should be seen as a temporary measure to stabilize the patient for definitive surgery. Alternatively, a Camino intracranial pressure monitor can be inserted; this takes less than 5 minutes and can be performed at bedside, such as in the CT suite or emergency department. If intracranial pressure is elevated, a ventriculostomy is then inserted. If rebleeding occurs, the catheter should be clamped, as continued drainage may worsen the extent of hemorrhage. Once inserted attempts should be made to wean the ventriculostomy, because the risk of infection increases with time (5 days). Therefore, Hasan and colleagues [82•] have advocated serial lumbar punctures to a closing pressure of 15 cm H_2O. Although most patients improved neurologically, overall outcome was not improved [82•]. The rebleed rate was not increased, however, and only 4% of the patients required ventriculoperitoneal shunts. Most reports indicate that half the patients with acute clinical hydrocephalus eventually require a ventriculoperitoneal shunt. Obviously, lumbar punctures cannot be performed in patients with raised intracranial pressure, but they may be a useful adjunct for weaning a ventriculostomy once intracranial pressure is controlled or decreasing the risk of shunt failure by removing red blood cell breakdown products.

About half the patients with acute hydrocephalus following SAH eventually require long-term shunting for chronic hydrocephalus. This results from blood-induced meningeal thickening, damage to arachnoid villi and ependymal cells, and blockage of normal cerebrospinal fluid pathways. Chronic hydrocephalus is more common after large hemorrhages in poor-grade patients. Even though ventricular pressure is often normal, cerebral blood flow is attenuated, and significant improvement can be expected after the insertion of a ventriculoperitoneal shunt [24].

VASOSPASM

Following surgery, vasospasm poses the greatest threat to the poor-grade patient. Both clinical and experimental studies demonstrate that the severity of vasospasm correlates with the amount of SAH. In turn, the severity of SAH also predicts clinical grade [34,83•]. Significant vasospasm is three times more likely in poor-grade patients [2,8•,29,34].

Pathogenesis

Despite numerous investigations, the exact pathogenesis of vasospasm is not clear, although it is certain that prolonged contact with red blood cells and oxyhemoglobin (derived from red blood cell lysis) are key factors in its genesis. This has been confirmed in a primate model of SAH. After infusion of oxyhemoglobin or red blood cell supernatant around the cerebral vessels, vessel narrowing with the same angiographic and morphologic changes seen in clinical vasospasm is observed [84••]. Some ultrastructural studies reveal a proliferative vasculopathy and endothelial convolutions. By contrast, immunohistochemical analysis of vasospastic vessels demonstrates no increase in either extracellular matrix (principally collagen) or cytoskeletal elements [85••]. In addition, hydroxyproline (indicating collagen synthesis) is not elevated, suggesting that, at least initially, vasoconstriction may be the basis of vasospasm. This is consistent with *in vitro* studies that demonstrate that oxyhemoglobin is a vasoconstrictor. Ultrastructural changes, including collagen deposition or rearrangement and myonecrosis, may occur later as a response to injury. These changes may be particularly relevant since the advent of balloon angioplasty.

Recent studies also suggest that the damaged endothelium can contribute to vasospasm through an imbalance in endothelian (ET-1, a vasoconstrictor) and endothelium-derived relaxing factor (EDRF, a vasodilator). For example, Suzuki and colleagues [86••] measured ET-1 levels in SAH patients. Five to 7 days after hemorrhage plasma levels were elevated eightfold, whereas cerebrospinal fluid levels were elevated only in those patients with vasospasm. Edwards and colleagues [87••], in a series of eloquent experiments, observed that cGMP levels (a marker of EDRF activity) were reduced in pig middle cerebral artery

vessels, after chronic exposure to hemoglobin *in vivo*. Similar effects could be seen *in vitro* after endothelial denudation, adventitial placement of hemoglobin, or nitric oxide synthesis inhibition (nitric oxide and EDRF appear to be the same substance). Cerebral vessels have large adventitial pores; it is thus possible that oxyhemoglobin diffuses through these pores and scavenges EDRF, leading to vasoconstriction [87••].

The initial phase of smooth muscle contraction is mediated by an influx of calcium that modulates protein kinase second messengers [88••]. *In vitro* oxyhemoglobin increases intracellular calcium concentration. These levels decrease when the vessel is returned to a more normal environment [89••]. Minami and colleagues [88••] tested this hypothesis further and found that protein kinase inhibition dilates vasospastic basilar arteries *in vivo*. Calcium may also increase phospholipases and free radicals, which in turn can damage cell membranes. However, Macdonald and colleagues [90•] found that the free radical scavengers superoxide dismutase and catalase did not attenuate vasospasm and therefore suggested that free radicals may not be involved in its pathogenesis. Further evidence for the role of calcium comes from observations by Ram and colleagues [91•]. When topical magnesium sulfate is added to spastic rat basilar arteries, dilatation results. Magnesium is a competitive calcium antagonist and may mediate calcium influx at the N-methyl-D-aspartate channel. An imbalance of dilatatory and constricting prosta-glandins has also been implicated in vasospasm. O'Neill and colleagues [92•], however, found that even though prostaglandin levels may increase after SAH in humans, there is no correlation with the amount of hemorrhage, vasospasm, or delayed ischemic deficits. Inflammation may also play a role in the pathogenesis of vasospasm. Support for this proposal is provided by Yamamoto and colleagues [93•], who used a serine protease, FUT-145, in patients with SAH and found that vasospasm was prevented, even in patients with large bleeds. FUT-145 inhibits protein-derived inflammation and the complement pathway. Further study may be necessary in light of previous investigations that have demonstrated the effectiveness of high-dose steroids and/or cyclosporine in select patients with vasospasm. Steroids may benefit poor-grade patients for three reasons: 1) attenuation of edema formation, 2) less risk of hydrocephalus because of decreased meningeal inflammation, and 3) partial amelioration of vasospasm. In this last action, steroids may attenuate the increased number of white cells associated with meningeal inflammation. At low concentrations, white cells release nitric oxide (EDRF), but at high concentrations, release superoxide anions that destroy EDRF.

Clinical management

Perhaps the most effective treatment of vasospasm is its prevention. Therefore, attempts have been made to remove clot from around vessels. Experimental studies suggest that this should be accomplished within 48 hours. Extensive saline irrigation can prevent vasospasm [94•], but more recently fibrinolysis, tissue plasminogen activator in particular, has been used with some success. Excellent clot lysis, on postoperative CT scan, and an almost complete absence of severe vasospasm, even in patients with large hemorrhages, has been demonstrated in three separate preliminary reports. Tissue plasminogen activator provides clot-specific fibrinolysis, and so systemic coagulopathies have not been found. The aneurysm should be obliterated before the use of tissue plasminogen activator; early surgery is thus essential [95••,96••,97•].

Aneurysm obliteration is also necessary to institute hypervolemic, hypertensive therapy safely, which currently is accepted as the most effective management of vasospasm. By improving collateral flow, it ameliorates the ischemic complications, rather than prevent or treat vasospasm directly. Hemodilution is a secondary gain, which may improve tissue oxygen delivery. Care must be taken not to decrease the hematocrit below 30% because hemoglobin and oxygen dissociation may be attenuated. Hypervolemia should be instituted as soon as possible after hemorrhage and is safest once the aneurysm is occluded. A combination of albumin and normal saline can effectively increase intravascular volume, which is best assessed with a Swan-Ganz catheter (pulmonary capillary wedge pressure 16 to 18 mm Hg). Cardiac output should be maintained at 6.0 L/min or more; if not, dobutamine may be added. Fludrocortisone and occasionally vasopressin, which must be used with caution because pulmonary edema can be precipitated, may attenuate the associated diuresis. Cardiorespiratory complications may also occur; therefore, meticulous cardiovascular monitoring (*ie,* Swan-Ganz catheter) is needed. Care must be taken not to exacerbate intracranial pressure when using hypervolemic therapy. If intracranial pressure rises, treatment of cerebral hypertension may necessitate reduction in the hypervolemic therapy.

Calcium channel blockers, particularly nimodipine, also ameliorate the effects of vasospasm. Several large, controlled studies have demonstrated that nimodipine improves the number of patients having a good outcome in both good-grade and poor-grade patients [98,99]. The mechanism of action is not known. It is postulated that the effect may be mediated through pial vessels or neuronal protection because basal vessels in spasm do not show angiographic change. The best effect is observed when calcium channel blockers are used synergistically with hypervolemia [100•]. In addition, normoglycemia is necessary, as even mild hyperglycemia can attenuate the protective effect provided by calcium channel blockers [101••].

Although both hypervolemia and nimodipine are useful in minimizing the effects of cerebral ischemia, they are less effective once a neurologic deficit develops. We now use transfemoral, transluminal angioplasty (Figure 10.5) if a patient becomes symptomatic despite maximal hypervolemia and in the presence of calcium channel blockers [102•,103]. Silicone

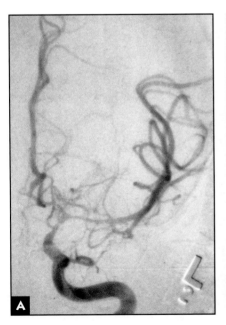 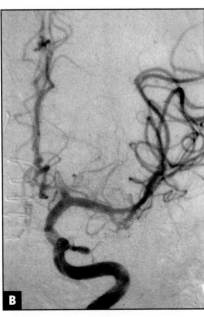

Figure 10.5

Vasospasm commonly complicates the course of the poor-grade aneurysm patient. If the patient develops a neurologic deficit despite maximal hypervolemia and the use of calcium channel blocks, angioplasty may restore vessel patency. **A,** Left internal carotid anteroposterior angiogram showing severe vasospasm in the supraclinoid carotid and middle cerebral arteries. **B,** Patency of the vessels is restored after angioplasty.

microballoons are preferable. The balloon size must be carefully selected to prevent endothelial damage or vessel rupture. Furthermore, the aneurysm should be obliterated before attempting angioplasty because aneurysm rupture can occur when blood flow is increased after mechanical dilatation. Angioplasty is indicated when a neurologic deficit, not related to other causes and not responsive to optimal hypervolemia and hypertension, develops. In addition, there should be no evidence of infarction on CT. Angiography is first performed to document vasospasm in the vascular distribution consistent with the deficit before performing angioplasty. The mechanism by which mechanical dilatation counteracts vasospasm is not known. Experimental studies suggest that the collagen architecture of the vessel is disrupted [104•]. The effect is sustained, and the pathogenic process is reversed. For example, transcranial Doppler studies have demonstrated marked improvement of flow in vessels that have been mechanically dilated whereas continued spasm is observed in those vessels that were not dilated [103,104•]. Preliminary results of angioplasty are encouraging [102•,103]; angiographic improvement is almost invariable. Furthermore, improvement in both the level of consciousness or focal neurologic findings is observed in 60% to 70% of patients.

The successful management of vasospasm in poor-grade patients is centered on early surgery, calcium channel blockers, hypervolemic hypertensive therapy, and judicious use of angioplasty. In the future, potentially intraoperative clot lysis with tissue plasminogen activator may play a role. Despite these therapeutic advances, careful hemodynamic monitoring and ongoing evaluation of cerebral physiology underly the successful management of vasospasm.

Monitoring

Secondary deterioration in the poor-grade patient can be caused by many factors, including increased intracranial pressure, hydrocephalus, vasospasm, postoperative hematoma or swelling, infarction, seizures, meningitis (both aseptic and bacterial), hypotension, hypoxia, and hyponatremia (Table 10.3). In addition, other complications, such as deep vein thrombosis, pulmonary embolus, gastrointestinal hemorrhage, and sepsis can occur and adversely affect outcome [24,65]. The key to management of these problems is their prevention, which requires constant assessment. The clinical examination in the unconscious patient, however, can be difficult to interpret. Therefore, all patients must be cared for in the intensive care unit and invasive monitoring implemented.

Careful attention should be paid to cardiorespiratory function and volume status. This is best monitored through an intra-arterial blood pressure monitor; Swan-Ganz catheter to assess pulmonary capillary wedge pressure, pulmonary artery diastolic pressure, cardiac output, and cardiac index; and chest film and analysis of arterial blood gas. Central venous pressure, especially in patients older than 40 years, is not sufficient to assess volume status. Frequent assessment of electrolytes, osmolality, glucose, hematocrit, and urine output supplement invasive monitoring. An intracranial pressure monitor is essential in all patients; this might be augmented with a retrograde jugular catheter to determine venous oxygen saturation, arteriovenous difference of oxygen ($AVDO_2$), and lactate. In head injury, these parameters have been

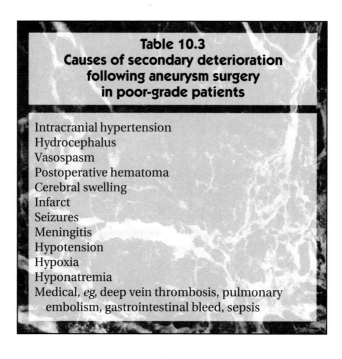

Table 10.3
Causes of secondary deterioration
following aneurysm surgery
in poor-grade patients

Intracranial hypertension
Hydrocephalus
Vasospasm
Postoperative hematoma
Cerebral swelling
Infarct
Seizures
Meningitis
Hypotension
Hypoxia
Hyponatremia
Medical, *eg*, deep vein thrombosis, pulmonary
    embolism, gastrointestinal bleed, sepsis

found to be useful in identifying patients with compensated hypoperfusion who are at risk for ischemia. Moreover, the $AVDO_2$ difference guides the rational adjustment of $PaCO_2$ and systemic arterial blood pressure to maximize cerebral blood flow [106•,107••]. In the future, cerebral metabolic function may be assessed by the use of microdialysis catheters. [108••]. However, microdialysis only allows assay of a small area. Frequent CT scans should supplement monitoring. In some circumstances, electrophysiologic monitoring may prove useful [109•]. Cortical microcirculation can also be assessed continuously in the intensive care unit by laser Doppler flowmetry [110•].

As more effective treatments of vasospasm have developed, it has become necessary to accurately diagnose vasospasm and assess the effects of management. Until recently, the diagnosis was by exclusion. Confirmation was possible only with angiography. A noninvasive test, transcranial Doppler (Figure 10.6), can now be used to diagnose patients with vasospasm [105•,111•,112••,113•]. The recent development of transcranial color-coded Doppler should further enhance diagnostic specificity in the future [114•]. The changes in blood flow velocity detected by transcranial Doppler correlate with the severity of vasospasm; velocities greater than 120 cm/s indicate spasm, whereas velocities greater than 200 cm/s are usually associated with symptoms. A rapid increase in velocity (> 50 cm/s/d) indicates a patient at high risk for developing ischemic symptoms [112••]. Relative flow velocity is also important, as blood flow velocity may increase with increased flow volume. To differentiate spasm and hyperdynamic flow, assessment of the middle cerebral artery-to-internal carotid artery ratio is necessary. A ratio greater than 3 indicates spasm is present; greater than 6 is associated with severe spasm; and greater than 8 is invariably symptomatic. These values apply best to the middle cerebral artery and may be different for other vessels. A decrease in velocity has also been seen after calcium channel blockers are given, even when there are no angiographic changes. This decrease may reflect dilatation

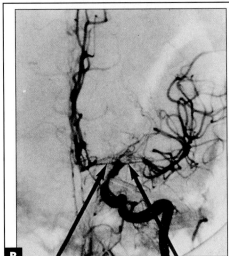
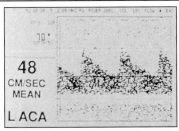
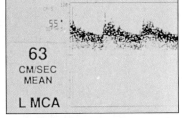
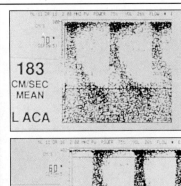

Figure 10.6

Transcranial Doppler (TCD) can be used to diagnose patients with vasospasm. A velocity of greater than 200 cm/s is usually associated with symptoms. **A,** Angiogram and TCD findings shortly after early surgery in a patient with a ruptured aneurysm (*arrows*). **B,** Angiogram and TCD findings (*arrows*) in the same patient after patient developed symptoms of delayed ischemia. (*From* Seiler and Newell [126]; with permission.)

of the microcirculation or improved collateral flow. In turn flow through the spastic vessel is decreased. Transcranial Doppler offers numerous advantages: it is noninvasive, repeatable, and can be performed at the bedside. All poor-grade patients should have daily transcranial Doppler examinations. In addition, transcranial Doppler can be used to determine when hypervolemic therapy can be weaned in the asymptomatic patient. If velocities decrease on two consecutive days, we begin weaning hypervolemic therapy, but reinstitute it if velocities increase.

Transcranial Doppler, however, does not accurately evaluate the distal (*ie*, third order) vessels and the microcirculation. Both may be a factor in the development of symptoms and may be addressed by studies of cerebral blood flow. SPECT examination is most commonly used (Figure 10.7). Correlation between SPECT findings and transcranial Doppler velocities is high but not 100% [111•,113•]. For example, when transcranial Doppler reflects severe symptomatic vasospasm, regional hypoperfusion is detected by SPECT in only 70% to 80% of cases. Normal SPECT is found in all patients with abnormal transcranial Doppler velocities but normal neurologic examinations. Thus, SPECT appears useful in identifying a subgroup of patients with compensated hypoperfusion. Xenon-133 CT may also be used to detect hypoperfusion. Several studies indicate that a cerebral blood flow less than 15 mL/100 g/min is always associated with symptomatic vasospasm [115•]. Xenon, however, can cause respiratory depression, thus limiting its use. Whereas transcranial Doppler is readily repeated, neither SPECT nor xenon studies can be repeated on a regular basis. Measurement of cerebral blood flow by both SPECT and xenon methods requires moving the patient from the intensive care unit, therefore, other bedside tests may be useful. For example, EEG abnormalities have been found to predict and correlate with vasospasm [116•]. We obtain baseline SPECT studies immediately after surgery and interpret this study in conjunction with a postoperative CT scan. SPECT studies are repeated if transcranial Doppler velocities exceed 200 cm/s or when angioplasty is contemplated. Following successful angioplasty, improvement in both transcranial Doppler velocities and SPECT can be observed [105•,113•]. Furthermore, transcranial Doppler can be used to monitor the progress of vasospasm in vessels that were not dilated.

OUTCOME

Coma on admission after SAH has been well documented to adversely affect outcome [1,2,5,6•,7••,8•,9•, 65]. In the first studies that addressed natural history of ruptured cerebral aneurysms, patients who were

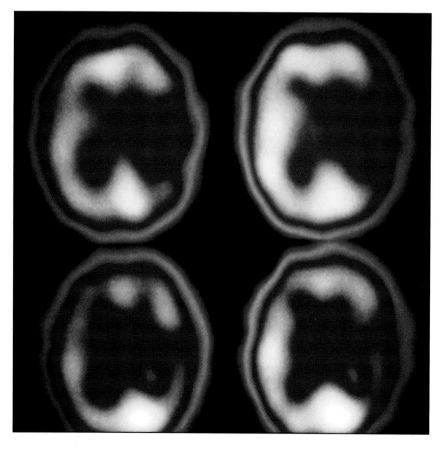

Figure 10.7

Top, Single-photon emission computed tomographic (SPECT) study showing regional hypoperfusion secondary to vasospasm. **Bottom,** Following angioplasty and restoration of vessel patency, SPECT study demonstrates improved regional hypoperfusion.

unconscious at admission had a greater than 90% mortality, three times that of those who were alert. In the first Cooperative Study, 7% of grade V patients survived 1 year. By contrast 54% of grade I or II patients survived [2]. These findings are also evident in the second Cooperative Study [65]. Whereas 75% of patients who were alert at admission had a good outcome, only 11% of those in coma did well (Table 10.2). The management of SAH, however, has changed dramatically in the last decade. Recent experience indicates that an intensive management policy may substantially improve outcome in poor-grade patients [11,18]. Early surgery and aggressive prevention and management of vasospasm are central to this success. The management results of poor-grade patients from several series are compiled in Table 10.4.

In the past, a delay prior to surgery was advocated for poor-grade patients. Many poor-grade patients who initially survived succumbed from either intracranial hematoma or rebleeding before surgery. It is thus important to look at management results rather than surgical results as a delayed surgery population is highly selective [24,117].

Many deaths that occur while waiting for surgery are attributed to rebleeding. To prevent this, early surgery is advocated. The recent Cooperative Study attempted to answer whether early surgery improves overall management results [65]. A total of 3251 patients were evaluated in a multicenter, prospective, observational epidemiologic study. Overall management results were similar for both early and late surgery; however, patients who were alert at admission did better following early surgery. Fifty-eight percent of good-grade patients at admission were able to return to their premorbid state. A separate analysis of the North American Centers involved in the Cooperative Study revealed that alert patients treated with early surgery had a significant increase in good outcome [67••]. By contrast, this advantage was not evident in poor-grade patients. Poor-grade patients, however, are at high risk for vasospasm, which was found to be the leading cause of death or disability. The Cooperative Study, however, reflected care in the early 1980s before the use of transcranial Doppler, hypervolemia, calcium channel blockers, or angioplasty. In the late 1980s and early part of this decade a policy of early surgery and aggressive vasospasm treatment has emerged as an acceptable management strategy of SAH. Improved outcome results related to a lower incidence of delayed ischemic neurologic deficit are now reported. For example, among 238 patients admitted to a single institution within 72 hours of SAH, 25% suffered a poor outcome [14••]. Most deaths were due to the effect of the initial hemorrhage, particularly if an intracerebral hematoma was found; only 0.5% were due to a delayed ischemic neurologic deficit. Although clinical grade remained a strong predictor of outcome, 89% of grade IV patients, particularly if no intracranial hematoma was identified, had a good outcome. These results were attributed to the aggressive management of vasospasm. Taylor and colleagues [9•] recently reviewed 295 patients treated for SAH in Glasgow. Poor grade, intracranial hematoma, and delayed ischemic neuro-

Table 10.4
Outcome in poor-grade (Hunt and Hess IV and V) subarachnoid hemorrhage patients*

Study	Cases, n	Follow-up, mo	Results, %†			
			Good	Fair	Poor	Dead
Hunt and Hess [3]	47	3	–	–	–	78.7
Adams et al. [120]	61	3	18	–	24.6	57.4
Ljunggren et al. [121]	21	7	9.5	19	14.3	57.1
Hijdra et al. [122]	42	3	0	5	23	71
Chyatte et al. [123]	80	–	16	9	29	46
Inagawa et al. [124]	157	12	3.8	5.7	15.2	75.2
Petruk et al. [98]	108	3	12.0	13	21.3	53.7
Bailes et al. [11]	54	3	35.2	7.4	7.4	50
Winn et al. [18]	56	6	37.5	–	25	37.5
Auer et al. [125]	52	6	21	21	10	48
Säveland et al. [7••]	110	3–6	19	36‡		45

*Modified from Bailes et al. [11]; with permission.
†Good–independent lifestyle; fair–partly dependent; poor–totally dependent.
‡Results were pooled as morbidity.

logic deficit all adversely affected outcome, although 76% of patients who developed a delayed ischemic deficit improved with hypervolemia and nimodipine. Furthermore, early surgery was found to improve outcome in good-grade patients. Grade V patients, however, were not admitted to neurosurgical care. However, 28 grade IV or V patients were treated, and 70% had a favorable outcome. In a prospective study from Sweden in which early surgery and hypervolemia were used in 325 patients, 81% of the good-grade patients were able to return to their premorbid state. Only 5.5% developed a delayed ischemic neurologic deficit [7••]. Furthermore, 33% of grade V patients achieved a good outcome. Again, the presence of an intracranial hematoma adversely affected outcome.

Two recent reports have specifically addressed poor-grade patients. In both, management policy was centered on early surgery, control of intracranial pressure, and aggressive vasospasm management. Bailes and colleagues [11] evaluated 54 grade IV or V patients. Nineteen patients were not actively treated for various reasons including elevated intracranial pressure despite ventricular drainage, extensive damage on CT, or poor vessel filling on angiography—all died. Of the remaining patients, 22.9% died and 43% survived with no or moderate disability only. Winn and colleagues [18] treated 66 grade IV or V patients; none were excluded from treatment. Mortality was 35% and 41% among grade IV and grade V patients, respectively. In both series, the presence of an intracerebral hematoma, especially if accompanied by shift, was correlated with a poor outcome. In the study by Winn and colleagues [18], 59% of patients with intracranial hematoma and midline shift died whereas only 13% of patients without CT evidence of midline shift died. Consequently, we [118•] have altered our approach to patients with a large intracranial hematoma and now perform immediate surgery on grade V patients with evidence of brainstem compression from the intracranial hematoma. Rather than delay for angiography, infusion CT scanning is used. We have used this approach in 25 patients. Whereas previous reports have advocated no treatment, or reported a 100% mortality, 48% of the patients in our series survived. More importantly, 32% of the initially moribund grade V patients are independent and living at home. There were no preoperative factors that predicted outcome. This, however, became apparent in the 72 hours following surgery.

Although coma at admission after SAH (grade IV and V) is unquestionably associated with a poor outcome, it should not be the sole basis for exclusion from active treatment. Consideration should be made of the patient's age, medical history, and family wishes. A management policy centered on early surgery, control of intracranial pressure, and aggres-sive treatment of vasospasm may lead to a favorable outcome in many poor-grade patients. This is a substantial improvement over the natural history.

MANAGEMENT POLICY FOR THE POOR-GRADE ANEURYSM PATIENT

Outlined below is our present approach to patients with SAH secondary to ruptured aneurysm and is based on our experience with 500 patients admitted to Harborview Medical Center and the University of Washington, Seattle. All patients with suspected aneurysmal SAH are evaluated by a member of the neurosurgery team on arrival in the emergency department. A guide to the initial assessment and management of poor-grade aneurysm patients is depicted in Figure 10.3. When the patient is stabilized, an unenhanced CT scan, followed by an infusion CT scan are obtained. In a deteriorating patient with a mass lesion, the patient is taken directly to the operating room for intracranial hematoma evacuation and aneurysm clipping based on the infusion scan alone. In patients with mass lesions, who are neurologically stable, an angiogram tailored to the infusion scan is obtained before surgery. In these patients an intracranial pressure monitor is placed before angiography. Intracranial pressure should be treated judiciously with mannitol when greater than 20 mm Hg. If intracranial pressure remains elevated or clinical deterioration occurs, immediate surgery based on the infusion scan becomes necessary. Similarly, in patients demonstrating ventricular enlargement on CT, an intracranial pressure monitor is inserted and a ventriculostomy placed if the intracranial pressure is greater than 20 mm Hg. The drainage gradient should be set at 15 cm H_2O to minimize overdrainage and possible aneurysm rupture.

Apart from those patients going directly to the operating room, the poor-grade patient should be transferred directly to the neurosurgery intensive care unit once the diagnosis of SAH is made. All patients who have a depressed level of consciousness should be intubated and mechanically ventilated to maintain PaO_2 greater than 80 mm Hg and $PaCO_2$ 30 to 35 mm Hg. Preferably this should have been achieved in the field or emergency department. We routinely monitor our poor-grade patients with an arterial catheter, Swan-Ganz catheter, and Foley catheter as well as an intracranial pressure monitor. Hypertension is often present in these patients and may be associated with increased intracranial pressure. Any decision to treat hypertension should not be taken lightly; there is no evidence that decreasing blood pressure protects against rebleeding and instead it may aggravate cerebral ischemia. Systemic arterial blood pressure greater than 240 mm Hg, however, can be carefully lowered, initially with sedation, paralysis, and mechanical ventilation. If these methods are not successful, a short-acting agent such as nitroprusside or labetalol can be continuously titrated to control systemic arterial blood pressure and cerebral perfusion pressure. Diuretics and longer acting agents such as hydralazine should be avoided if possible. Because beta-blockers can have a negative inotropic effect, cardiac output requires assessment. Normovolemia must be ensured before attempting to lower the systemic arterial blood pressure, and can be achieved by administering alternate volumes of albumin and normal saline. Ringer's lactate should be avoided because it is hypotonic, and dextrose should not be given because even moderate hyperglycemia (> 200) may aggravate cerebral ischemia. Pulmonary capillary wedge pressure and cardiac output should be maintained between 10 and 12 mm and 6 L/min, respectively. Medications frequently used in these patients include dexamethasone, dilantin, nimodipine, and H_2 blockers, such as ranitidine. Baseline transcranial Doppler studies, electrocardiogram, a chest film, arterial blood gas, electrolytes, osmolality, glucose, coagulation screen, and hematocrit are obtained. Cardiac enzymes are ordered dependent on the electrocardiogram. Deep vein thrombosis prophylaxis using intermittent compression stockings is started.

Once intracranial pressure is controlled and normovolemia, hemodynamic stability, and adequate oxygenation ensured, four-vessel angiography is carried out. Surgical obliteration of the aneurysm is achieved as soon as possible in the next 24 hours. Intravascular volume must be maintained during surgery. A retrograde jugular catheter can be inserted for monitoring jugular venous oxygen saturation. Judicious lumbar cerebrospinal fluid drainage and mannitol are given to provide brain relaxation. When temporary clips are used, cerebral protection is provided by giving isoflurane, thiopentone or additional mannitol. Following surgery, baseline CT, SPECT, and angiography are obtained.

On return to the intensive care unit (Table 10.5), hypervolemia is instituted with albumin and crystalloid boluses to maintain the pulmonary capillary wedge pressure between 16 to 18 mm Hg and the cardiac output greater than 6 to 8 L/min. We do not favor the use of low molecular weight dextran or hetastarch because coagulopathies may be associated with their use. If cardiac output falls, β-adrenergic agonists such as dobutamine can be used provided there is no evidence of pulmonary edema. Fludrocortisone is sometimes required to maintain intravascular volume. On occasion, vasopressin may be given to prevent diuresis but should be used with caution, as pulmonary edema can be precipitated. Hourly assessment of pulmonary capillary wedge pressure or pulmonary artery diastolic pressure and 6-hour cardiac output assessment by thermodilution are necessary. Calculation of central venous pressure alone is insufficient. Electrolytes, arterial blood gas, and osmolality are assessed at 6-hour intervals. Hyponatremia should not be treated by fluid restriction. If serum sodium, however, is less than 125 mEq, 3% normal saline may be given. Hematocrit is maintained at 30% to 33% to prevent a deleterious shift in the hemoglobin/oxygen dissociation curve. Mechanical ventilation is maintained using morphine

---

Table 10.5
Postsurgical care for poor-grade aneurysm patients

Intensive care unit
Intracranial pressure monitor
Frequent computed tomography and single photon emission
    computed tomography
Daily transcranial Doppler
Angiogram (four-vessel)
Mechanical ventilation: PaO_2 > 80 mm Hg
                      $PaCO_2$ 25–30 mm Hg
Medication, *eg*, dexamethasone, dilantin, nimodipine,
    ±fludrocortisone, ±ventriculostomy
Hypervolemic therapy
    Swan-Ganz catheter
    Saline-albumin boluses to maintain pulmonary capillary wedge
        pressure 16–18 mm Hg and cardiac output > 6.0 L/min
    Desired hematocrit 30%
    Dopamine or dobutamine as clinically indicated
Angioplasty as indicated

sulfate, midazolame, and pancuronium as needed. PEEP monitoring must be used cautiously because it can decrease cardiac output. By contrast, intracranial pressure should not be affected unless PEEP is greater than 15 cm H_2O. Nutritional support should be implemented within 48 hours of surgery to minimize the deleterious effects of a negative nitrogen balance. Enteral feeding is preferred to parenteral nutrition as the risk of gastrointestinal ulcer or bleeding is less. Furthermore, parenteral nutrition is often associated with hyperglycemia, hyposmolality, and other metabolic abnormalities that can worsen cerebral ischemia.

Daily transcranial Doppler examinations are carried out. If a neurologic deficit, attributable to vasospasm, develops a bolus of 500 mL of albumin is given and the volume increased to tolerable levels. If this is not effective, systemic arterial blood pressure is increased by administering dopamine. The dose is titrated to the minimum necessary to reverse any deficits but not to cause systemic arterial blood pressure to increase greater than 240 mm Hg. Significant hypertension may cause breakthrough edema or hemorrhage. The effects of hypervolemic therapy should be observed within 1 to 2 hours. If there is no response, a SPECT study is obtained and angioplasty indicated. Hypervolemia should be maintained for a minimum of 10 days and tapered according to transcranial Doppler velocities. In the long-term, patients may require a ventriculoperitoneal shunt, tracheostomy, and feeding jejunostomy. Physical therapy should be instituted in the immediate postoperative period. Complications such as deep vein thrombosis, pulmonary embolus, pneumonia, and infection must be constantly considered, actively prevented, and treated.

The effective management of the poor-grade aneurysm patient has its foundation in the prevention, early diagnosis, and correction of any complications. Successful outcome in these very compromised patients requires close monitoring and meticulous attention to detail.

REFERENCES AND RECOMMENDED READING

Papers of particular interest, published within the annual period of review, have been highlighted as:
• Of special interest
•• Of outstanding interest

1. Rosenorn J, Eskesen V, Schmidt K, *et al.*: Clinical features and outcome in 1076 patients with ruptured intracranial saccular aneurysms: a prospective consecutive study. *Br J Neurosurg* 1987, 1:33–46.

2. Sahs AL, Nibbelink DW, Torner JC: *Aneurysmal Subarachnoid Hemorrhage: Report of the Cooperative Study.* Philadelphia: Urban & Schwarzenberg; 1981.

3. Hunt WE, Hess RM: Surgical risk as related to time of intervention in the repair of intracranial aneurysms. *J Neurosurg* 1968, 28:14.

4. Drake CG: Report of World Federation of Neurological Surgeons Committee on a universal subarachnoid hemorrhage grading scale. *J Neurosurg* 1989, 68:985.

5. Alvord EC, Loeser JD, Bailey WL, *et al.*: Subarachnoid hemorrhage due to ruptured aneurysms: a simple method of estimating prognosis. *Acta Neurol* 1972, 27:273–284.

6. • Deruty R, Mottolese C, Pelissou-Guyotat I, *et al.*: Management of the ruptured intracranial aneurysm: early surgery, late surgery, or modulated surgery? *Acta Neurochir (Wien)* 1991, 113:1–10.

A total of 468 SAH patients were analyzed. After instituting a policy of selected early surgery, overall management results improved and mortality decreased. The study included poor-grade patients less than 50 years of age.

7. •• Säveland H, Hillman J, Brandt L, *et al.*: Overall outcome in aneurysmal subarachnoid hemorrhage. *J Neurosurg* 1992, 76:729–734.

A management protocol of early surgery and aggressive anti-ischemia therapy was used in 270 patients; 81% made a good recovery, and only 5.5% suffered delayed ischemic deficit. Poor outcome was associated with poor admission grade and the presence of an intracranial hemorrhage.

8. • Solomon RA, Onesti ST, Klebanoff L: Relationship between the timing of aneurysm surgery and the development of delayed cerebral ischemia. *J Neurosurg* 1991, 75:56–61.

In 145 patients with SAH undergoing surgery followed by prophylactic postoperative volume expansion, the incidence of cerebral infarction or poor outcome was not affected by the timing of surgery.

9. • Taylor B, Harries P, Bullock R: Factors affecting outcome after surgery for intracranial aneurysm in Glasgow. *Br J Neurosurg* 1991, 5:591–600.

Poor outcome in 295 SAH patients was correlated with poor admission clinical grade, intracranial hematoma, or delayed ischemic deficit. Early surgery, especially in good-grade patients, was associated with improved outcome. Two thirds of patients who developed ischemic deficits made a good recovery by using hypervolemia and calcium channel blockers.

10. Pakarinen S: Incidence, etiology and prognosis of primary subarachnoid hemorrhage: a study based on 589 cases diagnosed in a defined population during a defined period. *Acta Neurol Scand* 1967, 43(suppl 29):1–128.

11. Bailes JE, Spetzler RS, Hadley MN, *et al.*: Management morbidity and mortality of poor grade aneurysm patients. *J Neurosurg* 1990, 72:559–596.

12. Hayashi M, Marukawa S, Fujii H, *et al.*: Intracranial hypertension in patients with ruptured intracranial aneurysms. *J Neurosurg* 1978, 46:584–590.

13. Voldby B, Enevoldsen EM: Intracranial pressure changes following aneurysm rupture. Part 1: clinical and angiographic correlations. *J Neurosurg* 1982, 56:186–196.

14. •• Auer LM: Unfavorable outcome following early surgical repair of ruptured cerebral aneurysms: a critical review of 238 patients. *Surg Neurol* 1991, 35:152–158.

Two hundred patients underwent early surgical repair of ruptured cerebral aneuryms; poor outcome occurred in 25% and was most often related to the effects of the initial hemorrhage, poor clinical grade, and intracranial hematoma. Delayed ischemic deficit occurred in only one patient. The use of nimodipine was thought to attenuate the effects of vasospasm.

15. Heiskanen O, Poranen A, Kuurne T, *et al.*: Acute surgery for intracerebral hematomas caused by rupture of an intracranial arterial aneurysm: a prospective randomized study. *Acta Neurochir (Wien)* 1988, 90:81–83.

16. Pasqualin A, Bazzan A, Cavazzani P, *et al.*: Intracranial hematomas following aneurysmal rupture: experience with 309 cases. *Surg Neurol* 1986, 25:6–17.

17. Wheellock B, Weir B, Watts R, *et al.*: Timing of surgery for intracerebral hematomas due to aneurysm rupture. *J Neurosurg* 1983, 58:476–481.

18. Winn HR, Newell DW, Mayberg MR, *et al.*: Early surgical management of poor grade patients with intracranial aneurysms. *Clin Neurosurg* 1990, 36:289–298.

19. Black P: Hydrocephalus and vasospasm after subarachnoid hemorrhage from ruptured intracranial aneurysms. *Neurosurgery* 1986, 18:12–16.

20. Graff-Redford MR, Torner JC, Adams HP, *et al.*: Factors associated with hydrocephalus after subarachnoid hemorrhage: a report of the cooperative aneurysm study. *Acta Neurol* 1989, 46:744–752.

21. •• Hasan D, Tanghe HLJ: Distribution of cisternal blood in patients with acute hydrocephalus after subarachnoid hemorrhage. *Ann Neurol* 1992, 31:374–378.

Hydrocephalus after SAH is associated with intraventricular hemorrhage or the presence of large amounts of blood in the ambient cisterns.

22. Mohr G, Ferguson G, Khan M, *et al.*: Intraventricular hemorrhage from ruptured aneurysm: retrospective analysis of 91 cases. *J Neurosurg* 1983, 58:482–487.

23. • Rajshekhar V, Harbaugh RE: Results of routine ventriculostomy with external ventricular drainage for acute hydrocephalus following subarachnoid haemorrhage. *Acta Neurochir (Wien)* 1992, 115:8–14.

Hydrocephalus occurred in 27% of 194 patients with SAH and was treated with ventriculostomy drainage. Fifty percent showed definite clinical improvement within 24 hours.

24. Yasargil MG: *Microneurosurgery.* Stuttgart: Georg Thieme Verlag; 1984.

25. • Kamiya K, Inagawa T, Yamamoto M, *et al.*: Subdural hematoma due to ruptured intracranial aneurysm. *Neurol Med Chir (Tokyo)* 1991, 31:82–86.

Subdural hematoma were observed in 15 of 484 cases of aneurysmal rupture, commonly middle cerebral artery or anterior cerebral artery aneurysms. Five of seven patients undergoing surgery made a good recovery.

26. Crompton MR: Cerebral infarction following the rupture of cerebral berry aneurysms. *Brain* 1964, 87:263–279.

27. Graham DF, MacPherson F, Pitts LH: Correlation between angiographic vasospasm, hematoma and ischemic brain damage following SAH. *J Neurosurg* 1983, 59:223–230.

28. Brouwers PJAM, Wijdicks EFM, Van Gijn J: Infarction after aneurysm rupture does not depend on distribution of clearance rate of blood. *Stroke* 1990, 23:374–379.

29. Adams HP, Kassell NF, Torner JC: Predicting cerebral ischemia after aneurysmal subarachnoid hemorrhage: influences of clinical condition CT and antifibrinolytic therapy. *Neurology* 1987, 37:1586–1591.

30. Jakubowski J, Bell BA, Symon L, *et al.*: A primate model of subarachnoid hemorrhage: change in regional cerebral blood flow, autoregulation, carbon dioxide reactivity and central conduction time. *Stroke* 1982, 13:601–611.

31. Nornes H, Magnas B: Intracranial pressure in patients with ruptured intracranial aneurysm. *J Neurosurg* 1972, 36:537–547.

32. • Brinker T, Seifert V, Dietz H: Cerebral blood flow and intracranial pressure during experimental subarachnoid haemorrhage. *Acta Neurochir (Wien)* 1992, 115:47–52.

Intracranial pressure increases acutely after experimental SAH in cats and temporarily arrests cerebral circulation. The Cushing response does not improve cerebral circulation.

33. •• Fazl M, Houlden DA, Weaver K: Correlation between cerebral blood flow, somatosensory evoked potentials, CT scan grade, and neurologic grade in patients with subarachnoid hemorrhage. *Can J Neurol Sci* 1991, 18:453–457.

Cerebral blood flow (xenon inhalation) is lowest in poor-grade aneurysm patients. Central conduction time (SSEP) correlates only with a cerebral blood flow that is less than 30 mL/100 g/min and is unable to detect marginal ischemia.

34. Fisher CM, Kistler JP, Davis JM: Relation of cerebral vasospasm to subarachnoid hemorrhage visualized by computerized tomographic scanning. *Neurosurgery* 1990, 6:1–9.

35. • Mountz JM, McGillicuddy JE, Wilson MW, *et al.*: Pre- and postoperative cerebral blood flow changes in subarachnoid haemorrhage. *Acta Neurochir (Wien)* 1991, 109:30–33.

Cerebral blood flow (portable xenon inhalation) is higher in good-grade SAH patients (44.2 ± 0.71) than in poor-grade patients (34.1 ± 1.7). After surgery, there is improvement in cerebral blood flow in good-grade but not poor-grade patients.

36. •• Carpenter DA, Grubb RL Jr, Tempel LW, *et al.*: Cerebral oxygen metabolism after aneurysmal subarachnoid hemorrhage. *J Cereb Blood Flow Metab* 1991, 11:837–844.

Positron emission tomography measurements in 11 patients with aneurysmal SAH indicated that the initial rupture produced a primary reduction in cerebral metabolic rate of oxygen and that vasospasm contributed to secondary ischemia.

37. Grubb RL, Raichle ME, Eichling JO, *et al.*: Effects of subarachnoid hemorrhage on cerebral blood volume, blood flow and oxygen utilization in humans. *J Neurosurg* 1977, 44:446–452.

38. Dernbach PD, Little JR, Jones SC, *et al.*: Altered cerebral autoregulation and CO_2 reactivity after aneurysmal subarachnoid hemorrhage. *Neurosurgery* 1988, 22:822–826.

39. Tenjin H, Hirakawa K, Mizukawa N, *et al.*: Dysautoregulation in patients with ruptured aneurysms: cerebral blood flow measurements obtained during surgery by a temperature- controlled thermoelectrical method. *Neurosurgery* 1988, 23:705–709.

40. Voldby B, Enevoldsen EM, Jensen FT: Cerebrovascular reactivity in patients with ruptured intracranial aneurysms. *J Neurosurg* 1985, 62:59–67.

41. • Klingelhöfer J, Sander D: Doppler CO_2 test as an indicator of cerebral vasoreactivity and prognosis in severe intracranial hemorrhages. *Stroke* 1992, 23:962–966.

A significantly reduced carbon dioxide reactivity, particularly in those with increased intracranial pressure, was seen in patients with SAH. Low carbon dioxide reactivity ($0.8 \pm 0.3\%$) indicated a poor outcome.

42. • Shinoda J, Kimura T, Funakoshi T, *et al.*: Acetazolamide reactivity on cerebral blood flow in patients with subarachnoid haemorrhage. *Acta Neurochir (Wien)* 1991, 109:102–108.

Acetazolamide-activated SPECT is a means of evaluating cerebral vasodilatory capacity. Decreased reserve is seen in all poor-grade SAH patients.

43. • Handa Y, Hayashi M, Takeuchi H, *et al.*: Time course of the impairment of cerebral autoregulation during chronic cerebral vasospasm after subarachnoid hemorrhage in primates. *J Neurosurg* 1992, 76:493–501.

Cerebral autoregulation is impaired in experimental primate SAH. The lower limit of autoregulation recovers during the remitting phase of vasospasm.

44. •• Vollmer DG, Takayasu M, Dacey R: An *in vitro* comparative study of conducting vessels and penetrating arterioles after experimental subarachnoid hemorrhage in the rabbit. *J Neurosurg* 1992, 77:113–119.

In vitro SAH produced increased basilar artery contraction and attenuated relaxation. Intracerebral resistance vessels of the microcirculation were not similarly affected.

45. • Nakao N, Itakura T, Uematsu Y, *et al.*: A possible involvement of central atrial natriuretic peptide in cerebral cortical microcirculation. *Neurosurgery* 1992, 30:236–240.

The administration of atrial natriuretic factor produced a dose-dependent reduction in cerebral blood flow assessed by cortical laser Doppler in rats.

46. Rossenwasser RH, Delgado TE, Bucheit WA, *et al.*: Control of hypertension and prophylaxis against vasospasm in cases of subarachnoid hemorrhage. *Neurosurgery* 1983, 12:658–661.

47. •• Nelson RJ, Roberts J, Rubin C, *et al.*: Association of hypovolemia after subarachnoid hemorrhage with computed tomographic scan evidence of raised intracranial pressure. *Neurosurgery* 1991, 29:178–182.

Plasma volume was measured in 15 patients within 96 hours of SAH. Those with CT evidence of increased intracranial pressure were at particular risk for systemic hypovolemia.

48. Solomon RA, Post KD, McMurtry JG III: Depression of circulating blood volume in patients after subarachnoid hemorrhage: implications for the management of symptomatic vasospasm. *Neurosurgery* 1984, 15:354–361.

49. Wijdicks EFM, Vermeulen M, Hijdra A, *et al.*: Hyponatremia and cerebral infarction in patients with ruptured intracranial aneurysms: is fluid restriction harmful? *Ann Neurol* 1985, 17:137–140.

50. • Diringer MN, Lim JS, Kirsch JR, *et al.*: Suprasellar and intraventricular blood predict elevated plasma atrial natriuretic factor in subarachnoid hemorrhage. *Stroke* 1991, 22:577–581.

Atrial natriuretic factor concentration was measured in 26 patients with SAH and found to be higher in patients with intraventricular or suprasellar blood. A relationship between atrial natriuretic factor and sodium concentration was not found.

51. •• Wijdicks EFM, Ropper AH, Hunnicutt EJ, *et al.*: Atrial natriuretic factor and salt wasting after aneurysmal subarachnoid hemorrhage. *Stroke* 1991, 22:1519–1524.

Diurnal, plasma atrial natriuretic factor levels were measured for 5 days in 14 patients with SAH. An increased atrial natriuretic factor level was found to precede natriuresis and volume depletion. Patients with natriuresis were at increased risk for delayed cerebral infarction.

52. • Nelson RJ, Perry S, Burns ACR, *et al.*: The effects of hyponatremia and subarachnoid haemorrhage on the cerebral vasomotor responses of the rabbit. *J Cereb Blood Flow Metab* 1991, 11:661–666.

In rabbits, hyponatremia and SAH impaired cerebral blood flow autoregulation. The combined effects are not additive.

53. Brouwers PJAM, Wijdicks EFM, Hasan D, *et al.*: Serial electrocardiographic recording in aneurysmal subarachnoid hemorrhage. *Stroke* 1989, 20:1162–1167.

54. •• Davies KR, Gelb AW, Manninen PH, *et al.*: Cardiac function in aneurysmal subarachnoid haemorrhage: a study of electrocardiographic and echocardiographic abnormalities. *Br J Anaesth* 1991, 67:58–63.

Electrocardiographic changes are evident in half the patients with cerebral aneurysms but do not accurately predict myocardial function. Myocardial dysfunction is more closely related to the severity of SAH.

55. Marion DW, Segal R, Thompson ME: Subarachnoid hemorrhage and the heart. *Neurosurgery* 1986, 18:101.

56. Weir BKA: Pulmonary edema following fatal aneurysm rupture. *J Neurosurg* 1978, 49:502–507.

57. •• Adams HP Jr, Kassell NF, Boarini DJ, *et al.*: Clinical spectrum of aneurysmal subarachnoid hemorrhage. *J Stroke Cerebrovasc Dis* 1991, 1:3–8.

Among 268 patients with SAH, 40.5% had a classic clinical presentation. Sixty-eight had altered consciousness, but only 15% presented with coma. Nuchal rigidity (59%) was the most common clinical finding. A delay in diagnosis occurred in 56 patients (19%).

58. • Ramirez-Lassepas M, Ahmed A: Cardiorespiratory arrest in aneurysmal subarachnoid hemorrhage. *J Stroke Cerebrovasc Dis* 1991, 1:49–56.

Retrospective review of 95 patients with SAH. Fifteen presented with cardiorespiratory arrest. Risk factors included female sex, posterior circulation aneurysm, intraventricular hemorrhage, or intracranial hematoma. One patient survived hospitalization.

59. Newell DW, Le Roux PD, Dacey RG, *et al.*: CT infusion scanning for the detection of cerebral aneurysms. *J Neurosurg* 1989, 71:175–179.

60. Juvela S: Rebleeding from ruptured intracranial aneurysm. *Surg Neurol* 1989, 32:323–326.

61. Kassell NF, Torner JC: Aneurysmal rebleeding: a prelimi-

nary report from the cooperative aneurysm study. *Neurosurgery* 1983, 13:479.

62. Inagawa T, Kamiya K, Ogasawara H, *et al.*: Rebleeding of ruptured intracranial aneurysms in the acute stage. *Surg Neurol* 1987, 28:93–99.

63. Torner JC, Kassell NF, Wallace RB, *et al.*: Preoperative prognostic factors for rebleeding and survival in aneurysm patients: report of the Cooperative Study. *Neurosurgery* 1981, 9:506–511.

64. Voldby B, Enevoldsen E: Intracranial pressure changes during aneurysm rupture: recurrent hemorrhages. *J Neurosurg* 1982, 56:784–789.

65. Kassell NF, Torner JC, Haley EC, *et al.*: The International Cooperative Study on the timing of aneurysm surgery. *J Neurosurg* 1990, 73:18–46.

66. •• Haley EC Jr, Kassell NF, Torner JC, *et al.*: International Cooperative Study on the Timing of Aneurysm Surgery: the North American experience. *Stroke* 1992, 23:205–214.

A total of 772 patients admitted within 3 days of SAH were treated in 27 North American centers as part of the International Cooperative Study. Patients undergoing early surgery (<72 hours) had significantly improved rates of good recovery than those undergoing late surgery (70.9% versus 61.7%).

67. •• Findlay JM, Macdonald L, Weir BKA, *et al.*: Surgical manipulation of primate cerebral arteries in established vasospasm. *J Neurosurg* 1991, 75:425–432.

Established vasospasm in a primate model of SAH was not aggravated by surgical manipulation. The surgical risk to patients with documented vasospasm may be secondary to hypotension, hypoxia, or brain retraction.

68. Lam AM, Nicholas JF, Manninen PH: Influence of succinylcholine in lumbar cerebral spinal pressure in man. *Anesth Analg* 1984, 63:240.

69. Cote CJ, Greenhow E, Marshall BE: The hypotensive response to rapid intravenous administration of hypertonic solutions in man and rabbit. *Anesthesiology* 1979, 50:30.

70. Ravussin P, Archer DP, Meyer E, *et al.*: The effect of rapid infusion of saline and mannitol on cerebral blood volume and intracranial pressure in dogs. *Can Anaesth Soc J* 1985, 32:506–515.

71. Sullivan HG, Kennan RL, Isrow L: The critical importance of $PaCO_2$ during intracranial aneurysm surgery. *J Neurosurg* 1980, 52:426–432.

72. •• Giannotti SL, Oppenheimer JH, Levy ML, *et al.*: Management of intraoperative rupture of aneurysm without hypotension. *Neurosurgery* 1991, 28:531–536.

During 276 surgical procedures, aneurysm rupture occurred 41 times. Hypotension did not protect against rupture and was associated with a worse outcome than when tamponade alone was used to control bleeding.

73. • Bailes JE, Deeb ZL, Wilson JA, *et al.*: Intraoperative angiography and temporary balloon occlusion of the basilar artery as an adjunct to surgical clipping: technical note. *Neurosurgery* 1992, 30:949–953.

Four patients underwent combined interventional neuroradiologic and surgical techniques to clip basilar aneurysms. Proximal control was achieved with a nondetachable endovascular balloon, and intraoperative angiography was used to confirm aneurysm obliteration and vessel patency.

74. Busto R, Dietrich WD, Globus M-T: The importance of brain temperature in cerebral ischemic injury. *Stroke* 1989, 20:1113.

75. Minamisawa H, Nordstrom C-H, Smith M-L: The influence of mild body and brain hypothermia on ischemic brain damage. *J Cereb Blood Flow Metab* 1990, 10:365.

76. • Meyer FB, Muzzi DA: Cerebral protection during aneurysm surgery with isoflurane anesthesia. *J Neurosurg* 1992, 76:541– 543.

The combination of high-concentration isoflurane, temporary vessel occlusion, and maintenance of normal blood pressure was found to be protective in six patients undergoing aneurysm surgery.

77. •• Watson JC, Drummond JC, Patel PM, *et al.*: An assessment of the cerebral protective effects of etomidate in a model of incomplete forebrain ischemia in the rat. *Neurosurgery* 1992, 30:540–544.

The protective effects of etomidate were most marked in CA1 and CA3 in the hippocampus of rats undergoing incomplete forebrain ischemia. The results suggest that the protective effect of etomidate is best in tissue in which cerebral blood flow reduction is of intermediate severity.

78. •• Friedman WA, Chadwick GM, Verhoeven FJS, *et al.*: Monitoring of somatosensory evoked potentials during surgery for middle cerebral artery aneurysms. *Neurosurgery* 1991, 29:83–88.

Patients undergoing middle cerebral artery aneurysm surgery who demonstrate reversible SSEP changes after clip readjustment, removal of temporary clips, or induction of hypertension are less likely to suffer postoperative neurologic deficits.

79. • Mizoi K, Yoshimoto T: Intraoperative monitoring of the somatosensory evoked potentials and cerebral blood flow during aneurysm surgery. *Neurol Med Chir (Tokyo)* 1991, 31:318–325.

Somatosensory evoked potential monitoring was useful in detecting ischemia after middle cerebral artery occlusion but not internal carotid artery or anterior cerebral artery occlusion. Rapid disappearance of N_{20} signal was the strongest predictor of ischemia.

80. • Ogawa A, Sato H, Sakurai Y, *et al.*: Limitation of temporary vascular occlusion during aneurysm surgery. *Surg Neurol* 1991, 36:453–457.

Temporary clips were used in 39 cases of ruptured cerebral aneurysm. Permanent neurologic deficits occurred in two and transient deficits in four patients. Prolonged occlusion, even if the residual flow was relatively high, internal carotid artery occlusion or trapping increased the risk of ischemic defects. Occlusion times of less than 10 minutes are recommended.

81. • Paré L, Delfino R, Leblanc R: The relationship of ventricular drainage to aneurysmal rebleeding. *J Neurosurg* 1992, 76:422–427.

Among 128 patients suffering SAH, 15 rebled. The rate of rerupture was significantly higher in poor-grade patients or those who underwent ventricular drainage, particularly if there was hydrocephalus.

82. • Hasan D, Lindsay KW, Vermeulen M: Treatment of acute hydrocephalus after subarachnoid hemorrhage with serial lumbar puncture. *Stroke* 1991, 22:190–194.

Seventeen patients who developed acute hydrocephalus after SAH underwent serial lumbar punctures. Rebleeding was not precipitated. Clinical improvement was observed in 12 patients, and only four required an internal shunt. Overall outcome, however, was not improved.

83. • Ram Z, Sahar A, Hadani M: Vasospasm due to massive subarachnoid haemorrhage: a rat model. *Acta Neurochir (Wien)* 1991, 110:181–184.

In the rat, the amount of SAH predicts the severity of cerebral vasospasm.

84. •• Macdonald RL, Weir BKA, Runzer TD, *et al.*: Etiology of cerebral vasospasm in primates. *J Neurosurg* 1991, 75:415–424.

Significant vasospasm occurred in primates who received intrathecal oxyhemoglobin or red blood cell supernatant. Animals who received methemoglobin or bilirubin demonstrated little evidence of vasospasm.

85. •• Macdonald RL, Weir BKA, Young JD, *et al.*: Cytoskeletal and extracellular matrix proteins in cerebral arteries following subarachnoid hemorrhage in monkeys. *J Neurosurg* 1992, 76:81–90.

Apart from fibronectin, there was no significant increase of extracellular matrix or cytoskeletal elements, identified immunohistochemically in cerebral arteries in primate SAH. Collagen deposition, therefore, may not significantly contribute to lumen narrowing observed in vasospasm.

86. •• Suzuki R, Masaoka H, Hirata Y, *et al.*: The role of endothelin-1 in the origin of cerebral vasospasm in patients with aneurysmal subarachnoid hemorrhage. *J Neurosurg* 1992, 77:96–100.

Levels of cerebrospinal fluid and plasma ET-I (an endothelium-derived vasoconstrictor) were significantly higher in patients who developed vasospasm after SAH.

87. •• Edwards DH, Byrne JV, Griffith TM: The effect of chronic subarachnoid hemorrhage on basal endothelium-derived relaxing factor activity in intrathecal cerebral arteries. *J Neurosurg* 1992, 76:830–837.

In vitro denudation of endothelium; inhibition of nitric oxide synthetase, adventitial application of hemoglobin, and prolonged *in vivo* exposure of pig cerebral vessels to hemoglobin decreased endothelium-derived relaxing factor activity. Loss of endothelium-derived relaxing factor activity may contribute to cerebral vasospasm.

88. •• Minami N, Tani E, Maeda Y, *et al.*: Effects of inhibitors of protein kinase C and calpain in experimental delayed cerebral vasospasm. *J Neurosurg* 1992, 76:111–118.

Calcium modulation of protein kinases may underlie smooth muscle contraction in cerebral vasospasm. The use of protein kinase inhibitors can attenuate vessel spasm in primates.

89. •• Takanashi Y, Weir BKA, Vollrath B, *et al.*: Time course of changes in concentration of intracellular free calcium in cultured cerebrovascular smooth muscle cells exposed to oxyhemoglobin. *Neurosurgery* 1992, 30:346–350.

When exposed to oxyhemoglobin *in vitro*, smooth muscle cells derived from monkey middle cerebral artery demonstrated increased intracellular calcium, vasoconstriction, and phospholipase activation. Membrane disruption results.

90. • Macdonald RL, Weir BKA, Runzer TD, *et al.*: Effect of intrathecal superoxide dismutase and catalase on oxyhemoglobin-induced vasospasm in monkeys. *Neurosurgery* 1992, 30:529–539

In the primate, intrathecal superoxide dismutase and catalase do not prevent oxyhemoglobin-induced vasospasm.

91. • Ram Z, Sadeh M, Shacked I, *et al.*: Magnesium sulfate reverses experimental delayed cerebral vasospasm after subarachnoid hemorrhage in rats. *Stroke* 1991, 22:922–927.

In a rat model of SAH, intracisternal injection of magnesium sulfate caused dramatic dilatation of the basilar artery. Intravenous administration dilated the vessel to 75% of its baseline diameter.

92. • O'Neill P, Walton S, Foy PM, *et al.*: Role of prostaglandins in delayed cerebral ischemia after subarachnoid hemorrhage. *Neurosurgery* 1992, 30:17–22.

In patients suffering SAH, no significant correlation was found between the level of plasma or cerebrospinal fluid prostaglandins (prostaglandin E_2, prostaglandin $F_{2\alpha}$, and thromboxane B_2) and admission clinical grade; amount of CT subarachnoid blood; vasospasm; delayed ischemic deficits; or outcome.

93. • Yamamoto H, Kikuchi H, Sato M, *et al.*: Therapeutic trial of cerebral vasospasm with the serine protease inhibitor, FUT-175, administered in the acute stage after subarachnoid hemorrhage. *Neurosurgery* 1992, 30:358–363.

The incidence of delayed ischemic deficits after SAH decreased from 55% in control patients to 13% in patients treated with a synthetic serine protease inhibitor (FUT-175).

94. • Aydin IH, Önder A: The effect of very early cisternal irrigation on basilar artery spasm after SAH in the rat model. *Acta Neurochir (Wien)* 1991, 113:69–73.

Saline irrigation within 15 minutes of experimental SAH in rats prevented vasospasm.

95. •• Findlay JM, Weir BKA, Kassell NF, *et al.*: Intracisternal recombinant tissue plasminogen activator after aneurysmal SAH. *J Neurosurg* 1991, 75:181–188.

Fourteen of 15 patients who received cisternal tissue plasminogen activator, within 48 hours of severe SAH, demonstrated partial or complete resolution of the clot on postoperative CT. The patient who did not demonstrate clot reduction was the only patient to develop symptomatic vasospasm.

96. •• Öhman J, Servo A, Heiskanen O: Effect of intrathecal fibrinolytic therapy on clot lysis and vasospasm in patients with aneurysmal subarachnoid hemorrhage. *J Neurosurg* 1991, 75:197–201.

The amount of blood observed on postoperative CT and severity of angiographic vasospasm was decreased, in a dose-dependent fashion, in 30 patients treated with tissue plasminogen activator after aneurysmal SAH.

97. • Zabramski JM, Spetzler RF, Lee KS, *et al.*: Phase I trial of tissue plasminogen activator for the prevention of vasospasm in patients with aneurysmal subarachnoid hemorrhage. *J Neurosurg* 1991, 75:189–196.

No systemic evidence of fibrinolysis occurred in 10 patients who received tissue plasminogen activator after SAH. Minor, local bleeding complications occurred in patients who received larger doses.

98. Petruk KC, West M, Mohr G, *et al.*: Nimodipine treatment in poor grade aneurysm patients: results of a multicenter double-blind placebo-controlled trial. *J Neurosurg* 1988, 68:505.

99. Pickard JD, Murray GD, Illingworth R, *et al.*: Effect of oral nimodipine on cerebral infarction and outcome after subarachnoid haemorrhage: British Aneurysm Nimodipine Trial. *BMJ* 1989, 298:636–642.

100. • Medlock MD, Dulebohn SC, Elwood PW: Prophylactic hypervolemia without calcium channel blockers in early aneurysm surgery. *Neurosurgery* 1992, 30:12–16.

Forty-seven patients received hypervolemia after SAH. A reduction in morbidity and mortality compared with historical controls was not evident. Calcium channel blockers were not used. The effect of hypervolemia and calcium channel blockers may be synergistic in ameliorating the effects of cerebral vasospasm.

101. •• Chew W, Kucharczyk J, Moseley M, et al.: Hyperglycemia augments ischemic brain injury: in vivo MR imaging/spectroscopic study with nicardipine in cats with occluded middle cerebral arteries. *AJNR* 1991, 12:603–609.

After middle cerebral artery occlusion in cats, hyperglycemia reduced high-energy phosphates, increased infarct size, and attenuated the protective effect provided by calcium channel blockers.

102. • Higashida RT, Halbach VV, Dowd CF, et al.: Intravascular balloon dilatation therapy for intracranial arterial vasospasm: patient selection, technique, and clinical results. *Neurosurg Rev* 1992, 15:89–95.

Transfemoral, microballoon angioplasty was performed in 99 cerebral vessels in 28 patients for vasospasm after SAH. Angiographic improvement was seen in all vessels and clinical improvement in 17 cases.

103. Newell DW, Eskridge JM, Mayberg MR, et al.: Angioplasty for the treatment of symptomatic vasospasm following subarachnoid hemorrhage. *Neurosurgery* 1989, 71:654.

104. • Yamamoto Y, Smith RR, Bernanke DH: Mechanism of action of balloon angioplasty in cerebral vasospasm. *Neurosurgery* 1992, 30:1–6.

Mechanical balloon dilatation of vasospastic cerebral arteries altered the normal collagen structure and disrupted connective tissue in the vessel wall.

105. • Newell DW, Eskridge JM, Lewis D, et al.: Transcranial Doppler usefulness in balloon angioplasty. In *Advances in Neurosonology.* Edited by Oka M, Von Reutern GM, Furuhata H, et al. New York: Elsevier Science Publishers; 1992:101–103.

Thirty-one patients underwent angioplasty for vasospasm after SAH. Transcranial Doppler velocities improved in all but one patient. The angioplastic effect was sustained and interrupted the pathogenic process.

106. • Robertson CS, Contant CF, Narayan RK, et al.: Cerebral blood flow, AVD0$_2$, and neurologic outcome in head-injured patients. *J Neurotrauma* 1992, 9(suppl):S349–S358.

Jugular venous oxygen desaturation occurred more commonly in patients with reduced cerebral blood flow and correlated with widened AVD0$_2$ and poor neurologic outcome.

107. •• Sheinberg M, Kanter MJ, Robertson CS, et al.: Continuous monitoring of jugular venous oxygen saturation in head-injured patients. *J Neurosurg* 1992, 76:212–217.

Episodes of jugular venous oxygen desaturation were commonly observed in severely head-injured patients, even when they received intensive care. Patients demonstrating oxygen desaturation had a high mortality.

108. •• Persson L, Hillered L: Chemical monitoring of neurosurgical intensive care patients using intracerebral microdialysis. *J Neurosurg* 1992, 76:72–80.

Intracerebral microdialysis was used in four patients. There was a 25-fold increase in excitatory amino acids, high lactate-to-pyruvate ratio and increased hypoxanthine, following cerebral ischemia or hypoxia.

109. • Dauch WA: Prediction of secondary deterioration in comatose neurosurgical patients by serial recording of multimodality evoked potentials. *Acta Neurochir (Wien)* 1991, 111:84–91.

Decreased amplitude, or disappearance of the primary cortical SSEP peak, precedes clinical deterioration in comatose patients.

110. • Meyerson BA, Gunasekera L, Linderoth B, et al.: Bedside monitoring of regional cortical blood flow in comatose patients using laser Doppler flowmetry. *Neurosurgery* 1991, 29:750–755.

Laser Doppler flowmetry may be used continuously in comatose patients to assess cortical microcirculation. Cerebral hemodynamics are accurately reflected.

111. • Davis SM, Andrews JT, Lichtenstein M, et al.: Correlations between cerebral arterial velocities, blood flow, and delayed ischemia after subarachnoid hemorrhage. *Stroke* 1992, 23:492–497.

In patients who did not develop delayed neurologic deficit after SAH, SPECT demonstrated normal cerebral blood flow even in the face of transcranial Doppler evidence of vasospasm. In patients who developed symptoms, SPECT identified hypoperfusion concordant with transcranial Doppler velocities.

112. •• Grosset DG, Straiton J, du Trevou M, et al.: Prediction of symptomatic vasospasm after subarachnoid hemorrhage by rapidly increasing transcranial Doppler velocity and cerebral blood flow changes. *Stroke* 1992, 23:674–679.

Peak blood flow velocity, middle carotid artery-to-internal carotid artery ratio, and maximal velocity increase over 24 hours were all increased in patients demonstrating symptomatic vasospasm after SAH. Regional hypoperfusion, identified by SPECT imaging, correlated with transcranial Doppler velocities.

113. • Lewis DH, Hsu S, Eskridge J, et al.: Brain SPECT and transcranial Doppler ultrasound in vasospasm-induced delayed cerebral ischemia after subarachnoid hemorrhage. *J Stroke Cerebrovasc Dis* 1992, 2:12–21.

Brain SPECT can evaluate the effects of vasospasm on cerebral blood flow and supplements transcranial Doppler in the diagnosis of clinical vasospasm. SPECT, transcranial Doppler, and frequent neurologic examination should be used in combination for optimal, noninvasive diagnosis of vasospasm.

114. • Becker G, Greiner K, Kaune B, et al.: Diagnosis and monitoring of subarachnoid hemorrhage by transcranial color-coded real-time sonography. *Neurosurgery* 1991, 28:814–820.

Transcranial color-coded Doppler provided a dynamic complement to the fine structural resolution of other imaging modalities in diagnosing SAH, aneurysms, and vasospasm.

115. • Fukui MB, Johnson DW, Yonas H, et al.: Xe/CT cerebral blood flow evaluation of delayed symptomatic cerebral ischemia after subarachnoid hemorrhage. *AJNR* 1992, 13:265–270.

Xenon-CT cerebral blood flow studies can identify patients at risk for cerebral infarction following SAH.

116. • Rivierez M, Landau-Ferey J, Grob R, et al.: Value of electroencephalogram in prediction and diagnosis of vasospasm after intracranial aneurysm rupture. *Acta Neurochir (Wien)* 1991, 110:17–23.

Electroencephalographic abnormalities can be both predictive and diagnostic of cerebral ischemia following vasospasm. The degree of arterial narrowing correlates with the electroencephalographic abnormalities.

117. Ljunggren B, Säveland H, Brandt L: Causes of unfavorable outcome after early aneurysm operation. *Neurosurgery* 1983, 13:629–633.

118. • Le Roux PS, Dailey A, Newell DW, *et al.*: Emergent aneurysm clipping without angiography in the moribund patient with intracerebral hemorrhage: the use of CT infusion scans. *Neurosurgery* 1993.

Twenty-five moribund, grade V patients underwent craniotomy for aneurysmal intracranial hemorrhage based on CT infusion scan alone. Eight are independent at follow-up.

119. • Spencer MP: Detection of cerebral arterial emboli.: In *Transcranial Doppler*. Edited by Newell DW, Aaslid R. New York: Raven Press; 1992: 215–230.

120. Adams Jr HP, Kassell NF, Torner JC, *et al.*: Early management of aneurysmal subarachnoid hemorrhage: a report of the Cooperative Aneurysm Study. *J Neurosurg* 1981, 54:141–145.

121. Ljunggren B, Säveland H, Brandt L, *et al.*: Aneurysmal subarachnoid hemorrhage: total annual outcome in a 1.46 million population. *Surg Neurol* 1984, 22:435–438.

122. Hijdra A, Braakman R, van Gijn J, *et al.*: Aneurysmal subarachnoid hemorrhage: complications and outcome in a hospital population. *Stroke* 1987, 18:1061–1067.

123. Chyatte D, Fode NC, Sundt Jr TM: Early versus late intracranial aneurysm surgery in subarachnoid hemorrhage. *J Neurosurg* 1988, 69:326–331.

124. Inagawa T, Takahashi M, Aoki H, *et al.*: Aneurysmal subarachnoid hemorrhage in Izumo City and Shimane Prefecture of Japan: outcome. *Stroke* 1988, 19:176–180.

125. Auer LM, Schneider GH, Auer T: Computerized tomography and prognosis in early aneurysm surgery. *J Neurosurg* 1986, 65:217–221.

126. Seiler RR, Newell DW: Subarachnoid hemorrhage and vasospasm. In *Transcranial Doppler*. Edited by Newell DW, Aaslid R. New York: Raven Press; 1992: 101–107.

Chapter 11

Radiosurgery for Arteriovenous Malformations

William A. Friedman
Frank J. Bova

Lars Leksell [1,2], in 1951, coined the term *radiosurgery* to describe his method of stereotactically directing multiple 200 kV x-ray beams toward a common intracranial target. The radiation source was subsequently replaced with proton beams from a synchrocyclotron. During the same time period (1950s), groups at Berkeley and in Boston also began research on the use of proton beams for this purpose [3,4]. In 1980, the Berkeley group began to use helium ion beams for radiosurgical treatments. Proton and helium beams have a physical property, called the *Bragg peak* effect, in which the majority of their energy is deposited at a predictable depth in tissue. This property has obvious theoretical advantages. Unfortunately, a cyclotron is necessary for the production of such particle beams. The expense involved (>$20 million) and physical limitations in the actual application of the particle beam to brain lesions have limited the availability and practical application of this radiosurgical modality.

In 1968, Leksell's group began to use the device known as the *gamma knife*. The first unit used 179 cobalt sources to provide finely collimated radiation beams, all directed toward a common focal point. The spontaneous decay of cobalt creates photon radiation, called *gamma rays*. This unit was originally intended as a functional neurosurgical tool to create very small elliptical lesions in the brain. Subsequently, the gamma unit was redesigned to include 201 cobalt sources, with circular collimators, such that spherical lesions, more appropriate for treating anatomic brain problems (*ie*, arteriovenous malformations, tumors), could be created. Multiple gamma units have been installed, mainly during the last 5 years, and mainly in the United States and Japan.

Most recently (1980s), multiple groups have developed radiosurgery units using conventional linear accelerators (LINACs) as the radiation source [5–8]. The LINAC is a device, long used in conventional radiation therapy, which produces high-energy photons, called *x-rays*, by accelerating electrons to nearly the speed of light and colliding them with a heavy metal. These x-rays are virtually equivalent in energy and character to the photons produced in the gamma unit by the spontaneous decay of cobalt. Neither x-rays nor gamma rays have the Bragg peak associated with particle beams (protons, helium nuclei). LINAC radiosurgery systems rely on a treatment paradigm wherein multiple noncoplanar arcs of radiation are focused on one spot within the brain. The large number of radiation pathways through normal brain result in minimal dose to the normal brain, with a tremendous concentration of radiation at the target.

A large number of pathologic entities have been treated with radiosurgery, including acoustic schwannomas, meningiomas, metastatic tumors, gliomas, craniopharyngiomas, and pituitary tumors. It is safe to say, however, that the treatment of deep-seated arteriovenous malformations is the single most solidly established indication for radiosurgery. A large amount of long-term follow-up data concerning efficacy and complications is available on this topic.

In this chapter, we describe the radiosurgical technique used at the University of Florida as a detailed example of a common radiosurgical methodology. We then review our results and discuss all other reports in the literature.

ARTERIOVENOUS MALFORMATION RADIOSURGERY AT THE UNIVERSITY OF FLORIDA

In 1985, the Departments of Neurosurgery and Radiation Oncology decided to institute radiosurgery at the University of Florida. After reviewing the other existing radiosurgical options, it was decided to develop a new, LINAC-based radiosurgical system [7–10]. Our goal was to build a system with the following design criteria: highest possible accuracy, state-of-the-art computer hardware and software for dose planning, and a large number of collimators, such that any lesion between 5 and 35 mm in diameter could be treated with a homogeneous field of radiation. A team that included neurosurgeons, radiation physicists, and computer programmers engaged in a 2-year research, development, and testing process.

Radiosurgical treatment system

The University of Florida radiosurgical system has been described in detail in several publications [7–11]. Briefly meeting the first goal of our program, to provide the highest possible accuracy of radiation beam delivery, required a mechanical system independent of the relatively inaccurate (1 to 2 mm) LINAC gantry and patient support systems (Figure 11.1). The motions that required precise control were the arcing movements of the LINAC and the movements of the patient during repositioning for new arcs. To solve this problem, high-precision bearings were assembled in house. One bearing controls the isocentric accuracy of the collimator. A second bearing controls the rotation of the patient. These two bearing systems are coupled mechanically so the rotational axes coincide. However, this system alone cannot produce the desired accuracy if rigidly attached to the LINAC head. To avoid any torque transfer from the LINAC head to the collimator, a gimbal-type bearing, with a sliding collimator mount, was developed. This allows the collimator to tilt and slide by minute increments, so it remains in precise alignment with the isocenter defined by the mechanical bearing system without being dragged off by the "sagging" LINAC gantry. In addition, all standard stereotactic pieces were remachined to provide the accuracy desired for radiosurgery. The accuracy of radiation beam delivery in this system is 0.2±0.1 mm, which is as high as that reported for any other radiosurgical device [7,8].

The second design goal was to use state-of-the-art computer hardware and software for dose planning. Because every lesion is different in location, size, shape, and so on, every dose plan must be modified to optimize the treatment. An accurate and rapid dose planning system is, therefore, essential. We currently use a SUN 4/280 (SUN Microsystem, Inc., Mountain View, CA), with an 80-megaflop array processor. The general approach is to create and evaluate a three-dimensional treatment plan through the use of interpolated, reformatted computed tomographic (CT) images, a database with which neurosurgeons are quite familiar.

The third design goal was to provide a sufficiently large number of collimators, such that any lesion between 5 and 35 mm in diameter could be treated with a homogeneous field of radiation. Although its value in radiosurgery is debated currently, target dose homogeneity has been a primary goal in radiation treatment planning for decades. Accordingly, a series of cerrobend collimators was constructed, 15 cm in length and ranging in diameter from 5 to 35 mm (by 2-mm increments). Single beam profiles were obtained for each collimator, using standard dosimetric techniques.

Radiosurgical treatment paradigm

With the exception of the first few cases, all of our radiosurgery has been performed on an outpatient basis. The patient reports to the neurosurgical clinic at 8:15 AM. There a stereotactic head ring is applied with the patient under local anesthesia. No skin shaving or preparation is required. The patient is transported to the angiography suite, where a stereotactic angiogram is performed. Subsequently, stereotactic CT scanning is performed. A bolus of intravenous contrast material is given just before imaging through the lesion to maximize resolution. Because the stereotactic angiogram is a relatively poor three-dimensional database [12,13••,14], we also rely on the appearance of the nidus on contrast-enhanced CT scans for treatment planning. After CT scanning, the patient is transported to the outpatient radiology area for postangiographic observation.

The stereotactic angiogram and the stereotactic CT scan (now on magnetic tape) are taken to the radiation physics suite for dosimetry. The nidus of the arteriovenous malformation is outlined on the angiogram, which is then mounted on a digitizer board. A mouselike device is used to identify the stereotactic fiducial markers and to trace the nidus; they simultaneously appear on the computer screen. The computer then generates anteroposterior, lateral, and vertical coordinates of the center of the lesion as well as its demagnified diameter. Next the computer quickly determines the position of all of the CT images within the stereotactic coordinate system. The angiographic target center point is displayed on the CT image. Dosimetry then begins and continues until the neurosurgeon, radiation therapist, and radiation physicist

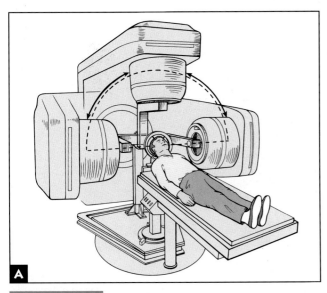
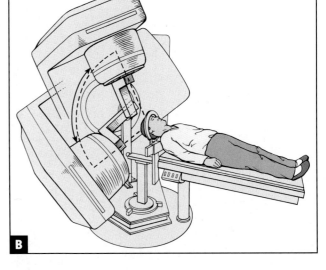

Figure 11.1

A linear accelerator (LINAC) produces high-energy photons (called x-rays) by accelerating electrons to nearly the speed of light and colliding them with a heavy metal alloy. **A,** The resultant radiation is collimated and focused on the target, which, in this application, is stereotactically positioned at the central point of the LINAC gantry rotation. **B,** The patient is rotated to new couch positions in between LINAC arcs. Typically, five to 11 separate arcs are performed. This paradigm produces a series of noncoplanar radiation arcs that only coincide at the target point. The unmodified LINAC has a tendency, because of its weight, to sag as it rotates from the vertical to the horizontal position. The University of Florida system couples several high-precision bearings to the LINAC to produce a radiation beam accuracy of 0.2±0.1 mm.

are satisfied that an optimal dose plan has been developed (Figure 11.2). A final computer printout shows all of the treatment parameters in a checklist format.

Patients rest comfortably until the end of the normal radiation therapy treatment day (around 4:30 PM). The radiosurgical device is attached to the LINAC. The patient then is attached to the device and treated. The actual radiation treatment time averages approximately 15 minutes. Afterward the head ring is removed, and, after a few minutes of observation, the patient is discharged. The radiosurgical device is disconnected from the LINAC, which is then ready for conventional usage.

Patient population

Between 5/18/88 and 8/18/92, 195 patients were treated on the University of Florida radiosurgery system. Of these patients, 119 had arteriovenous malformations. There were 61 men and 58 women in the series. The mean patient age was 40 years (range, 13 to 67 years). Presenting symptoms included hemor-

rhage (53), seizure (42), headache/incidental (22), and progressive neurologic deficit (two). Nineteen patients had undergone prior surgical attempts at arteriovenous malformation excision. Thirteen patients had undergone at least one embolization procedure. All patients were screened by a vascular neurosurgeon before consideration of radiosurgery.

The mean radiation dose to the periphery of the lesion was 1610 cGy (range, 1000 to 2500 cGy). This treatment dose was almost always delivered to the 80% isodose line (range, 70% to 90%). The mean lesion diameter was 24 mm (range, 10 to 35 mm). The diameter of the 80% isodose line almost always equaled the collimator size, which equaled the diameter of the lesion. One hundred eight patients were treated with one isocenter, seven patients with two isocenters, and four patients with three isocenters.

Follow-up consisted of clinical examination and magnetic resonance (MR) imaging every 3 to 6 months after treatment [15]. If possible, follow-up was performed in Gainesville; otherwise scan and examination results were forwarded by the patient's local physician. All patients were initially asked to

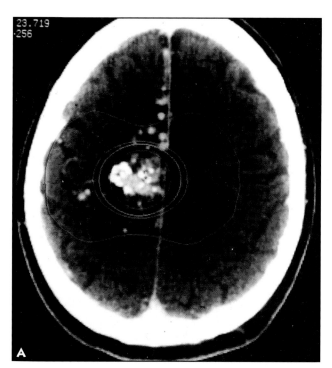

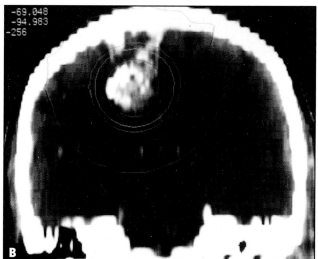

Figure 11.2

After stereotactic angiography, treatment planning proceeds on a background of reformatted computed tomographic (CT) scans or magnetic resonance images. The final treatment plan for this arteriovenous malformation shows the 80%, 40%, 16%, and 8% isodose lines, superimposed on contrast-enhanced, thin-section CT scans (**A,** axial view; **B,** coronal view). A dose of 1500 cGy was prescribed to the 80% isodose line. A 28-mm collimator was used. CT scans are routinely used for arteriovenous malformation dosimetry planning because they represent an anatomic-radiographic database that is easily understood by neurosurgeons, and because of the inherent limitations of stereotactic angiography.

undergo angiography at yearly intervals, regardless of the MR imaging findings, until complete occlusion of the arteriovenous malformation was demonstrated. More recently, since our 1-year thrombosis rate was established at approximately 40% overall [9], we have elected to follow up on patients with MR imaging until that study suggested complete thrombosis, before performing a follow-up angiogram. In this manner, the number of posttreatment angiograms can be limited to one for most patients.

One-year angiographic occlusion rate

Follow-up information was obtained on 118 of 119 patients in this series. Mean follow-up was 22 months (range, 1 to 51 months). Eighty-three patients have been followed up for 1 year or longer. Of these 83 patients, 49 have had 1-year angiograms (Figure 11.3). Thirty-four patients did not undergo 1-year angiography for the following reasons: one was lost to follow-up, two refused, and the 31 latest patients have been followed up pending MR imaging thrombosis. The results of the 49 1-year follow-up angiograms are as follows: total occlusion, 22 (45%); greater than 90% occlusion, 11 (22.5%); 50% to 90% occlusion, 11 (22.5%); and less than 50% occlusion, five (10%). There was a significant correlation between 1-year occlusion rate and arteriovenous malformation size, with smaller arteriovenous malformations more likely to thrombose.

Two-year angiographic occlusion rate

Forty-eight patients have been followed up for 2 years or longer. Of these 48 patients, 37 have had follow-up angiography (Figure 11.4). Eleven patients did not have 2-year follow-up angiography for the following reasons: four refused, one was lost to follow-up, and six have been delayed due to scheduling conflicts. The results in the 37 patients who underwent follow-up angiography are as follows: total occlusion, 31 (84%); greater than 90% occlusion, two (5%); 50% to 90% occlusion, three (8%); and less than 50% occlusion, one (3%). There was no significant correlation between 2-year occlusion rates and arteriovenous malformation size.

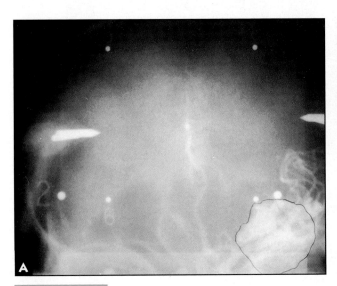

Figure 11.3

This 49-year-old man presented with a history of seizures. He was found to have a deep left frontal arteriovenous malformation and was referred for radiosurgery. **A,** Lateral angiogram. **B,** Anteroposterior angiogram. He was treated with 1500 cGy to the 80% iso-dose line, with a 28-mm collimator. These follow-up 1-year angiograms show complete thrombosis.

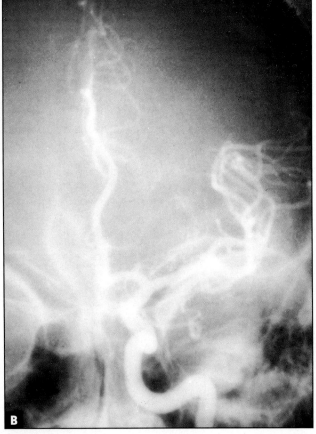

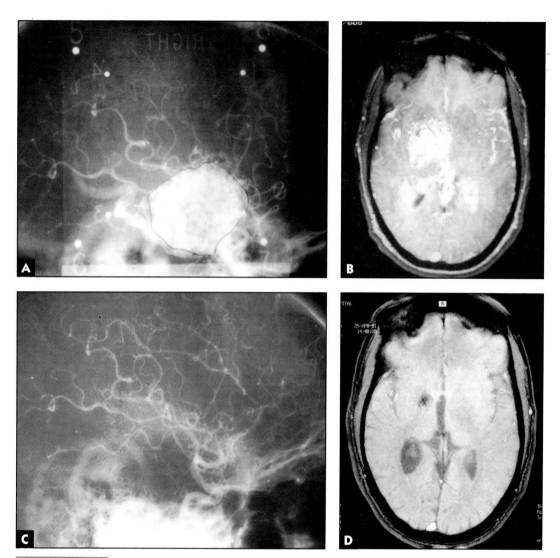

Figure 11.4

This 39-year-old man presented with a history of headaches, seizures, and a progressive visual field cut. He was referred for radiosurgery, and received 1000 cGy to the 70% isodose line through a 35-mm collimator. **A,** Lateral view pretreatment angiogram; **B,** Pretreatment magnetic resonance image. One-year angiogram revealed substantial but incomplete thrombosis of the lesion. Two-year angiogram revealed complete nidus thrombosis. **C,** Lateral view posttreatment angiogram; **D,** Posttreatment magnetic resonance image.

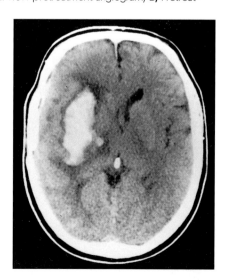

Figure 11.5

Image of a 61-year-old man 3 months after he underwent middle cerebral aneurysm clipping and partial excision of a right motor strip area arteriovenous malformation. The residual arteriovenous malformation nidus was treated with radiosurgery (1500cGy, 80% isodose line, 22-mm collimator). Three months after radiosurgery, he experienced an intracerebral hemorrhage, accompanied by hemiparesis and dysphasia. After prolonged rehabilitation he recovered to his preradiosurgical functional level. One-year angiography showed partial thrombosis. Two-year angiogram is pending.

Complications

Acute morbidity

Two patients, both early in the series, experienced seizures within 48 hours of radiosurgery. Both had originally presented with a seizure disorder. In subsequent patients with a history of seizures, anticonvulsant levels have been optimized in the high normal range before radiosurgical therapy, and no further posttreatment seizures have been observed. No other acute morbidity has been seen after radiosurgery.

Hemorrhage

Three patients (2.5%) experienced intracerebral hemorrhages after radiosurgical treatment. One patient had undergone partial surgical excision of a parietal arteriovenous malformation before radiosurgery. Three months after radiosurgery, he experienced an intracerebral hemorrhage, accompanied by hemiparesis and dysphasia. After prolonged rehabilitation, the patient recovered to his preradiosurgical functional level. The second patient underwent five attempts at embolization of a thalamic arteriovenous malformation before radiosurgery (Figure 11.5). Two months after radiosurgical treatment, he experienced a severe intraventricular hemorrhage, necessitating prolonged in-patient treatment, including a ventriculoperitoneal shunt. He made a substantial recovery and is currently undergoing further rehabilitation. The third patient presented with a longstanding seizure disorder and underwent radiosurgical treatment of a frontal arteriovenous malformation. He experienced a severe intracerebral-intraventricular hemorrhage 4 months after treatment, from which he eventually made a good recovery. None of these three patients had originally presented with a hemorrhage.

Radiation edema and necrosis

Five patients (4.2%) have experienced delayed complications directly attributable to radiosurgery. The first patient was treated with 2500 cGy to the 80% isodose line for a 24-mm arteriovenous malformation. Her 1-year angiogram showed complete thrombosis. One month later, she experienced a flurry of seizure activity. MR imaging revealed a 24-mm lesion, consistent with radionecrosis, as well as considerable surrounding edema. She responded to large doses of dexamethasone, and, after months, the medication was tapered off. She currently has only a minor limp.

In the second patient, a 30-mm brain stem arteriovenous malformation was treated with 1750 cGy to the 80% isodose line. Approximately 10 months after treatment, Parinaud's syndrome and obstructive hydrocephalus developed. MR imaging showed edema throughout the mesencephalon. He was treated with a ventriculoperitoneal shunt and steroids. After several months, the steroids were successfully tapered off. He has done well, with only a residual Parinaud's syndrome.

The third patient had a 16-mm arteriovenous malformation, which was treated with 1750 cGy to the 80% isodose line. Her 1-year angiogram showed complete thrombosis. Shortly thereafter, she reportedly developed dysphasia, which corresponded to edema on her MR image. She responded to a short course (1 month) of steroids and is now entirely well, with a normal MR image.

The fourth patient underwent radiosurgical treatment of a 26-mm motor strip area arteriovenous malformation, with 1500 cGy to the 80% isodose line (Figure 11.6). Her 1-year angiogram showed greater than 90% thrombosis. Two months later, she presented with complaints of headache. Subsequent MR imag-

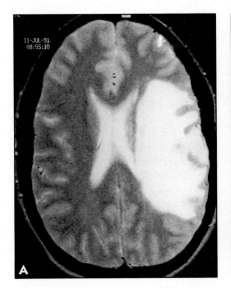
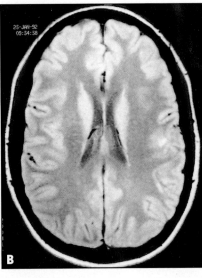

Figure 11.6

This 30-year-old woman developed a grand mal seizure disorder and was discovered to have a left frontoparietal arteriovenous malformation. She was treated with 1500 cGy to the 80% isodose line through a 26-mm collimator. One-year angiogram showed more than 90% thrombosis. One month later she presented with complaints of headache. T_2-weighted magnetic resonance (MR) image revealed an area of probable radiation necrosis in the exact area treated with radiosurgery, surrounded by considerable edema (**A**). She was treated with steroids, which produced a prompt and dramatic clinical improvement. After months of therapy, her MR image normalized (**B**). Two-year angiogram revealed complete arteriovenous malformation thrombosis.

ing revealed an area of gadolinium enhancement in the treatment area, surrounded by edema. After several months of steroid therapy, her MR image normalized. A subsequent angiogram revealed complete arteriovenous malformation thrombosis.

The fifth patient underwent radiosurgical treatment of a 30-mm left parietooccipital arteriovenous malformation with 1500 cGy to the 80% isodose line. His 1-year angiogram showed 50% thrombosis. Three months later, he presented with headache and mild dysphasia. An MR image revealed an area of gadolinium enhancement in the treatment area, surrounded by edema. This resolved after 3 months of steroid therapy.

In summary, two patients (1.7%) have experienced minor but permanent neurologic deficits as a result of radiation. Another three patients (2.5%) have experienced transient complications. Figure 11.7 shows the treatment dose and lesion size of all patients with radiation-induced complications. Lesion volume, treatment dose, and patient age did not significantly correlate with the occurrence of complications.

DISCUSSION AND LITERATURE REVIEW

Multiple studies have demonstrated a substantial (3% to 4% per year) risk of hemorrhage, often associated with morbidity or mortality, in patients harboring arteriovenous malformations [16,17]. Refinements in microsurgical technique as well as the development of increasingly effective endovascular treatments render many of the lesions amenable to successful, safe, surgical cure [18,19]. Those arteriovenous malformations that are not suitable for surgical removal are often considered for radiosurgical management.

Angiographic thrombosis rates

Radiosurgery appears to produce arteriovenous malformation thrombosis by inducing a pathologic process in the arteriovenous malformation nidus, leading to gradual thickening of the vessels until thrombosis occurs [16]. Several radiosurgical series have systematically evaluated this process by obtaining 1-year and 2-year follow-up angiograms. Steiner and coworkers [20••,21–24] have published multiple reports on gamma knife radiosurgery for arteriovenous malformations. They have reported 1-year occlusion rates ranging from 33.7% to 39.5% and 2-year occlusion rates ranging from 79% to 86.5%. However, these results were "optimized" by retrospectively selecting patients who received a minimum treatment dose. For example, in a recent report, he stated, "...a large majority of patients received at least 20 to 25 Gy of radiation.... Of the 248 patients treated before 1984, the treatment specification placed 188 in this group." The reported thrombosis rates in this paper applied only to these 188 patients (76% of his total series) [20••]. Interestingly, Yamamoto and coworkers [25] recently reported on 25 Japanese patients treated on the gamma unit in Stockholm but followed up in Japan. The 2-year thrombosis rate in those arteriovenous malformations that were completely covered by the radiosurgical field was 64%.

Kemeny and coworkers [26••] reported on 52 arteriovenous malformation patients treated with gamma knife radiosurgery. They all received 2500 cGy to the 50% isodose line. At 1 year, 16 patients (31%) had complete thrombosis, and 10 patients (19%) had "almost complete" thrombosis. They found that the results were better in younger patients and in patients with relatively lateral locations of arteriovenous mal-

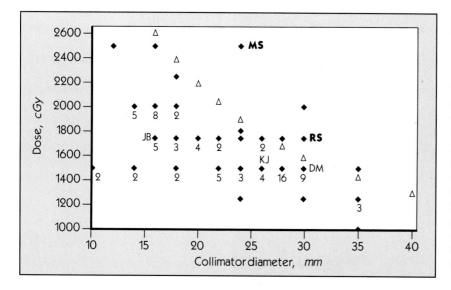

Figure 11.7

Lesion size for all the arteriovenous malformations in our series plotted against the prescribed irradiation dose (*diamonds*). The number of lesions treated at each data point is indicated. The *triangles* represent the 1% risk for radionecrosis according to Kjellberg *et al.* (*N Engl J Med* 1983, 309:269–274). The bold print initials (**RS** and **MS**) indicate the two patients who experienced permanent, minor neurologic deficits. These two patients received doses that fell well above Kjellberg's line. The regular print initials (JB, DM, and KJ) indicate the three patients who have experienced transient difficulties. They received doses well below Kjellberg's line.

formations. There was no difference in outcome between small (<2 cm^3), medium (2 to 3 cm^3), and large (>3 cm^3) arteriovenous malformations.

Recently, Lunsford and coworkers [27] reported on 227 arteriovenous malformation patients treated with gamma knife radiosurgery. The mean dose delivered to the arteriovenous malformation margin was 21.2 Gy. The Pittsburgh gamma knife was the first to use an 18-mm secondary collimator, which was reported as "...invaluable for the treatment of larger arteriovenous malformations." Multiple isocenters were used in 48% of the patients. Seventeen patients underwent 1-year angiography, which confirmed complete thrombosis in 76.5%. As indicated in the paper, "this rate may be spurious since many of these patients were selected for angiography because their MR image had suggested obliteration." Among 75 patients who were followed up for at least 2 years, 2-year angiography was performed in only 46 (61%). Complete obliteration was confirmed in 37 of 46 (80%). This thrombosis rate strongly correlated with arteriovenous malformation size, as follows: less than 1 cm^3, 100%; 1 to 4 cm^3, 85%; 4 to 10 cm^3, 58%.

Steinberg and coworkers [28], in an analysis of 86 arteriovenous malformations treated with a particle-beam radiosurgical system, reported a 29% 1-year thrombosis, 70% 2-year thrombosis, and 92% 3-year thrombosis rate. The best results were obtained with smaller lesions and higher doses. Initially a treatment dose of 34.6 Gy was used, but a higher than expected neurologic complication rate (20% for the entire series) led to the currently used dose range of 7.7 to 19.2 Gy [18]. No patients treated with the lower dose range had complications.

Betti [5] and Betti and coworkers [29] reported on the results of 66 arteriovenous malformations treated with a LINAC radiosurgical system. Doses of "no more than 40 Gy" were used in 80% of patients. They found a 66% 2-year thrombosis rate. The percentage of cured patients was highest when the entire malformation was included in the 75% isodose line (96%) or the maximum diameter of the lesion was less than 12 mm (81%).

Colombo and coworkers [6,30] reported on 97 arteriovenous malformation patients treated with a LINAC system. Doses from 18.7 to 40 Gy were delivered in one or two sessions. Of 56 patients who were followed up for longer than 1 year, 50 underwent 12-month follow-up angiography. In 26 patients (52%), complete thrombosis was demonstrated. Fifteen of 20 patients (75%) undergoing 2-year angiography had complete thrombosis. Colombo and coworkers reported a definite relationship between arteriovenous malformation size and thrombosis rate, as follows. Lesions less than 15 mm in diameter had a 1-year obliteration rate of 76% and a 2-year rate of 90%.

Lesions 15 to 25 mm in diameter had a 1-year thrombosis rate of 37.5% and a 2-year rate of 80%. Lesions greater than 25 mm in diameter had a 1-year thrombosis rate of 11% and a 2-year rate of 40%.

Souhami and coworkers [31] reported on 33 arteriovenous malformations treated with a LINAC system. The prescribed dose at isocenter varied from 50 to 55 Gy. A complete obliteration rate of 38% was seen on 1-year angiography. For patients whose arteriovenous malformation nidus was covered by a minimum dose of 25 Gy, the total obliteration rate was 61.5%, whereas none of the patients who had received less than 25 Gy at the edge of the nidus obtained a total obliteration.

Loeffler and coworkers [32] reported on 16 arteriovenous malformations treated with a LINAC system. The prescribed dose was 15 to 25 Gy, typically to the 80% to 90% line. The total obliteration rate was five of 11 (45%) at 1 year and eight of 11 (73%) at 2 years after treatment.

We reported on 119 patients treated with the University of Florida radiosurgery system. A 45% 1-year thrombosis rate and an 84% 2-year thrombosis rate were identified. Although the 1-year thrombosis rate did correlate with arteriovenous malformation size, the 2-year thrombosis rate did not.

Complications

Hemorrhage

Multiple series report that the hemorrhage rate for arteriovenous malformations treated, but not yet obliterated, with radiosurgery is the same as if they had not been treated [6,16,21,27,29]. Most recently, Steiner and coworkers [33] analyzed clinical outcomes in 247 consecutive cases of arteriovenous malformation treated with the gamma knife. No patient with angiographically proven thrombosis had a hemorrhage. The protective effect of radiosurgery against hemorrhage in incompletely obliterated lesions was evaluated, using both the person-year and Kaplan-Meier life table methods of analysis. The person-year method showed a rebleed rate of 2% to 3% per year—very similar to the known natural history of the disease. The Kaplan-Meier analysis showed a risk of 3.7% per year until 5 years after radiosurgery. At that point, the risk seemed to "plateau." As discussed by the authors, this plateau, which has long been the source of controversy in the radiosurgery literature, is very likely an artifact of this statistical method when applied to a relatively small group of patients. In general, most authors believe that radiosurgery provides no protective effect against hemorrhage until the arteriovenous malformation has thrombosed. This is, in fact, the major known drawback of radiosurgery compared with microsurgery.

Radiation-induced complications

Several authors have previously reported that radio-surgery can acutely exacerbate seizure activity [16,27]. After observing this phenomenon in two of our early patients, we systematically optimized anticonvulsant levels in those patients with a seizure history, before radiosurgical treatment. Since adopting this policy, we have not observed any further treatment-related seizures. Others have reported nausea, vomiting, and headache occasionally occurring after radiosurgical treatment [27,34].

Delayed radiation-induced complications have been reported by all groups performing radiosurgery. Steiner [21,22] found symptomatic radiation necrosis in approximately 3% of his patients. Statham and coworkers [35] described one patient who developed radiation necrosis 13 months after gamma knife radiosurgery of a 5.3-cm^3 arteriovenous malformation with 25 Gy to the margin [10]. Lunsford and coworkers [27] reported that 10 patients in their series (4.4%) developed new neurologic deficits thought secondary to radiation injury. Symptoms were location-dependent and developed between 4 and 18 months after treatment. All patients were treated with steroids, and all improved. Only two patients were reported to have residual deficits that appeared permanent. The radiation dose and isodose line treated did not correlate with this complication. As they noted, the failure of correlation of dose and complications may very well relate to the fact that the dose was selected to fall below Flickinger's [36, 37] computed 3% risk line. This is a mathematically derived line that prescribes lower doses for larger lesions.

Steinberg and coworkers [28] reported a definite correlation between lesion dose and complications.

The initial treatment dose of 34.6 Gy led to a relatively high complication rate [3]. No patients treated with the subsequently used lower dose range had complications. In an earlier report on 75 arteriovenous malformation patients treated with helium particles at a dose of 45 Gy, seven of 75 patients (11%) experienced radiation-induced complications [3]. Kjellberg and Abbe [4] and Kjellberg and coworkers [38], using a compilation of animal and clinical data, constructed a series of log-log lines, relating prescribed dose and lesion diameter. His 1% isorisk line is quite similar to Flickinger's mathematically derived 3% risk line.

In Colombo *et al.*'s series [6], three of 97 (3%) patients experienced symptomatic radiation-induced complications. Loeffler and coworkers [39] reported that one of 21 arteriovenous malformation patients developed a similar problem, which responded well to steroids. Souhami and coworkers [31] reported "severe side effects" in two of 33 (6%) patients. Marks and Spencer [40] recently reviewed six radiosurgical series and found a 9% incidence of clinically significant radiation reactions. Seven of 23 cases received doses below Kjellberg's 1% risk line.

Others have reported that asymptomatic radiation-induced changes appear frequently (24% in Lunsford's series) on MR images [27,41]. We have also observed this phenomenon. These changes tend to be asymptomatic if the lesion is located in a relatively "silent" brain area and symptomatic if the lesion is located in an "eloquent" brain area. Thus, lesion location may be another important consideration in radiosurgical treatment planning and dose selection.

Most radiosurgical series report their radiation-induced complications as a percentage of the total patient population treated. Because most radiation-

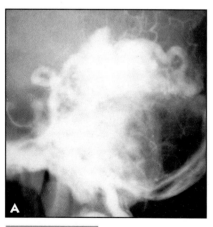 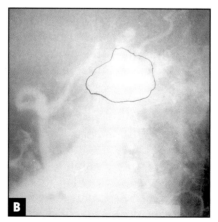 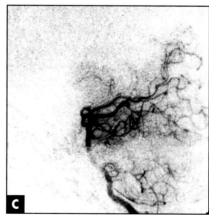

Figure 11.8

This 40-year-old man presented with a history of headaches and seizures. He underwent multiple endovascular treatments for a large left occipitoparietal arteriovenous malformation. **A,** Preembolization lateral angiogram. **B,** Postembolization lateral angiogram, with nidus outlined, shows the residual nidus, which was treated with radiosurgery (1500 cGy, 80% isodose line, 28-mm collimator). **C,** One-year posttreatment lateral digital angiogram shows complete thrombosis.

induced complications do not appear for 12 to 18 months after treatment, this results in a systematic underestimate of the true complication rate.

SPECIAL ISSUES

Multimodality arteriovenous malformation treatment

Radiosurgery may be used alone in the treatment of arteriovenous malformations less than 3.5 cm in diameter. Occasionally larger arteriovenous malformations are treated with a combination of endovascular therapy, surgery, and radiosurgery. The following case examples illustrate the potential usefulness of such multimodality treatment.

Case 1. A 40-year-old white man presented with a 5-year history of headaches and seizures. Work-up disclosed a large left parietooccipital arteriovenous malformation, which was initially treated with embolization (Figure 11.8). Several months later, he underwent radiosurgical treatment of a substantially

reduced nidus, with 1500 cGy applied to the 80% iso-dose line of a 28-mm collimator. An arteriogram performed 1 year after radiosurgery revealed complete arteriovenous malformation thrombosis.

Comment. Embolization and radiosurgery have been applied with increasing frequency. Many questions remain to be answered regarding this combination of therapies. For example, what type of embolic material is best? Currently we treat the nidus that remains after embolization. Because radiosurgery frequently takes 2 years to produce nidus thrombosis, the possibility exists that the embolic material will "wash out" during this latent period [42•].

It does seem reasonably clear at this point that radiosurgery combined with embolization exposes the patient to the risk of both procedures. Because embolization alone rarely produces a cure, it should be used only when the arteriovenous malformation is too large to be safely treated with radiosurgery alone.

Case 2. A 30-year-old woman presented after an intraventricular hemorrhage from a posterior left sylvian area arteriovenous malformation (Figure 11.9). She underwent multiple embolization procedures,

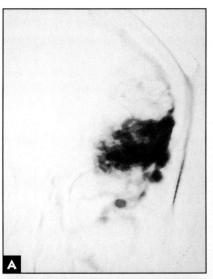

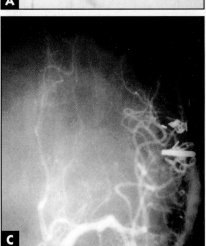

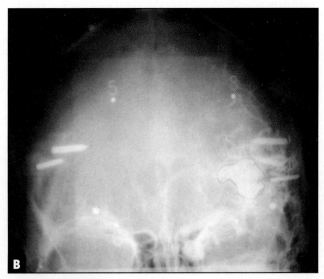

Figure 11.9

A, Anteroposterior pretreatment angiogram of a 30-year-old woman who presented after an intraventricular hemorrhage secondary to a left sylvian arteriovenous malformation. She underwent multiple embolization procedures, followed by craniotomy and partial arteriovenous malformation excision. **B,** Preradiosurgery anteroposterior angiogram. The remaining nidus was treated with radiosurgery (1500 cGy, 80% isodose line, 28-mm collimator). **C,** One-year follow-up arteriogram showed disappearance of the shunt, with minimal remaining abnormal vascularity. Two-year angiogram is pending.

followed by a craniotomy with partial arteriovenous malformation resection. Subsequently, the remaining nidus was treated with 1500 cGy to the 80% isodose line of a 28-mm collimator. An arteriogram performed 1 year after radiosurgery showed disappearance of the vascular shunt, with minimal remaining abnormal vascularity. Two-year angiography is pending.

Comment. This case illustrates the potential combination of embolization, surgery, and radiosurgery.

Case 3. A 33-year-old woman presented after recovering from an intracerebral hemorrhage. She underwent surgical resection of a large right frontoparietal arteriovenous malformation (Figure 11.10). Postoperative angiography revealed a small residual nidus. This nidus was treated with 2000 cGy to the 80% isodose line of a 16-mm collimator. One-year follow-up angiography showed complete obliteration of the nidus.

Comment: This case illustrates the potential combination of surgery, followed by radiosurgery for persistent nidus.

Case 4. A 28-year-old white man presented with a seizure disorder. He underwent partial surgical resection of a right temporal arteriovenous malformation. The postoperative arteriogram revealed residual nidus in the posteromedial temporal lobe, with questionable residual nidus in the anterior temporal lobe. The posterior nidus was treated with radiosurgery (1500 cGy, 80% isodose line, 26-mm collimator). Two-year follow-up angiography revealed total occlusion of the targeted lesion but persistence of the anterior

temporal abnormality. He underwent repeat craniotomy, and the anterior temporal component was easily resected.

Comment. This case illustrates the potential combination of radiosurgery for a deep arteriovenous malformation component, followed by surgical resection of the more accessible component.

Cavernous malformations

The advent of MR imaging as a neurologic screening test has resulted in the identification of substantial numbers of cavernous malformations. This vascular malformation differs pathologically from true arteriovenous malformations. The role of radiosurgery in the treatment of angiographically occult vascular malformations is not well defined. Kondziolka and coworkers [43] reported on 24 patients treated on the gamma knife at the University of Pittsburgh. Radiosurgery was used conservatively; each patient had sustained two or more hemorrhages and had an MR imaging–defined angiographically occult vascular malformation located in a region of the brain where microsurgical removal was judged to pose an excessive risk. Fifteen malformations were in the medulla, pons, or mesencephalon, and five were located in the thalamus or basal ganglia. Follow-up ranged from 4 to 24 months. Nineteen patients either improved or remained clinically stable and did not hemorrhage again during the follow-up interval. One patient suffered another hemorrhage 7 months after radio-

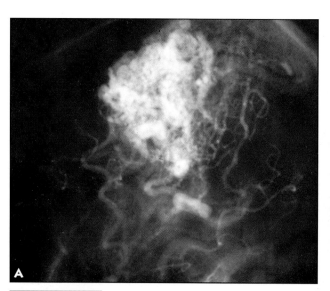
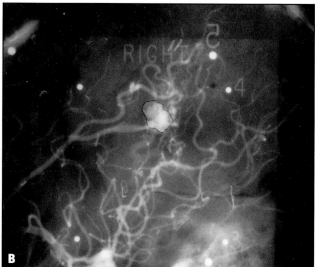

Figure 11.10

This 33-year-old woman presented with a large right frontoparietal arteriovenous malformation. **A,** Lateral arteriogram. **B,** Postsurgery arteriogram revealed a small residual area of nidus. This nidus was treated with radiosurgery (2000 cGy, 80% isodose line, 16-mm collimator). One-year follow-up angiogram showed complete thrombosis.

surgery. Five patients experienced temporary worsening of preexisting neurologic deficits that suggested delayed radiation injury. MR imaging demonstrated signal changes and edema surrounding the radiosurgical target.

This report clearly indicates a significantly higher complication rate for radiosurgical treatment of cavernous malformations than for true arteriovenous malformations. In addition, the fact that they are angiographically occult means that no objective criteria for "successful" treatment exist. Only by following up on patients with a proven propensity for hemorrhage and demonstrating a significant decrease in hemorrhage rate can benefit be shown. Proof of such benefit does not currently exist. At the University of Florida, aggressive surgical therapy is used on the majority of symptomatic cavernous malformations. Radiosurgery is regarded as a last resort.

CONCLUSIONS

Radiosurgery, using particle beam, gamma knife, and LINAC systems, is becoming widely available. Many reports indicate that approximately 80% of arteriovenous malformations in the "radiosurgery size range" will be angiographically obliterated 2 years after radiosurgical treatment. Permanent neurologic complications are very rare (2% to 3%). The major drawback of this treatment method is that patients are unprotected against hemorrhage during the 2-year latent period. Although radiosurgery has been used primarily as a single modality of treatment in previous studies, more recently it has been increasingly employed as part of a multimodality treatment approach incorporating surgical and endovascular methods.

REFERENCES AND RECOMMENDED READING

Papers of particular interest, published within the annual period of review, have been highlighted as:
• Of special interest
•• Of outstanding interest

1. Leksell L: The stereotaxic method and radiosurgery of the brain. *Acta Chir Scand* 1951, 102:316–319.

2. Leksell L: *Stereotaxis and Radiosurgery.* Springfield, IL: Charles C. Thomas; 1971.

3. Hosobuchi Y, Fabrikant JI, Lyman JT: Stereotactic heavy-particle irradiation of intracranial arteriovenous malformations. *Appl Neurophysiol* 1987, 50:248–252.

4. Kjellberg RN, Abbe M: Stereotactic Bragg peak proton beam therapy. In *Modern Stereotactic Neurosurgery.* Edited by Lunsford LD. Boston: Martinus Nijhoff; 1988:463–470.

5. Betti OO: Treatment of arteriovenous malformations with the linear accelerator. *Appl Neurophysiol* 1987, 50:262.

6. Colombo F, Benedetti A, Pozza F, *et al.*: External stereotactic irradiation by linear accelerator. *Neurosurgery* 1985, 16:154–160.

7. Friedman WA: LINAC radiosurgery. *Neurosurg Clin North Am* 1990, 1:991–1008.

8. Friedman WA, Bova FJ: The University of Florida radiosurgery system. *Surg Neurol* 1989, 32:334–342.

9. Friedman WA, Bova FJ: LINAC radiosurgery for arteriovenous malformation. *J Neurosurg* 1992, 77:832–841.

10. Friedman WA, Spiegelmann R: LINAC radiosurgery. *Neurosurg Clin North Am* 1992, 3:141–166.

11. Bova FJ: Radiation physics. *Neurosurg Clin North Am* 1990, 1:909–931.

12. Bova FJ, Friedman WA: Stereotactic angiography: an inadequate database for radiosurgery? *Int J Radiat Oncol Biol Phys* 1991, 20:891–895.

13. •• Phillips MH, Kessler M, Chuang FY, *et al.*: Image correlation of MRI and CT in treatment planning for radiosurgery of intracranial vascular malformations. *Int J Radiat Oncol Biol Phys* 1991, 20:881–889.
    Summarizes the University of Florida radiosurgery experience with arteriovenous malformations and reviews the literature on the subject.

14. Spiegelmann R, Friedman WA, Bova FJ: Limitations of angiographic target localization in radiosurgical treatment planning. *Neurosurgery* 1992, 30:619–624.

15. Quisling RG, Peters KR, Friedman WA, *et al.*: Persistent nidus blood flow in cerebral arteriovenous malformation after stereotactic radiosurgery: MR imaging assessment. *Radiology* 1991, 180:785–791.

16. Ogilvy CS: Radiation therapy for arteriovenous malformations: a review. *Neurosurgery* 1990, 26:725–735.

17. Ondra SL, Troupp H, George ED, *et al.*: The natural history of symptomatic arteriovenous malformations of the brain: a 24-year follow-up assessment. *J Neurosurg* 1991, 73:387–391.

18. Heros RC, Korosue K, Diebold PM: Surgical excision of cerebral arteriovenous malformations: late results. *Neurosurgery* 1990, 26:570–578.

19. Spetzler RF, Martin NA: A proposed grading system of arteriovenous malformations. *J Neurosurg* 1986, 65:476–483.

20. •• Lindquist C, Steiner L: Stereotactic radiosurgical treatment of malformations of the brain. In *Modern Stereotactic Neurosurgery*. Edited by Lunsford LD. Boston: Martinus Nijhoff; 1988:491–506.

Reviews the University of Pittsburgh experience with the radiosurgical treatment of angiographically occult vascular malformations. It is the largest series currently in the literature.

21. Steiner L: Treatment of arteriovenous malformations by radiosurgery. In *Intracranial Arteriovenous Malformations*. Edited by Wilson CB, Stein BM. Baltimore: Williams & Wilkins; 1984:295–313.

22. Steiner L: Radiosurgery in cerebral arteriovenous malformations. In *Cerebrovascular Surgery*, vol 4. Edited by Fein JM, Flamm ES. Wien: Springer-Verlag; 1985:1161–1251.

23. Steiner L, Leksell L, Forster DM, *et al.*: Stereotactic radiosurgery in intracranial arterio-venous malformations. *Acta Neurochir* 1974, 21(suppl):195–209.

24. Steiner L, Leksell L, Greitz T, *et al.*: Stereotaxic radiosurgery for cerebral arteriovenous malformations: report of a case. *Acta Chir Scand* 1972, 138:459–464.

25. Yamamoto M, Jimbo M, Kobayashi M, *et al.*: Long-term results of radiosurgery for arteriovenous malformation: neurodiagnostic imaging and histological studies of angiographically confirmed nidus obliteration. *Surg Neurol* 1992, 37:219–230.

26. •• Kemeny AA, Dias PS, Forster DM: Results of stereotactic radiosurgery of arteriovenous malformations: an analysis of 52 cases. *J Neurol Neurosurg Psychiatry* 1989, 52:554–558.

Reviews the University of Pittsburgh experience with the radiosurgical treatment of arteriovenous malformations.

27. Lunsford LD, Kondziolka D, Flickinger JC, *et al.*: Stereotactic radiosurgery for arteriovenous malformations of the brain. *J Neurosurg* 1991, 75:512–524.

28. Steinberg GK, Famkant JI, Marks MP, *et al.*: Stereotactic heavy-charged particle Bragg peak radiation for intracranial arteriovenous malformations. *N Engl J Med* 1990, 323:96–101.

29. Betti OO, Munari C, Rosler R: Stereotactic radiosurgery with the linear accelerator: treatment of arteriovenous malformations. *Neurosurgery* 1989, 24:311–321.

30. Colombo F, Benedetti A, Pozza F, *et al.*: Linear accelerator radiosurgery of cerebral arteriovenous malformations. *Neurosurgery* 1989, 24:833–840.

31. Souhami L, Olivier A, Podgorsak EB, *et al.*: Radiosurgery of cerebral arteriovenous malformations with the dynamic stereotactic irradiation. *Int J Radiat Oncol Biol Phys* 1990, 19:775–782.

32. Loeffler JS, Alexander E III, Siddon RL, *et al.*: Stereotactic radiosurgery for intracranial arteriovenous malformations using a standard linear accelerator. *Int J Radiat Oncol Biol Phys* 1989, 17:673–677.

33. Steiner L, Lindquist C, Adler JR, *et al.*: Clinical outcome of radiosurgery for cerebral arteriovenous malformations. *J Neurosurg* 1992, 77:1–8.

34. Colombo F, Benedetti A, Pozza F, *et al.*: Linear accelerator radiosurgery of three-dimensional irregular targets. *Stereotact Funct Neurosurg* 1990, 54-55:541–546.

35. Statham P, Macpherson P, Johnston R, *et al.*: Cerebral radiation necrosis complicating stereotactic radiosurgery for arteriovenous malformation. *J Neurol Neurosurg Psychiatry* 1990, 53:476–479.

36. Flickinger JC: An integrated logistic formula for prediction of complications from radiosurgery. *Int J Radiat Oncol Biol Phys* 1989, 17:879–885.

37. Flickinger JC, Schell MC, Larson DA: Estimation of complications for linear accelerator radiosurgery with the integrated logistic formula. *Int J Radiat Oncol Biol Phys* 1990, 19:143–148.

38. Kjellberg RN, Hanamura T, Davis KR, *et al.*: Bragg-peak proton-beam therapy for arteriovenous malformations of the brain. *N Engl J Med* 1983, 309:269–274.

39. Loeffler JS, Siddon RL, Wen PY, *et al.*: Stereotactic radiosurgery of the brain using a standard linear accelerator: a study of early and late effects. *Radiother Oncol* 1990, 17:311–321.

40. Marks LB, Spencer DP: The influence of volume on the tolerance of the brain to radiosurgery. *J Neurosurg* 1991, 75:177–180.

41. Marks MP, Delapaz RL, Fabrikant JI, *et al.*: Intracranial vascular malformations: imaging of charged-particle radiosurgery. Part II: complications. *Radiology* 1988, 168:457–462.

42. • Dawson RC, Tarr RW, Hecht ST, *et al.*: Treatment of arteriovenous malformation of the brain with combined embolization and stereotactic radiosurgery: results after 1 and 2 years. *AJNR* 1990, 11:857–864.

Surveys the clinical outcome of a large radiosurgically treated arteriovenous malformation patient population, including a detailed analysis of the risk of hemorrhage.

43. Kondziolka D, Lunsford LD, Coffey RJ, *et al.*: Stereotactic radiosurgery of angiographically occult vascular malformations: indications and preliminary experience. *Neurosurgery* 1990, 27:892–900.

Chapter 12

The Current Status of Carotid Endarterectomy

Jed P. Weber
Marc R. Mayberg

In the late 1980s, controversy arose regarding the efficacy and overuse of carotid endarterectomy [1]. This criticism stemmed largely from the lack of rigorous scientific studies comparing carotid endarterectomy with other forms of therapy for stroke prevention. Several major randomized trials have provided data that clearly define certain indications for carotid endarterectomy [2••–4••,5•]. In addition, technologic advances offer hope of improving preoperative evaluation, reducing operative risk, and expanding therapeutic alternatives. This new information has resulted in an exciting period of rapid redefinition and renewed confidence in carotid endarterectomy.

CLINICAL TRIALS FOR CAROTID ENDARTERECTOMY

Previous clinical trials investigating the therapeutic options for patients with carotid stenosis failed to meet the criteria enabling valid comparisons between appropriate groups [6]. To meet these criteria, six separate prospective randomized, multicenter clinical trials for carotid endarterectomy were initiated in the 1980s (Table 12.1) [2••–4••,5•,7,8•,9].

Trials for symptomatic stenosis

Three randomized, prospective multicenter clinical trials were designed to evaluate the role of carotid endarterectomy in patients with symptomatic carotid stenosis: the North American Symptomatic Carotid Endarterectomy Trial (NASCET) [2••], the European Carotid Surgery Trial [3••], and the Veterans Administration Symptomatic Stenosis Trial [4••]. In general, these studies were conducted similarly: each entered patients with neurologic symptoms clearly referable to an ipsilateral carotid stenosis and randomized them to receive either carotid endarterectomy and the best medical therapy, or the best medical therapy alone. The entry criteria for symptoms were similar for each study; they included transient ischemic attacks, amaurosis fugax, and small completed stroke ipsilateral to carotid stenosis. The length of time after onset of symptoms and prior to randomization varied from less than 120 days for NASCET and the Veterans Administration trial to 180 days for the European Carotid Surgery Trial. This difference is important because the risk of subsequent stroke has been shown to decrease with time after the initial event, *ie*, later randomization selects for patients with reduced risk [7].

The North American Symptomatic Carotid Endarterectomy Trial

The NASCET was designed to proceed until it had entered 1900 patients [2••]. However, randomization of the subgroup of patients with more than 70% carotid stenosis was prematurely terminated due to an overwhelming reduction in stroke risk in the operative group. At the point of termination, there were 659 patients with high-grade stenosis randomized to receive either surgical (n = 331) or nonsurgical (n =

Table 12.1
Comparison among six randomized prospective multicenter clinical trials for carotid endarterectomy*

Trial	Carotid stenosis, %	Time from event to study, d	Primary end-points	Patient sample size, n
Symptomatic				
NASCET	30–69 70–99[†]	≤120	Stroke Death	1900
ECST	<30[†] 30–69 70–99	≤180	Stroke (>7 days) Death	2000 minimum
VA Symptomatic	>50	≤120	Stroke Crescendo transient ischemic attacks Death	250 each group
Asymptomatic				
ACAS	>60		Stroke Retinal infarction Transient ischemic attacks Death	750 each group
VA Asymptomatic	>50		Stroke Transient ischemic attacks Death	250 each group
CASANOVA	50–90		Stroke Death	400 each group

Data from NASCET (North American Symptomatic Carotid Endarterectomy Trial) [2••], ECST (European Carotid Surgery Trial) [3••], Veterans Administration Symptomatic Stenosis Trial, ACAS (Asymptomatic Carotid Atherosclerosis Study) [11], Asymptomatic Carotid Stenosis Veterans Administration Study, and CASANOVA (Carotid Artery Stenosis With Asymptomatic Narrowing: Operation Versus Aspirin) [5•]; with permission.

[†]Indicates completed stenosis.

328) therapy. At a mean follow-up of 24 months, the rate of ipsilateral stroke was 26% in the nonsurgical group and 9% in the surgical group (P < 0.001) (Figure 12.1A). This difference amounts to an absolute risk reduction of 17%, or a relative risk reduction of 71%. The perioperative morbidity and mortality within 30 days after surgery was 5.8%, after which there were few events in the surgical group. However, the non-surgical group experienced a continuing incidence of stroke in which treatment failures exceeded those in the surgical group by 3 months. Patient accrual continues in this trial for patients with intermediate ranges (30% to 70%) of carotid stenosis [8•].

The European Carotid Surgery Trial

The European Carotid Surgery Trial enrolled patients with mild (less than 30%), moderate (30% to 69%), and severe (70% to 99%) carotid stenosis, and randomized them to receive surgical or nonsurgical treatment [3••]. Although the patients were to be observed for a minimum of 5 years, interim analysis of 2200 patients at 2.7 years' mean follow-up led to premature termination of entry into the mild and severe stenosis groups. For 374 patients with mild stenosis, there was no significant difference in ipsilateral stroke between the surgical and nonsurgical groups despite a low (2.3%) 30-day morbidity and mortality for surgical patients. However, patients with 70% to 99% stenosis who underwent carotid endarterectomy had a 10.3% stroke risk at 3 years as compared with 16.8% risk in the nonsurgical group (Figure 12.1B). More important, the risk of death or ipsilateral disabling stroke was reduced from 11% in the nonsurgical group to 6% in the surgical group. Randomization in this study continues for patients in the moderate (30% to 69%) stenosis group.

The Veterans Administration Symptomatic Stenosis Trial

The Veterans Administration Symptomatic Stenosis Trial randomized fewer patients than the other two symptomatic trials, but offered the advantages of a relatively uniform patient population and standardized protocols for evaluation and treatment in the Veterans Affairs health care system [4••]. This study screened 5000 patients and excluded 4807 through an extensive set of exclusionary criteria. The remaining uniform group of 193 men was randomized to receive carotid endarterectomy (n = 91) or the best medical treatment (n = 98).

The Veterans Administration trial was prematurely halted coincident with the publication of data from the other symptomatic stenosis trials. At a mean fol-

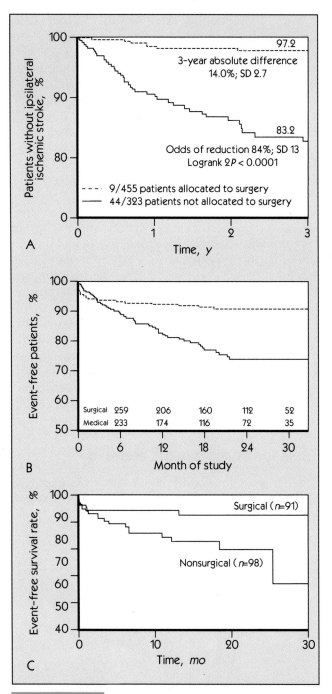

Figure 12.1

Kaplan-Meier curves showing cumulative event-free survival in the surgical and nonsurgical groups for the symptomatic trials. **A,** Percent without ipsilateral stroke in the European Carotid Surgery Trial 70% to 99% stenosis group. **B,** Proportion who were event-free in the North American Symptomatic Carotid Endarterectomy Trial 70% to 99% stenosis group. **C,** Proportion without cerebral ischemia in the Veterans Administration Symptomatic Trial 50% to 99% stenosis group. (*From* the North American Symptomatic Carotid Endarterectomy Trial Collaborators [2••] and Mayberg *et al.* [4••]; with permission.)

low-up of 11.9 months, there was a 7.7% risk of cerebral ischemia in the surgical group as compared with 19.4% ($P = 0.011$) for the nonsurgical group (absolute risk reduction of 11.7% or relative risk reduction of 60% (Figure 12.1C). Again, despite a perioperative risk of 6.6% (death or ipsilateral stroke after 30 days) among surgical patients, there was only one additional ipsilateral stroke during the study period.

Conclusions from symptomatic stenosis trials

In the symptomatic endarterectomy trials, several features were notable. Carotid endarterectomy provided significant protection against subsequent ipsilateral cerebral ischemia in patients with high-grade symptomatic stenosis. The stroke risk reduction provided by surgery occurred early, persisted over extended periods, and was independent of other risk factors. For all studies, annual stroke rates in the nonsurgical group ranged from 12% to 18%, considerably exceeding the 3% to 7% stroke rate estimated from prior studies. Surgical morbidity and mortality at acceptable levels were achieved at multiple centers. Data from the symptomatic endarterectomy trials suggest that all patients with symptoms or signs of anterior circulation ischemia should be rapidly evaluated for potential carotid endarterectomy.

Trials for asymptomatic stenosis

Three trials included only patients with asymptomatic carotid stenosis. These were the Carotid Artery Stenosis with Asymptomatic Narrowing Operation Versus Aspirin (CASANOVA) Study [5•], the Veterans Administration Asymptomatic Stenosis Study [9,10], and the Asymptomatic Carotid Atherosclerosis Study [11].

The CASANOVA Study Group trial [5•] randomized patients with asymptomatic carotid stenosis greater than 50% but less than 90% to receive either immediate carotid endarterectomy ($n = 206$) or no immediate surgery. These patients included some who underwent delayed surgery after developing new symptoms or severe, bilateral, or contralateral stenosis ($n = 204$). At 3-year follow-up, with death or new stroke as endpoints, there was no difference in outcome between the immediate surgery group and the other group (10.7% vs 11.3%). However, nearly half the patients in the "no immediate surgery" group eventually did have an endarterectomy for one of the reasons stated above. The unusual study design for this trial considerably lessens its statistical validity. The Veterans Administration Asymptomatic Trial randomized patients with asymptomatic carotid stenosis (more than 50%) to undergo surgery ($n = 211$) or receive nonsurgical therapy ($n = 233$) [9]. This study was completed in April 1991, and publication of the results is under way. A preliminary report presented the perioperative risk of morbidity (2.4%) and mortality (1.9%) for the surgical group [9]. The Asymptomatic Carotid Atherosclerosis Study randomized more than 1100 asymptomatic patients (the goal is 1500) with more than 60% carotid stenosis [11]. The results of this study should be available in the near future.

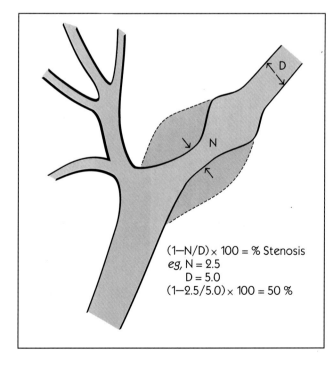

$(1-N/D) \times 100 = \%$ Stenosis
eg, $N = 2.5$
$D = 5.0$
$(1-2.5/5.0) \times 100 = 50\%$

Figure 12.2

For recent trials of carotid endarterectomy, carotid stenosis was measured by taking the ratio of the diameter at the site of the greatest narrowing (N) and the diameter of the normal artery beyond the diseased segment (D). The percentage of stenosis in the example shown is 50%. (*From* Barnett [8•]; with permission.)

ADVANCES IN PREOPERATIVE ASSESSMENT OF CAROTID STENOSIS

On the basis of the studies described above, determining accurately the degree of carotid stenosis is of paramount importance in selecting the appropriate therapy. Carotid arteriography has been considered the gold standard for carotid stenosis evaluation. However, new modalities are having a major impact on the preoperative assessment of carotid stenosis.

Carotid arteriography

Although it provides excellent images of the cervical carotid arteries, carotid arteriography depends heavily on observer interpretation [12•]. To standardize carotid artery measurements from arteriograms, most clinical trials used the ratio of the diameter of the maximal stenosis to that of the distal internal carotid artery (Figure 12.2) [13]. Although not as accurate as direct pathologic examination, standardized measurements may improve precision in describing stenotic lesions at the carotid bifurcation.

Carotid duplex scanning

Duplex scanning has become a widely used, noninvasive tool for screening carotid stenosis [14]. Retrospective reviews comparing arteriography with duplex scanning have yielded specificity ranging from 73% to 95% and sensitivity ranging from 80% to 99% [14–17]. On the basis of these results and the risk of complication associated with arteriography, several authors have suggested that carotid endarterectomy based on carotid duplex scanning alone is reasonable

for selected patients [15,16,18]. However, preliminary data from the Veterans Administration Study and NASCET cast doubt on this recommendation [2••,4••]. The Veterans Administration Study obtained prospective duplex scans and arteriography on all patients. Comparison of these modalities revealed that the accuracy of carotid duplex scanning was only 25% in patients with angiographic stenosis of 30% to 49%, and that stenosis was underestimated in 50% of patients in this range (Figure 12.3). These data suggest that patients with symptoms of cerebral ischemia should not necessarily be included in or excluded from consideration for carotid endarterectomy solely on the basis of duplex examination.

Magnetic resonance imaging

Magnetic resonance (MR) angiography is a powerful, noninvasive imaging technique well suited to the rapid laminar flow of the carotid artery [19•]. Based on standard MR principles, MR angiography uses special imaging coils and protocols for data analysis (eg, time-of-flight analysis). Two-dimensional MR angiography images are reconstructions of a series of thin transverse slices; they are very sensitive for low-flow states but have lower resolution and decreased contrast when flow is parallel to the slice [19•]. Three-dimensional MR angiography provides excellent resolution and high sensitivity to flow in any direction; however, there is poor contrast in low-flow states. Because the use of either image type alone results in problems with interpretation, it is recommendation that both two-and three-dimensional images be obtained for a full evaluation.

Despite its recent introduction, MR angiography

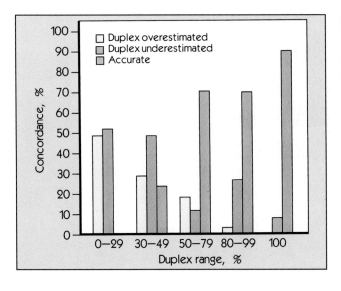

Figure 12.3

Accuracy of the duplex scans compared with angiography in determining carotid stenosis. (*Derived from* the Veterans Administration Symptomatic Stenosis Trial [4••]).

resolution has nearly equaled that of standard angiography for imaging carotid artery stenosis (Figure 12.4) [19•]. A study comparing MR angiography with conventional angiography of the internal carotid artery found a high correlation between the two modalities for determining the degree of stenosis. Differences, when they occurred, generally resulted from overestimation of stenosis by MR angiography. The improving accuracy and inherent safety of MR angiography suggest that it may soon become the imaging modality of choice for the carotid artery.

Transcranial Doppler scanning

Transcranial Doppler (TCD) scanning is a noninvasive modality that uses range-gated ultrasonographic assessments of intracranial artery velocities as an indirect measure of blood flow [20,21•]. Measurements can be obtained from all the large cerebral arteries, providing detailed information on blood flow patterns, such as collateral flow, intracranial stenosis, autoregulation, hemodynamic reserve, and emboli formation [20,21•,22,23].

Because of its ability to accurately determine changes in cerebral blood flow, TCD has been extensively evaluated as an intraoperative monitor during carotid endarterectomy [23]. However, TCD correlation with regional blood flow is not sensitive enough to permit strict ischemic limits to be established. Because TCD shows nearly instantaneous changes in flow, it has the advantage over electroencephalography (EEG) of providing an early indicator of a no-flow state [20]. Although TCD may find a place as an adjunct to intraoperative monitoring, it has not replaced EEG as a monitor of overall perfusion. However, TCD provides an excellent means for detection of intra-arterial emboli, which appear as transient aberrations in the TCD spectral display (Figure 12.5) [21•]. TCD may play a role in carotid surgery, both in the preoperative assessment of patients to localize the site of the embolic source [21•] and in the intraoperative detection of emboli.

Evoked potential monitoring

Intraoperative monitoring of somatosensory evoked potentials (SSEPs) has been evaluated as an alternative to EEG monitoring [24,25•]. Changes in SSEPs are more resistant to ischemia than are changes in EEG and are therefore more specific, although perhaps less sensitive for critical ischemia [25•]. In two clinical studies involving over 1300 patients, SSEP monitoring

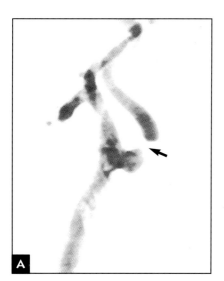
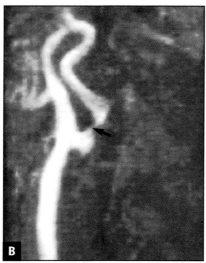

Figure 12.4

Comparison of imaging of the carotid artery bifurcation by magnetic resonance (MR) angiography and conventional angiography. **A,** Conventional angiographic demonstration of the critical stenosis of the internal carotid artery (*arrow*). **B,** Demonstration of the same stenosis (*arrow*) on sagittal three-dimensional MR angiography. (*From* Anderson *et al.* [19•]; with permission.)

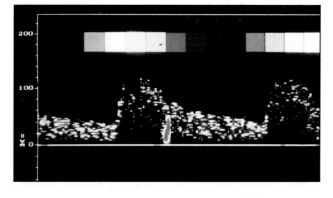

Figure 12.5

Middle cerebral artery embolus detection (*orange*) in a patient who had a cardiac embolic source. (*From* Russell [43]; with permission.)

provided a false-negative rate of 0.1% and a false-positive rate of 0.2% [24,25•]. Corresponding published rates for EEG are 0.9% and 8.1%, respectively [26]. These differences suggest that SSEP monitoring has equivalent sensitivity and greater specificity as compared with EEG in detecting true ischemic events.

PREOPERATIVE ASSESSMENT OF THE PATIENT

The considerable risk of stroke in patients with high-grade carotid stenosis mandates accurate diagnosis of potential causes, although the etiology of cerebral ischemia may be indeterminate in up to 40% of cases [27•]. Careful histories should be taken for all patients, including risk factors, family history, and the nature and timing of the presumed event. In many cases, ischemia from small vessel disease can be differentiated from large vessel pathology on the basis of clinical presentation, although the two disorders frequently coexist [28].

Assessment of perioperative risk

The efficacy of carotid endarterectomy depends on selecting patients with appropriate indications and minimizing perioperative risk. Owing to the concurrence of other significant medical disorders with carotid stenosis, all patients evaluated for carotid endarterectomy require a thorough preoperative medical evaluation (Table 12.2) [28]. Particular attention should be paid to cardiac status; cardiologic consultation for all patients is recommended. The initial car-

diac work-up should include electrocardiography and echocardiography, which also delineate potential cardiogenic sources of emboli [29••]. Medical therapy for existing medical disorders should be maximized prior to surgery. On the basis of medical, neurologic, and angiographic risk factors, patients can be categorized according to perioperative risk to determine those best suited for surgical intervention [30].

SURGICAL TECHNIQUE

Prospective trials have not standardized technique among participating surgeons, and analysis of technical factors associated with complications in these studies is retrospective. Also, the low rate of perioperative complications in those studies reporting detailed surgical results further limits any meaningful comparisons [2••–4••,5•,9]. In general, the surgeon's experience with a specific protocol supersedes other technical considerations in determining perioperative morbidity. With this consideration, the technique described in this section represents a general guideline for the operative and perioperative care of patients having endarterectomy.

Anesthetic considerations and positioning

Most surgeons perform carotid endarterectomy with the patient under general anesthesia, although excellent results have been presented for individual series using regional anesthesia [31]. The principal goal of

Table 12.2
Perioperative risk for carotid endarterectomy*

Grade	Neurologic status[†]	Medical risk[‡]	Angiographic risk[§]	Morbidity/mortality, %
I	Stable	No	No	<1
II	Stable	No	Yes	1.8
III	Stable	Yes	Yes or no	4.0
IV	Unstable	Yes or no	Yes or no	8.5

*Derived from Sundt et al. [30]; with permission.
[†]Neurologic instability includes progressive deficit, an infarct less than 7 days previously, transient ischemic attacks within 24 hours, crescendo transient ischemic attacks.
[‡]Medical risk factors include angina, recent myocardial infarction, congestive heart failure, severe hypertension, advanced chronic obstructive pulmonary disease age greater than 70 years, severe obesity.
[§]Angiographic risk factors include occlusion of opposite internal carotid artery, stenosis of ipsilateral internal carotid artery at siphon, extension of plaque proximally or distally from bifurcation, high cervical bifurcation, intraluminal thrombus.

anesthetic management is to maintain adequate cerebral and myocardial perfusion. Although most volatile anesthetics provide some protection from cerebral ischemia by depressing the cerebral metabolic rate, isoflurane has been shown to be modestly superior in decreasing the frequency of cerebral ischemia during carotid endarterectomy [32]. Although blood pressure should be maintained at or slightly above the patient's awake pressure, cardiac work may increase and lead to myocardial ischemia in some patients. If a barbiturate or etomidate is used to achieve cerebral metabolic protection at the time of carotid cross-clamping, it should be given well in advance to ensure adequate brain tissue levels of the drug [33]. Glucose-containing fluids should be avoided.

The patient is placed in the supine position, with the head turned away from the side of the operation (Figure 12.6). A small roll placed beneath the shoulders puts the neck in slight extension and facilitates full exposure of the carotid bifurcation. The operative field should extend from the mastoid process superiorly to the sternal notch inferiorly; care should be taken during preparation for surgery to avoid dislodging emboli by vigorous scrubbing. Instillation of local anesthetic into the superficial cervical plexus may reduce general anesthetic requirements. If a vein patch is used (*see* below), the ipsilateral leg is prepared for saphenous vein graft.

Operative procedure

The procedure is performed using loupe magnification and a headlight, although the operating microscope is an excellent alternative [33]. An incision is made along the anterior border of the sternocleidomastoid muscle, curving posteriorly toward the mastoid process about 1 cm below the angle of the mandible; this curve provides distal exposure of the internal carotid artery without injuring the mandibular ramus of the facial nerve (Figure 12.6). Meticulous hemostasis is maintained throughout the procedure using bipolar cautery. The platysma is incised and the dissection is carried along the generally avascular plane at the medial border of the sternocleidomastoid muscle. At this point the ansa cervicalis of the cervical plexus is frequently encountered. Although it is safe to section this nerve, we prefer to mobilize it medially to allow medial retraction of the hypoglossal nerve at its junction with the ansa when dissecting the distal internal carotid artery. Beneath the sternocleidomastoid muscle, the internal jugular vein is encountered, and the common facial branch of this vein is ligated and divided. Care must be taken in dissecting the carotid sheath because on rare occasion the vagus nerve is located anterior to the artery. Before manipulating the carotid artery in the region of the bifurca-

tion, 2% lidocaine without epinephrine is instilled into the carotid sinus and along the course of the nerve of Hering to minimize bradycardia and hypotension resulting from stimulation of these structures. The carotid sheath is opened along the anterior surface of the artery inferiorly to the level of the omohyoid muscle. Prior to further dissection, proximal control of the common carotid artery is obtained by carefully dissecting the posterior wall from the underlying vagus nerve and passing a vessel loop. Superiorly, the superior thyroid, external carotid, and internal carotid arteries are dissected in the region of the bifurcation (Figure 12.7).

Dissection is performed distally along the internal carotid artery. Extreme care must be taken to identify the hypoglossal nerve early in dissection because it crosses the distal internal carotid artery. On rare occasions it can be mobilized and gently retracted medially for better distal exposure. The carotid plaque can often be carefully palpated to determine its distal end; usually it extends further along the posterior wall of the artery compared with the anterior wall. Dissection must be carried out at least 1 cm distal to the end of the plaque to allow for posterior wall extension and placement of a shunt if necessary. Circumferential

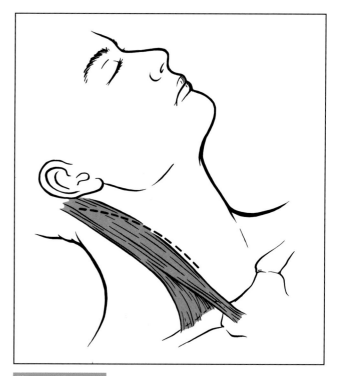

Figure 12.6

Carotid endarterectomy. The patient is in the supine position with the head turned away from the side of the operation. The incision runs along the anterior border of the sternocleidomastoid curving posteriorly approximately 1 cm below the angle of the mandible to avoid injury to the facial nerve. (*From* Ojemann *et al.* [44]; with permission.)

dissection around the internal carotid artery for placement of an umbilical tape is done only at the site of the tape position. A Rummel tourniquet is fashioned by passing the umbilical tapes on the internal carotid and common carotid arteries through a segment of rubber tubing. Dissection is then completed around the external carotid and superior thyroid arteries, which are isolated with vessel loops (Figure 12.7). At this point the anesthesiologist is instructed to give heparin (100 U/kg) as a bolus. The blood pressure is maintained at or slightly above awake baseline and the EEG is examined prior to clamping. The shunt tubing is filled with heparinized saline, clamped to prevent intraluminal bubbles, and compared with the internal carotid artery to ensure proper sizing. Clamps for the major arteries are tentatively placed without closing to ensure proper fit.

At 5 minutes after heparin administration the internal carotid artery is clamped; we prefer to use an aneurysm clip because it has a lower profile and is less traumatic to the vessel than other vascular clamps. The common carotid artery is then clamped using an angled or straight Fogarty Hydrogrip clamp (Baxter V. Mueller, Chicago). The external carotid and superior thyroid arteries are then clamped with aneurysm clips. An arteriotomy is started about 1 cm proximal to the bifurcation in the midline of the common carotid artery (Figure 12.8). The incision is carried through the arterial wall until plaque is encountered, and a smooth plan is developed between the plaque and the artery

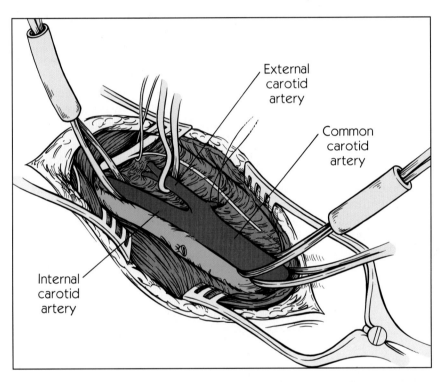

External carotid artery

Common carotid artery

Internal carotid artery

Figure 12.7

After division of the common facial vein, the carotid sheath is opened to expose the common, internal, and external carotid arteries. The hypoglossal nerve at the superior margin of the dissection can be gently retracted medially. (*From* Ojemann *et al.* [44]; with permission.)

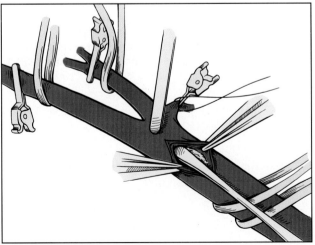

Figure 12.8

Clamps have been applied to the common, internal, and external carotid arteries and the superior thyroid artery. Note the tourniquets on the common carotid artery and internal carotid artery for potential shunt placement. The arteriotomy incision is initiated in the midline of the common carotid artery just below the bifurcation. (*From* Ojemann *et al.* [44]; with permission.)

wall. Some surgeons prefer to include the full thickness of the plaque in the arteriotomy incision; however, we believe that the dissection is more accurate if plaque is removed without being incised at this time. The EEG is then examined to determine whether shunt placement is necessary (*see* below). If no changes have occurred, dissection is carried distally along the plaque using a number 4 Penfield dissector (Codman & Shurtle, Randolph, MA), and the arteriotomy is completed with Potts scissors (Codman & Shurtle; Figure 12.9). The arteriotomy should extend along the anterior midline of the internal carotid artery until normal intima beyond the plaque is reached. Circumferential dissection of the plaque is then accomplished at the proximal end, a curved clamp is placed between the plaque and the artery wall, and the plaque is sharply incised with a scalpel (Figure 12.10). Care must be taken to ensure that the remaining plaque in the common carotid artery has a smooth edge. The plaque is then dissected free from the arterial wall using the Penfield dissector to the bifurcation and into the external carotid artery (Figure 12.10). It is frequently helpful to have the assistant release the external carotid artery clamp temporarily while dissection proceeds up that artery and the plaque is gently torn free from its distal attachment. A critical part of the dissection involves the distal attachment of the plaque to normal intima of the internal carotid artery. If gentle dissection and proximal traction are used, the plaque usually tears away from its distal attachment, leaving a firm, adherent, normal intima (Figure 12.11). If the intima at this site is not adherent, it should be resected or, less commonly, tacked to the arterial wall with a 6-0 proline suture.

Once the plaque is removed, the luminal surface is carefully inspected while the assistant irrigates continuously with heparinized saline. Small bits of debris

apparent during this maneuver should be meticulously removed under magnified vision to create a lumen that is as smooth as possible. The arteriotomy is then closed with a running 6-0 proline suture from the distal to proximal end (Figure 12.12). Extreme care must be taken to approximate the edges with small equivalent bites so that no regions of stenosis are created. Just prior to final suturing at the proximal end of the arteriotomy, the internal carotid artery clamp is briefly released. The resulting backflow of blood ensures that the artery is patent and flushes any residual debris from the lumen. We frequently remove the superior thyroid artery clamp as the final suture is placed to have continuous backflow of blood and prevent entraining of air into the lumen. The clamps are then removed in the following order: external carotid artery, common carotid artery, and internal carotid artery. Removal in this order ensures that any potential embolic material will be flushed into the external artery circulation. The arteriotomy is covered with oxidized cellulose and gentle pressure is applied to the wound with a sponge for about 1 minute. Meticulous hemostasis is maintained during closure; occasionally a small drain is placed in the superficial wound.

Intraoperative monitoring and shunt use

Intraoperative monitoring provides an assessment of cerebral blood flow during endarterectomy and may facilitate the decision of whether to use a shunt during carotid cross-clamping. Direct measurement of cerebral blood flow using diffusion modalities such as xenon-133 are cumbersome and require special operating room facilities. EEG is widely available and reflects diminished hemispheric cerebral blood flow, but may not reflect regional ischemia or embolic events [34]. SSEP monitoring appears to be as sensitive

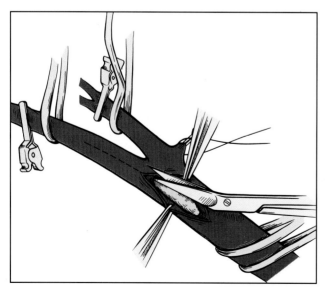

Figure 12.9

The arteriotomy is extended distally in the midline of the internal carotid artery using Potts scissors (Codman & Shurtle, Randolph, MA). The incision is continued until normal intima is encountered on the anterior wall of the artery. Plaque will usually extend slightly more distally on the posterior wall of the artery. (*From* Ojemann *et al.* [44]; with permission.)

but more specific in detecting true ischemia [25•]. Although internal carotid artery stump pressure is widely employed, it correlates poorly with cerebral blood flow and is not recommended as a sole measure of intraoperative monitoring [35]. Intraoperative monitoring demonstrates significant reductions in cerebral blood flow during carotid cross-clamping in 10% to 24% of cases depending on the modality used [35]. Presumably these patients would be at risk for hemodynamic ischemic infarction during cross-clamping, although short-acting barbiturates may attenuate cerebral metabolic demands at this time [33].

The use of a shunt during carotid endarterectomy is controversial, with proponents of no shunting [33], uniform shunting, and selective shunting on the basis of monitoring [34]. The potential disadvantages of shunts are dislodging of embolic material during placement, the necessity of additional distal exposure, and limited visualization at the critical distal margin of the plaque. For these reasons, we restrict use of a shunt to situations in which cerebral ischemia is demonstrated by EEG or other monitoring techniques. EEG changes occurring at the time of carotid artery cross-clamping (manifested by a decrease in higher

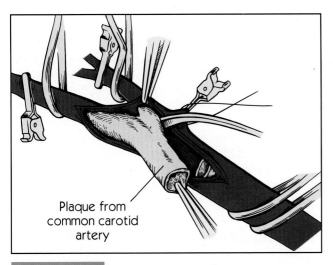

Figure 12.10

The plaque has been incised in the common carotid artery proximal to the bifurcation and dissection is carried distally into the internal and external carotid arteries using a Penfield dissector (Codman & Shurtle, Randolph, MA). A smooth plane can be developed between plaque and artery wall that facilitates removal. (*From* Ojemann *et al.* [44]; with permission.)

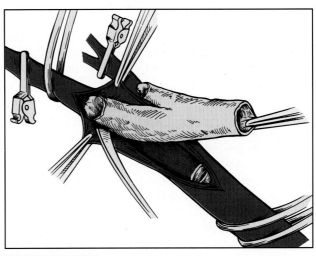

Figure 12.11

The distal margin of the plaque in the internal carotid artery is gently dissected from its attachment to normal intima on the posterior wall of the artery. Care must be taken to avoid creating an intimal flap at this site. (*From* Ojemann *et al.* [44]; with permission.)

Figure 12.12

The arteriotomy is closed using a running 6-0 proline suture. Care must be taken to ensure a precise approximation of the edges without compromising the lumen at any point. (*From* Ojemann *et al.* [44]; with permission.)

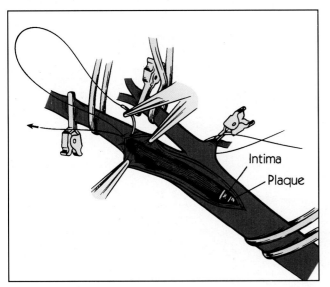

frequencies or in amplitude) will occasionally resolve spontaneously with elevation of the blood pressure. When changes persist more than 60 to 90 seconds, the arteriotomy is extended through the plaque along its entire length using Potts scissors to expose the normal intima of the distal internal carotid artery. The distal end of the saline-filled and clamped shunt tubing is carefully inserted into the internal carotid artery, which is briefly opened to permit shunt passage and then secured in place using a tourniquet. Backflow is ascertained by briefly removing the shunt clamp, and the proximal shunt is then inserted into the common carotid artery in a similar fashion (Figure 12.13). The shunt clamp is removed and flow through the shunt is documented using Doppler ultrasound. The midportion of the shunt is then retracted to the side to enable plaque removal, as described above. At the final stage of arteriotomy suturing, the shunt is removed by reversing the steps listed above for insertion.

POSTOPERATIVE CARE AFTER CAROTID ENDARTERECTOMY

The attention to detail necessary during the endarterectomy procedure must be maintained throughout the postoperative period because many complications occur during this time. All patients should be monitored in an intensive care unit for 24 to 48 hours after the procedure, with sequential neurologic examinations by nursing staff. Blood pressure should be rigidly controlled in the approximate preoperative range with continuous monitoring via arterial catheter [36]; hemodynamic parameters are similarly monitored by a Swan-Ganz catheter in selected patients. Intravenous fluids, pressors, inotropes, and antihypertensive agents are routinely administered to maximize these indices. Postoperative electrocardio-gram and chest radiographs should be performed for all patients. Urine output and serum electrolytes are monitored during the period of intensive care. The cervical wound is sequentially examined for enlargement or superficial bleeding. Aspirin therapy is initiated immediately after surgery and stable patients are generally discharged home within 3 to 5 days.

ALTERNATIVES TO CAROTID ENDARTERECTOMY

Medical therapy

Aside from risk reduction, the mainstay of medical therapy for carotid stenosis is aspirin [37]. The use of aspirin is based on several studies that reported reduced stroke risk in symptomatic patients [37,38]. However, most of these studies included myocardial infarction, other vascular events, or death as endpoints. When analyzed for stroke only, the effect of aspirin in these studies was found to be marginal. Ticlopidine, a new antiplatelet agent, was shown in a prospective trial to be slightly better than aspirin in reducing stroke incidence (the ticlopidine group experienced a 10% reduction versus 13% for the aspirin group) [38].

Percutaneous transluminal angioplasty

Percutaneous transluminal angioplasty has been applied to the treatment of carotid stenosis [39,40, 41•]. One review summarized the published results of this technique as applied to the carotid artery [41•]. Of 177 carotid arteries in which percutaneous transluminal angioplasty was attempted, the procedure succeeded in 93% of cases, with only 1.7% major complications. However, reduction in the risk of subsequent

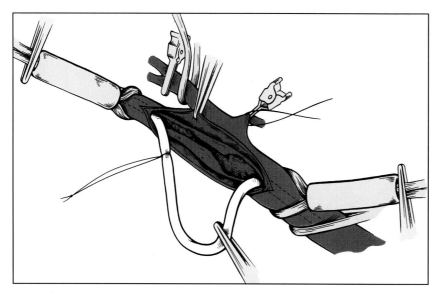

Figure 12.13

An intraluminal shunt is secured in the common and internal carotid arteries using tourniquets. The shunt tubing is retracted laterally during the plaque dissection. (*From* Ojemann *et al.* [44]; with permission.)

stroke and long-term patency have yet to be established by carefully controlled prospective trials. Transluminal angioplasty may play a role in the therapy of intracranial arterial stenosis not amenable to surgical treatment [42•].

CONCLUSIONS

Data from the recent trials for symptomatic carotid stenosis suggest that patients with transient ischemic attacks, amaurosis fugax, or small completed stroke ipsilateral to significant (more than 70%) carotid stenosis should be considered for carotid endarterectomy. The high rate of stroke in close proximity to presenting symptoms mandates that referral and evaluation should proceed with urgency. Both the Veterans Administration Trial and NASCET found inaccuracy of duplex ultrasonography in detecting high-grade carotid stenosis, suggesting that symptomatic patients should have definitive assessment by angiography (although MR angiography may become the assessment modality of choice in the near future). The benefit of surgery for patients with asymptomatic carotid stenosis or for symptomatic patients with intermediate (30% to 70%) degrees of carotid stenosis has not been fully determined. These patients should be carefully evaluated for endarterectomy or referred to ongoing randomized trials.

A growing consensus suggests that all surgical procedures should be tested according to the rigorous standards applied to new drugs. However, surgical procedures are not drugs and cannot necessarily be studied according to the same criteria. Clinical decision-making in surgery is a multifactorial process involving both subjective and objective evaluations, which are difficult to quantitate and standardize. Other factors, including referral patterns, fiscal concerns, and local variations in treatment can confound the best clinical trial design. Most important, there remains the profound ethical concern regarding the withholding of previously accepted therapy from one group of patients in a randomized trial of a surgical procedure. Nevertheless, the clinical trial has become the means by which existing and new surgical procedures may be judged in the near future, and the results of such trials may dictate surgical practice to some extent. For these reasons it is important that physicians become familiar with the methodology of clinical trials and examine these studies in a critical light.

REFERENCES AND RECOMMENDED READING

Papers of particular interest, published within the annual period of review, have been highlighted as:
• Of special interest
•• Of outstanding interest

1. Brook RH, Park RE, Chassin MR, et al.: Predicting the appropriate use of carotid endarterectomy, upper gastrointestinal endoscopy, and coronary angiography. N Engl J Med 1990, 323:1173–1177.

2. •• North American Symptomatic Carotid Endarterectomy Trial Collaborators: Beneficial effect of carotid endarterectomy in symptomatic patients with high-grade stenosis. N Engl J Med 1991, 325:445–453.
This prospective, randomized, multicenter trial for patients with symptomatic carotid stenosis showed a prominent reduction in stroke among patients receiving carotid endarterectomy for high-grade (70% to 99%) stenosis.

3. •• European Carotid Surgery Trialists' Collaborative Group: MRC European carotid surgery trial: interim results for symptomatic patients with severe (70-99%) or with mild (0-29%) carotid stenosis. Lancet 1991, 337:1235–1243.
This prospective randomized multicenter trial for patients with symptomatic carotid stenosis showed a prominent reduction in stroke among patients receiving carotid endarterectomy for high-grade (70% to 99%) stenosis, but no benefit for patients with mild (less than 30%) stenosis.

4. •• Mayberg MR, Wilson SE, Yatsu F, et al.: V.A. Cooperative Studies Program #309: the role of carotid endarterectomy in preventing stroke from asymptomatic carotid stenosis. JAMA 1991, 266:3289–3294.
This prospective randomized multicenter trial for patients with symptomatic carotid stenosis showed a prominent reduction in stroke among patients receiving carotid endarterectomy for 50% to 99% stenosis.

5. • The CASANOVA Study Group: Carotid surgery versus medical therapy in asymptomatic carotid stenosis. Stroke 1991, 22:1229–1235.
This prospective trial for patients with asymptomatic stenosis showed no benefit for those receiving carotid endarterectomy. However, the unusual study design prevents any definitive conclusions.

6. Fields WS, Maslenikov V, Meyer JS, et al.: Joint study of extracranial arterial occlusion: V: progress report of prognosis following surgery or nonsurgical treatment for transient cerebral ischemic attacks and cervical carotid artery lesions. JAMA 1970, 211:1993–2003.

7. Whisnant JP, Matsomoto N, Elveback LR: Transient cerebral ischemic attacks in a community. *Mayo Clin Proc* 1973, 48:194–198.

8. • Barnett HJM, Barnes RW, Clagett GP, *et al.*: Symptomatic carotid artery stenosis: a solvable problem. *Stroke* 1992, 23:1048–1053.

The symptomatic trials have demonstrated clear benefit of carotid endarterectomy for high-grade stenosis. However, the result for intermediate-grade stenosis is pending completion of NASCET and the European Carotid Surgery Trial. Assuming benefit of surgery for intermediate stenosis is inappropriate and jeopardizes completion of the symptomatic trials.

9. Towne JB, Weiss DG, Hobson RW: First place report of cooperative Veterans Administration Asymptomatic Carotid Stenosis Study: operative morbidity and mortality. *J Vasc Surg* 1990, 11:252–259.

10. A Veterans Administration Cooperative Study: Role of carotid endarterectomy in asymptomatic carotid stenosis. *Stroke* 1986, 17:534–539.

11. The Asymptomatic Carotid Atherosclerosis Study Group: Study design for randomized prospective trial of carotid endarterectomy for symptomatic atherosclerosis. *Stroke* 1989, 20:844–849.

12. • Estol C, Claassen D, Hirsch W, *et al.*: Correlative angiographic and pathologic findings in the diagnosis of ulcerated plaque in the carotid artery. *Arch Neurol* 1991, 48:692–694.

Comparison of angiographic findings with direct pathologic analysis of specimens from carotid endarterectomy demonstrated an overall accuracy of only 61% for angiography.

13. Barnett HJM: Stroke prevention by surgery for symptomatic disease in carotid territory. *Neurol Clin* 1992, 10:281–292.

14. Chant ADB, Thompson JF, Stranks GJ, *et al.*: Impact of duplex scanning on carotid endarterectomy. *Br J Surg* 1990, 77:188–189.

15. Farmilo RW, Scott DJA, Cole SEA, *et al.*: Role of duplex scanning in the selection of patients for carotid endarterectomy. *Br J Surg* 1990, 77:388–390.

16. Dawson DL, Zierler E, Kohler TR: Role of arteriography in the preoperative evaluation of carotid artery disease. *Am J Surg* 1991, 161:619–624.

17. Poindexter JM, Shah PM, Clauss RH, *et al.*: The clinical utility of carotid duplex scanning. *J Cardiovasc Surg (Torino)* 1991, 32:64–68.

18. Gelabert HA, Moore WS: Carotid endarterectomy without angiography. *Surg Clin North Am* 1990, 70:213–223.

19. • Anderson CM, Saloner D, Lee RE, *et al.*: Assessment of carotid artery stenosis by MR angiography: comparison with X-ray angiography and color-coded Doppler ultrasound. *AJNR* 1992, 13:989–1003.

Magnetic resonance angiography correlates well with conventional x-ray angiography, but tends to slightly overestimate the degree of stenosis. However, because of better spatial resolution and vessel wall imaging, MR angiography has advantages over conventional x-ray angiography in some cases.

20. Ringelstein EB, Otis SM: Physiological testing of vasomotor reserve. In *Transcranial Doppler*. Edited by Newell D, Aslid R. New York: Raven Press; 1992:83–100.

21. • Lash S, Newell D, Mayberg MM, *et al.*: Artery to artery cerebral emboli detection with transcranial Doppler: analysis of eight cases. *J Stroke Cerebrovasc Dis* 1993, 3:15–22.

The site of origin for embolic sources in the craniocervical circulation was determined using transcranial Doppler.

22. Aslid R: Developments and principles of transcranial Doppler. In *Transcranial Doppler*. Edited by Newell D, Aslid R. New York: Raven Press; 1992:1–8.

23. Aslid R: Cerebral hemodynamics. In *Transcranial Doppler*. Edited by Newell D, Aslid R. New York: Raven Press; 1992:49–56.

24. Haupt WF, Horsch S: Evoked potential monitoring in carotid surgery: a review of 994 cases. *Neurology* 1992, 42:835–838.

25. • Amantini A, Bartelli M, de Scisciolo G, *et al.*: Monitoring of somatosensory evoked potentials during carotid endarterectomy. *J Neurol* 1992, 239:241–247.

Somatosensory evoked potentials were obtained on 312 patients during carotid endarterectomy. Shunts were placed in 28 patients because of marked reduction in SSEPs. None of the patients who were not shunted developed postoperative neurologic deficits. However, four patients in the shunted group developed changes in SSEPs that persisted. All four patients had postoperative deficits. These data demonstrate that SSEP monitoring is a highly sensitive yet specific modality for detecting ischemic events during carotid endarterectomy.

26. Chiappa KH, Burke SR, Young RR: Results of electroencephalographic monitoring during 367 carotid endarterectomies. *Stroke* 1979, 10:381–388.

27. • Lanzino G, Andreoli A, Di Pasquale G, *et al.*: Etiopathogenesis and prognosis of cerebral ischemia in young adults: a survey of 155 treated patients. *Acta Neurol Scand* 1991, 84:321–325.

The cause of stroke was investigated in 155 young adults. Atherosclerosis was the most common cause (31%), followed by cardioembolic disorder (5.1%), spontaneous arterial dissection (4.5%), migraine (4%), puerperium (2.6%), and cervical trauma (2.6%). The etiology of the stroke remained obscure in 40% of cases.

28. Tegeler CH, Shi F, Morgan T: Carotid stenosis in lacunar stroke. *Stroke* 1991, 22:1124–1128.

29. •• Albers GW, Sherman DG, Gress DR, *et al.*: Stroke prevention in nonvalvular atrial fibrillation: a review of prospective randomized trials. *Ann Neurol* 1991, 30:511–518.

In three prospective randomized trials, anticoagulation with warfarin resulted in a reduction in stroke with only a slight risk of bleeding. One of the studies also demonstrated benefit with aspirin.

30. Sundt TM, Sandok BA, Whisnant JP: Carotid endarterectomy: complications and preoperative assessment of risk. *Mayo Clin Proc* 1975, 50:301–306.

31. Donato AT, Hill SL: Carotid arterial surgery using local anesthesia: a private retrospective study. *Am Surg* 1992, 58:446–450.

32. Michenfelder JD, Stundt TM, Fode N, *et al.*: Isoflurane when compared to enflurane and halothane decreases the frequency of cerebral ischemia during carotid endarterectomy. *Anesthesiology* 1987, 67:336–340.

33. Spetzler RF, Martin N, Hadley MN, *et al.*: Microsurgical endarterectomy under barbiturate protection: a prospective study. *J Neurosurg* 1986, 65:63–73.

34. Sundt TM: The ischemic tolerance of neural tissue and the need for monitoring and selective shunting during carotid endarterectomy. *Stroke* 1983, 14:93–98.

35. Sundt TM Jr, Sharbrough FW, Piepgras DG, *et al.*: Correlation of cerebral blood flow and electroencephalographic changes during carotid endarterectomy, with results of surgery and hemodynamics of cerebral ischemia. *Mayo Clin Proc* 1981, 56:533–543.

36. Towne JB, Bernhard VM: The relationship of post-operative hypertension to complications following carotid endarterectomy. *Surgery* 1980, 88:575–580.

37. Canadian Cooperative Stroke Study Group: A randomized trial of aspirin and sulfinpyrazone in threatened stroke. *N Engl J Med* 1978, 299:53–59.

38. Hass WK, Easton JD, Adams HP Jr, *et al.*: A randomized trial comparing ticlopidine hydrochloride with aspirin for the prevention of stroke in high-risk patients. *N Engl J Med* 1989, 321:501–507.

39. Brown MM, Butler P, Gibbs J, *et al.*: Feasibility of percutaneous transluminal angioplasty for carotid artery stenosis. *J Neurol Psychiatry* 1990, 53:238–243.

40. Vitek JJ: Angioplasty of arteries in the carotid territory. *AJNR* 1991, 12:1024.

41. • Kachel R, Basche S, Heerklotz I, *et al.*: Percutaneous transluminal angioplasty (PTA) of supra-aortic arteries especially the internal carotid artery. *Neuroradiology* 1991, 33:191–194.

Percutaneous transluminal angioplasty was performed on 105 patients with stenosis of supra-aortic arteries, 43 of which were carotid arteries. Overall there were only four minor complications. Of patients with carotid artery stenosis, 38 of 43 underwent successfully dilation.

42. • Rostomily RC, Mayberg MR, Eskridge J, *et al.*: Resolution of petrous internal carotid artery stenosis after transluminal angioplasty. *J Neurosurg* 1992, 76:520–523.

Successful percutaneous transluminal angioplasty of a severe stenosis of the petrous internal carotid artery with 2-year follow-up.

43. Russell D: The detection of cerebral emboli using Doppler ultrasound. In *Transcranial Doppler*. Edited by Newell D, Aslid R. New York: Raven Press; 1992:207–213.

44. Ojemann RG, Crowell RM, Heros R: *Surgical Management of Cerebrovascular Disease*. Baltimore: Williams & Wilkins; 1988.

Chapter 13

Cervical Spine Fusion

Volker K.H. Sonntag
Curtis A. Dickman

During the last few years, several operative techniques for internal fixation and new materials and instrumentation for cervical spine fusion have been reported. Modifications of fusion constructs and improvements in techniques have developed. Rigid cervical internal fixation with screws and screw plates has been refined and improved. Several reports emphasized biomechanical characteristics of fixations and compared techniques for internal fixation of the cervical spine. A rapid growth in clinical and basic scientific data for cervical fusion has occurred. Metal and titanium have been used in a variety of implants. The success of surgery ultimately depends on the use of autograft or allograft bone for the permanent fusion process. Multiple techniques for cervical spine fusion are discussed here, including the indications, advantages, and disadvantages.

Halifax interlaminar clamps

Technique

Halifax clamps are inserted by a posterior midline cervical exposure [1,2•]. A threaded clamp, an unthreaded clamp, and a screw are assembled and mounted on a clamp applicator forceps (Figure 13.1). Laminotomies are performed at the levels adjacent to the fixated levels so the clamps can fit into place. This approach is necessary because of the normal shingling and overlap of the cervical vertebrae. The ligamentum flavum must also be removed to avoid stenosis from the clamps. Bone struts are recommended (bicortical struts or wedge grafts at C1-2 or interspinous H grafts at subaxial levels) to prevent hyperextension and add stability to the construct.

The clamps are placed bilaterally and tightened in an alternating fashion with a 90°-angled locking adjustment wrench. Equal clamp tension should be achieved bilaterally. The clamps should be placed into position bilaterally then tightened sequentially. Fully tightening a unilateral clamp interferes with placement of the contralateral clamp if an alternating method is not used. Bilateral clamps are recommended to achieve rotational stabilization. The clamps must be inspected to ensure that they engage the lamina properly and are seated correctly.

Analysis

Aldrich and colleagues [1] treated 21 patients with titanium Halifax clamps to affix one or two motion segments between C-1 and C-7. Autogenous bone grafts were used to promote fusion. All cases attained fusion. No complications or mechanical failures occurred. However, the follow-up of the patients was short (average, 9 months). The authors concluded that the magnetic resonance imaging–compatible Halifax clamps produced minimal imaging artifact and provided an excellent fusion rate.

Halifax interlaminar clamps should be used with bone grafts to provide supplemental fixation and promote bone fusion. Halifax clamps do not rigidly fix the vertebrae in all directions of motion. These clamps serve as a compressive posterior cervical tension band that prevents flexion but poorly prevents

hyperextension. Bilateral clamps must be used to prevent rotation. Strut grafts or an H graft can prevent overreduction and inhibit extension. Bilateral Halifax clamps at C1-2 provide fixation comparable to the Brooks wire technique for atlantoaxial fusion [3••]. If multiple motion segments are spanned, no segmental fixation is achieved at intermediate levels.

Halifax clamps may be less effective for atlantoaxial arthrodesis than for other cervical levels because of the prominent rotation at C1-2 [2•]. Moskovich and Crockard [2•] placed wedges of bone beneath Halifax clamps at C1-2 to limit rotation and hyperextension in 25 patients. Fusion occurred in 20 patients (80%) within 3 months of surgery. Five patients required revision; three had nonunions, and two had early clamp failure. Failures were due to clamp loosening. This fusion rate is slightly lower compared with wiring techniques for atlantoaxial fusion [4•]. Clamp loosening is a problem that requires attention with a modified clamp design.

Rheumatoid patients have a high nonunion rate with this technique [2•]. Similar to other techniques of C1-2 fusion, when pseudarthrosis occurs, it is usually found between the bone graft and the posterior ring of C-1 [2•,4•]. Halifax clamps have the advantage of avoiding sublaminar wire passage. They cannot be used if the laminae are fractured. When the anterior and middle columns of the cervical spine are disrupted, Halifax clamps do not stabilize the spine adequately. The clamps can also reduce the bone surface area available for fusion.

Wiring and bone grafting for posterior atlantoaxial fusion

Technique

The interspinous method of posterior atlantoaxial arthrodesis has been developed as an alternative to the Brooks and Gallie techniques of fusion (Figure 13.2A) [4•,5]. This technique uses a curved, autologous, bicortical, iliac crest strut graft that is positioned between the posterior arches of C-1 and C-2 and secured in place by wire or multistranded cable. The bone graft is compressed between C-1 and C-2.

A routine posterior cervical exposure is performed. All soft tissue is removed from C-1 and C-2. The inferior surface of the posterior ring of C-1 and the supe-

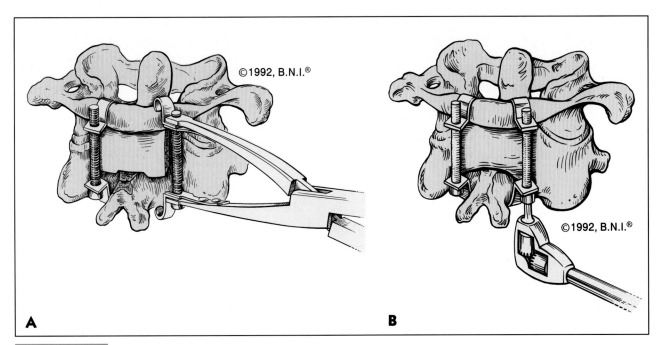

Figure 13.1

A, Halifax clamp placement at C1-2. A bicortical strut graft is positioned between C-1 and C-2 to prevent overreduction, add stability, and promote fusion. The clamps and screws are pre-

assembled and mounted on the clamp applicator forceps. **B,** A 90°-angle locking adjustment wrench is used to tighten the clamps sequentially and alternatingly.

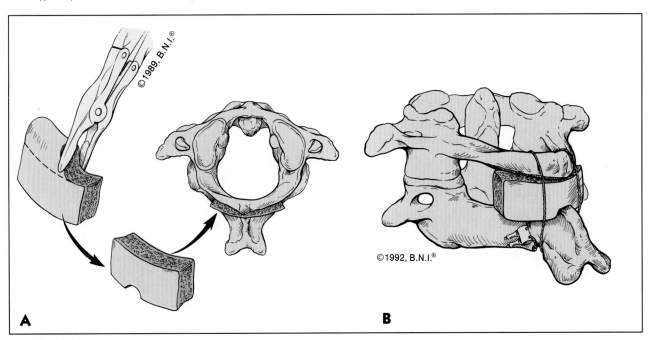

Figure 13.2

A, Autologous bone from the iliac crest is fashioned into a curved bicortical strut that is precisely fitted between C-1 and C-2. A notch is placed under the graft to fit the spinous process of C-2. **B,** The strut graft is compressed between C-1 and C-2. A braided

cable fixates the graft and prevents anterior and posterior displacement. (*Modified from* Sonntag and Dickman [5] and Dickman *et al.* [4●]; with permission.)

rior surface of the laminae of C-2 (areas of contact of C-1, C-2, and the graft) are decorticated with a drill or Kerrison rongeur. The sloping upper edge of the C-2 spinous process is leveled with a Leksell rongeur. Notches are made beneath the inferior edges of the C-2 spinous process–laminar junctions to seat the wire. The inferior edge of the bicortical strut graft is notched to match the contour of the C-2 spinous process.

A looped wire or braided cable is halved and passed sublaminar beneath the arch of C-1 directed cephalad. The graft is positioned between C-1 and C-2 as a strut. The loop is then passed behind the graft and fixed beneath the spinous process of C-2. The free ends of wire are passed anterior to the graft and beneath the spinous process of C-2. Accurate sizing of the bone graft prevents overreduction. As the wire is tightened, the graft is compressed between the posterior arches of C-1 and C-2 and is affixed anteriorly and posteriorly by wire (Figure 13.2*B*).

Analysis

Among 35 patients with various pathologies, a 97% union rate was achieved [4•]. Examination after a mean postoperative follow-up of 33.7 months revealed that 34 patients had a stable construct. There were 31 osseous unions, three fibrous unions, and one nonunion. The interspinous method of posterior atlantoaxial arthrodesis appears safe and technically simple and compares favorably with the fusion rates from other posterior atlantoaxial fusion techniques. The Gallie fusion cannot be used with posterior C-1 subluxations, but the interspinous method can. Compared with the Brooks fusion, multiple sublaminar wire passages, which carry a risk of neurologic injury, are avoided.

OCCIPITOCERVICAL FUSION

Threaded Steinman pin fusion

Technique

A wide-diameter, *threaded* Steinman pin (5/32-in diameter) is bent into a U shape, and secondary curves are placed to fit the occipitocervical contour. The pin is wired to the cervical lamina or facets and to the occiput (Figure 13.3) [5,6].

A routine posterior cervical exposure is performed. Bur holes are placed in the occiput. The posterior rim of the foramen magnum is enlarged with a Kerrison rongeur. The laminae are notched, and the ligamentum flavum is removed completely to facilitate sub-

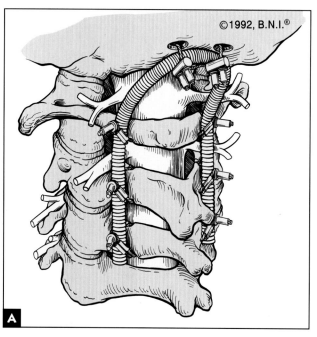

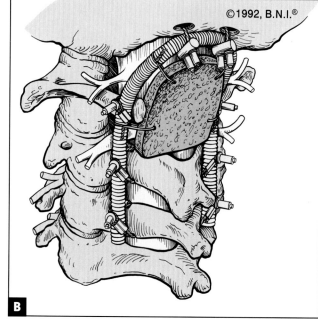

Figure 13.3

A, A 5/32-in diameter threaded Steinman pin is wired to the occiput and cervical laminae or facets. The pin should have smooth contours, fit precisely against the bone surfaces, and not extend across unfused segments. Bone grafts are used to promote fusion. **B,** A plate of cortical bone is wired to the Steinman pin after a posterior decompression. This bone plate provides a template for the fusion and preserves the decompression site. (*Modified from* Dickman *et al.* [6]; with permission.)

laminar wire passage. Wire or braided cables are passed between bur holes and the foramen magnum and sublaminar at the cervical levels to be fused. The Steinman pin should be contoured smoothly and should fit precisely against the bone surfaces. Sharp angles create stress risers where the pin may fracture. The pin is secured with wire and should be fixed rigidly against the bone. Gaps between the pin and bone result in inadequate fixation. The articular surfaces of the facets are roughened, the bone surfaces are decorticated, and autogenous bone grafts are added to promote fusion. A plate of cortical iliac crest bone can be fixated to the central portion of the pin to provide a template for the fusion. If a laminectomy has been performed, the pin can be wired to the facets.

Analysis

The wide-diameter threaded Steinman pin allows rigid fixation of the occipitocervical region and avoids settling or vertical translation of the construct. This technique was developed as an alternative to the Luque rectangle and to onlay graft or bone strut techniques. The smooth surfaces of the Luque rectangles can allow the construct to settle. Rib grafts or iliac crest bone grafts wired to the occiput and cervical laminae provide less rigid fixation. The grafts can fracture if enough force is applied. The Steinman pin technique must be used with supplemental bone grafts to promote osseous union. Among 28 patients treated with the Steinman pin fusion technique, 25 developed successful fusions with an average follow-up of 30 months.

Occipitocervical screw plate

Technique

A standard midline posterior cervical exposure is performed. Screws are placed into the facet joints at C1-2 using a technique originally described by Magerl and Seemann [7••]. These screws affix an inverted Y plate to the cervical spine and rigidly fixate C1-2. The upper limb of the plate is screwed into the midline of the occiput near the nuchal line. The screw-plate fixation is supplemented with autogenous bone grafts for fusion (Figure 13.4).

Analysis

Grob and colleagues [8•] reported their preliminary results with this screw-plate technique for occipitocervical fusion. Of 14 patients with occipitocervical instability, all achieved a solid fusion without major complications. Screw plates can provide rigid fixation if the bone is not osteoporotic. Posterior transarticular atlantoaxial facet screws provide the most rigid fixation available for C1-2 immobilization [3••,9,10].

This technique is more technically demanding than wire techniques. Surgeons must first be comfortable using drills and screws safely [11]. The thickness of the occipital bone must be measured individually to avoid intradural penetration. Short screws, which have relatively limited pullout strengths [11], are place in the occiput. Although this preliminary report is promising, more experience is needed with this technique before sound conclusions can be drawn. This technique is especially useful when a prior cervical laminectomy has been performed.

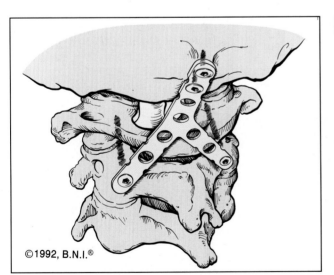

©1992, B.N.I.®

Figure 13.4

An inverted Y-shaped steel bone reconstruction plate is fixed with screws to the occiput and with C1-2 facet screws to the spine. (*Modified from* Dickman *et al.* [11]; with permission.)

WIRE FIXATION FOR POSTERIOR CERVICAL FUSION

Multistranded cables

Technique

Multistranded, flexible, braided cables have been introduced as an alternative to monofilament wire for spinal fixation (Figure 13.5) [12•,13]. The cables consist of two braided, 49-strand cables made of stainless steel or titanium. The proximal ends of the cables have a malleable blunt leader. The distal end has a small islet. When the multistranded flexible cables are placed, the tip of the leader wire is cut. The remaining leader is passed through the loop or eyelet in the cable, to form a noose. The free end of the cable is threaded into a crimp, held by the crimper device, and fed into the locking gear. The cable is tightened using a torque wrench. The wrench is preset to the desired tension (8 to 10 in-lbs is generally recommended). The crimp is fixated, and excess cable is cut flush with the crimp.

Analysis

Flexibility of the cable, excellent strength, and precise adjustment of the tension provide significant advantages compared with the monofilament wires [12•, 13]. Overtightening must be avoided so the cable does not pull through soft or osteoporotic bone. The crimp system irreversibly fixates the cable. If the spinal alignment is changed after the crimp is affixed, the cable may loosen. If the cable loosens after the crimp has been placed, the cable must be removed, and a new cable must be placed.

Stainless steel, multistranded cables are biomechanically superior to monofilament steel wire and titanium cables (for static and fatigue strength and for flexibility) [12•]. Biomechanical testing of Songer cables reveals that the yield strength of a single stainless steel cable is 2.85 to 2.94 times greater than that of a stainless steel wire of similar diameter [12•]. In fatigue tests, stainless steel cables require six to 22 times more cycles to cause failure than monofilament steel wire [12•]. Titanium multistranded cables are not as strong as stainless steel cables and can fail under high loads because of crimp failure. Titanium cables are comparable in strength to monofilament wire.

Braided cables are flexible, which allows the cable to conform to the undersurface of the laminae. The flexibility of the cable may help prevent neural injury during wire passage and tightening or during wire removal. The stiff, monofilament leader wire attached to the cables, however, can still potentially cause neural injury. The leader wire should be bent into a J shape for sublaminar passage. A preliminary surgical report of the use of sublaminar braided cables was favorable [12•].

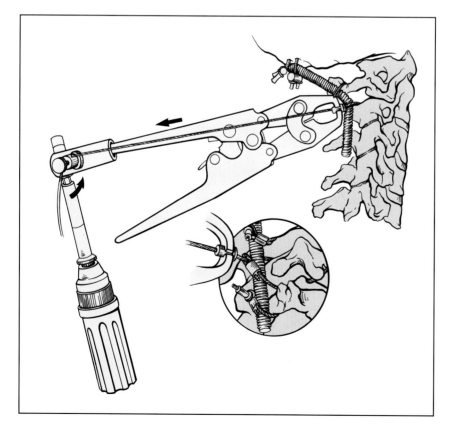

Figure 13.5

Braided, multistranded cables are threaded through a crimp, and the tension in the cable is adjusted with a torque wrench or tensioner device. The crimper is squeezed to fixate the crimp, and the cable is trimmed flush with the crimp (**inset**).

Wire without bone grafts for cervical fractures

Technique

A retrospective report evaluated posterior wiring without bone grafts for traumatic flexion injuries of the middle and lower cervical spine [14]. Patients had fractures of the facets or vertebral bodies associated with minimal deformity. Among 34 patients, three died postoperatively, and one was lost to follow-up. One patient required reoperation for early failure after redislocation from wire fracturing the spinous process. Posterior interspinous wiring was sufficient to allow healing in the remaining cases. The authors proposed that internal fixation alone was sufficient to allow certain cervical fractures to heal and to cause spontaneous fusion. Eight patients had late wire breakage (mean follow-up, 38 months); however, no patients had late spinal instability. Although wire fatigues with time, it can provide immediate internal stability during the time of osseous healing in selected cases.

Analysis

This technique is applicable only to a restricted subset of patients without neural compression or major spinal deformity. Obviously the posterior elements of the vertebrae (ie, lamina, spinous process, facets) have to be intact for wire application. Patients with major spinal deformities that have loss of architectural and structural support need supplemental reconstruction with bone grafts in addition to stabilization. Collapse of the vertebral bodies or anterior neural compression requires an anterior operative approach. Posterior wiring without grafts may be acceptable for facet fractures or vertebral body fractures associated with minimal deformity. These fractures heal satisfactorily with immobilization. Fractures associated with three-column ligament disruption or loss of architectural support (ie, major vertebral body collapse) should have bone graft added to reconstruct and fuse the injured segments. The patients in this series could also have healed satisfactorily without any surgery with just a halo brace.

TECHNIQUES OF SCREW FIXATION FOR THE CERVICAL SPINE

Overview and theory

Screw fixation techniques have been used extensively for long bone fractures and now have become popular for spinal fixation [11,15–25]. Titanium or stainless steel screws have been developed for rigid internal spinal fixation. Other alloys are being investigated. Screws may be used to fixate fractures directly, to reduce fracture fragments, and to fixate plates to the spine. Instrumentation and techniques for spinal screw placement have evolved rapidly.

Screw characteristics are divided into non–self-tapping screws and self-tapping screws [11]. These types differ primarily by the design of the screw threads and the methods of insertion. Self-tapping screws are sharp and have wide threads that can be inserted into a pilot hole without tapping the bone. Self-tapping screws are used in cancellous bone. Non–self-tapping screws have duller, narrower threads and are used for cortical bone fixation. The pilot hole must be tapped to cut threads into the bone before the non–self-tapping screw is inserted.

Lag screws place bone fragments under compression and thereby facilitate healing by restoring structural continuity of bone fragments [11]. The threads of the lag screw engage the distal bone fragment but not the proximal bone fragment and, under these circumstances, the bone fragments can be reduced and compressed. As the screw is tightened, a lag effect (ie, compression of the distal fragment) is generated as long as the functioning screw threads do not cross the fracture line. Screw purchase in the proximal bone is avoided by one of two mechanisms. Either the proximal screw shaft must have no threads, or the hole in the proximal bone must be drilled wider than the major screw diameter. The latter approach is useful with fully threaded screws. Such a wide proximal hole is called the *gliding hole.*

Cannulated screw systems consist of a long Kirschner wire and hollow instruments (eg, drills, taps, screws, and screw drivers) [11,18]. The Kirschner wire serves as a guide to thread the instrumentation and screws into the bone (Figure 13.6). The thin Kirschner wire allows the trajectory of the screw to be determined without destroying the adjacent bone. If a larger, wider screw is misdirected, the intended purchase of the screw would be lost by destroying the adjacent bone. Cannulated screw systems must be monitored with continuous fluoroscopic guidance to avoid inadvertent advancement of the Kirschner wire intradurally, which would cause neural injury.

The pullout strength of screws depends on the area of purchase of the screw within the bone [11]. Softened or diseased bone provides an inadequate purchase. Because metal screws are much stronger than bone, screws fail by a shearing mechanism and pull the bone from beneath the threads. Pullout strength of screws is determined primarily by the depth of screw insertion and the major screw diameter. Screws should be tightened using two fingers to turn the screwdriver. Overtightening strips the screw hole and results in inadequate screw purchase. The bending strength of screws is primarily a function of the minor screw diameter (*ie*, the shaft diameter beneath the threads). When screws bend or break, they fail at the site of the first screw thread, where the shaft and threaded portions join.

Direct screw fixation of fracture sites or vertebrae is useful for anterior or posterior cervical fusions. Direct anterior screw fixation of odontoid fractures has become popular. Anterior and posterior techniques for atlantoaxial facet screw fixation have also been developed.

ODONTOID SCREW FIXATION

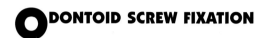

Technique

Odontoid fixation is performed by an anterior cervical exposure with the head extended. A transverse incision is made at the cricothyroid junction, and the platysma muscle is divided and undermined widely. The anterior border of the vertebral bodies is exposed up to the C2-3 disk space. The longus coli muscles are dissected from the anterior vertebral bodies.

Under biplanar fluoroscopy, pilot holes are drilled. The drills enter the anterior-inferior border of the C-2 body, and the tract is directed into the tip of the dens. The trajectory must be almost parallel to the anterior surface of the spine. The retractors and drill system developed by Apfelbaum (Aesculap, San Francisco, CA) are useful for access for odontoid screw fixation. Under fluoroscopic guidance, the anterior-inferior border of C-2 is exposed. The drill guide is inserted at the C2-3 interspace, and the drill is inserted at the anterior-inferior C-2 body. The odontoid is fixated with one or two lag screws with diameters of 3.5 mm, which are angled toward the midline 5° to 10°. The screws are inserted into the tip of the dens, avoiding intradural penetration. Cannulated or noncannulated screw systems may be used. Lag screws are preferred to place the fracture fragments under compression (Figure 13.6).

Analysis

Odontoid screw fixation is useful for directly fixating odontoid fractures and for preserving normal atlantoaxial motion [11,15,18,19]. This technique can be performed only when the transverse atlantal ligament is intact. If the transverse ligament is disrupted, fixating the odontoid does not fixate the atlas, and the spine remains unstable [26]. Anterior screw fixation is useful as an alternative to posterior cervical fixation,

especially when fractures preclude posterior wiring or when posterior fusions have failed. Preoperative computed tomographic (CT) studies are required to determine the extent of the fractures, to measure the size of the odontoid, and to assess for abnormalities that would preclude screw placement (*ie*, an anomalous course of the vertebral artery).

Anterior odontoid fixation is more difficult technically than posterior cervical fixation, and cannot be performed unless C1-2 alignment is restored. Chronic nonunions of odontoid fractures are problematic. With an anterior operation, it is difficult to remove the scar tissue to obtain the bone-bone contact that is required for the fracture to heal. Although two screws are recommended, no biomechanical data support the use of two screws or penetration of the tip of the dens for successful odontoid fixation. This procedure is very difficult or impossible to perform in patients with large chests or short necks.

Anterior screw fixation techniques and other cervical screw fixation techniques must be performed with anteroposterior and lateral fluoroscopy. The major limitation of anterior odontoid and C1-2 facet screw fixation techniques is the inability to add bone grafts to enhance fusion.

ANTERIOR ATLANTOAXIAL FACET SCREW FIXATION

Technique

Anterior C1-2 facet screw fixation is performed by an operative exposure identical to the odontoid screw fixation [11]. Before the screws are placed, the facet joints are decorticated with an angled curet to enhance fusion. Screws are placed into the groove between the C-2 vertebral body and the superior C-2 facet. The screws are directed rostrally and slightly laterally into the lateral masses of C-1. Single 3.5-mm diameter screws are placed into each facet under fluoroscopic guidance. Lag screws are preferred to compress the C1-2 facets (Figure 13.7).

Analysis

This technique has the same restrictions and problems as odontoid screw fixation. However, atlantoaxial motion is sacrificed with facet screws. The vertebral artery is at risk if the screws are misdirected laterally. An adequate exposure of the high cervical region can be difficult or impossible to achieve if the patient's neck is short and the chest is large.

POSTERIOR ATLANTOAXIAL FACET SCREW FIXATION

Technique

The posterior approach for atlantoaxial facet fixation requires controlled flexion of the patient's neck to obtain the proper trajectory for insertion of the drill and screws. Fluoroscopic visualization is also mandatory to assess the operative procedure and position of the drill and screws. The atlas and axis are realigned by manual reduction after exposing the vertebra subperiosteally by a standard posterior cervical incision. The C2-3 facet, the C-2 pedicle, and C1-2 articular surfaces are exposed. Bleeding can be bothersome from the venous plexus around the C-2 root. The ligamentum flavum adjacent to the C-2 pedicle is removed. A Kirschner wire is inserted along the upper surface of the C-2 pedicle into the C1-2 facet joint. The Kirschner wire is retracted superiorly to retract the C-2 nerve root so the trajectory of the screw may be visualized directly during the operative procedure.

Lateral fluoroscopic monitoring is used to adjust the drill and screws toward the anterior arch of C-1. In the anteroposterior direction, a trajectory of 0° to 10° medially is required to place the screw through the center of the pedicle. A trajectory too lateral or medial must be avoided to preserve the vertebral artery and dura. The posterior cortex of C-2 is penetrated with a bone or drill 2 to 3 mm lateral and 2 to 3 mm above the C2-3 facet joint. A 2.5-mm diameter drill enters this site and is directed to the posterior cortex of the anterior arch of C-1.

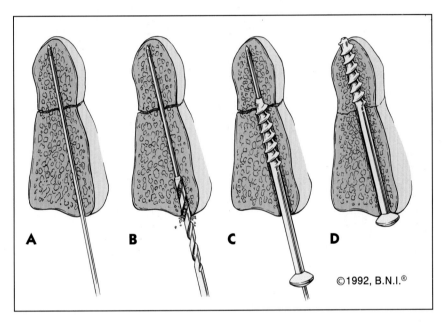

©1992, B.N.I.®

Figure 13.6

Cannulated screw fixation of an odontoid fracture. **A,** A threaded Kirschner wire is inserted into the dens. **B,** A 5-mm deep pilot hole is drilled into the proximal body of C-2 under fluoroscopic guidance. This hole allows the screw threads to purchase the bone. **C,** A self-tapping, partially threaded lag screw is placed over the Kirschner wire. Only the screw threads should engage the dens. **D,** The Kirschner wire is removed after the screw is inserted 1 or 2 mm beyond the cortex of the dens. (*Modified from* Dickman *et al.* [11]; with permission.)

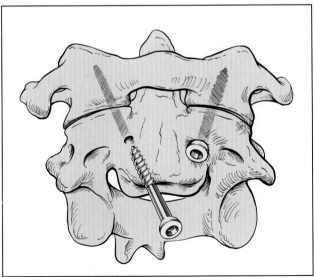

Figure 13.7

Anterior atlantoaxial facet screws are inserted in the groove between the C-2 body and superior facet and directed into the lateral mass of the atlas. (*Modified from* Dickman *et al.* [11]; with permission.)

Screws (3.5 mm in diameter) are placed through the C-2 pedicle, across the C1-2 facet, into the lateral masses of the atlas. As the screws cross the joint space into C-1, the atlas and axis become rigidly coupled (Figure 13.8).

Analysis

A supplemental bone graft is wired into position between the posterior arches of C1-2 to promote fusion and provide three-point fixation. A curettage or osteotomy can also be performed of the articular surfaces of C1-2 to promote fusion across the joint space. Posterior C1-2 screw fixation can be used when the posterior ring of the atlas is fractured or incompetent. This technique can be performed safely if the screws are placed precisely. A preoperative CT scan of C1-2 is essential to exclude an anomalous course of the vertebral artery. This is an excellent technique that provides the most rigid fixation of C1-2 available [3••,7••,9–11,27].

SCREW PLATE FIXATION

Screw plates can be used for anterior or posterior cervical fixation for the C-2 through C-7 segments [11,16,17,20–25,28,29]. The screw plates immobilize

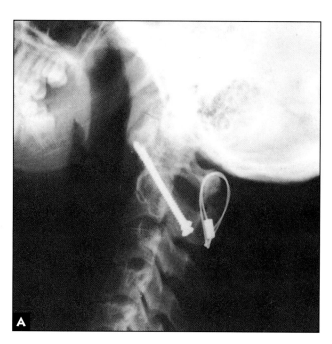

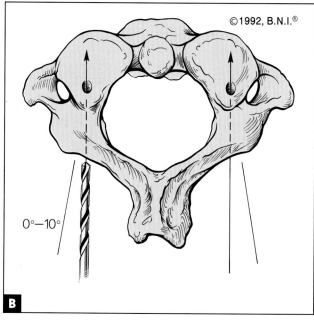

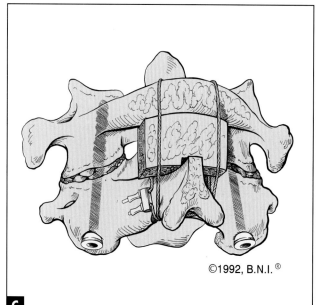

Figure 13.8

A, A lateral fluoroscopic image is used to adjust the drill and screw trajectory toward the posterior cortex of the anterior arch of C-1. **B,** The screws are placed through the center of the C-2 pedicle, with a trajectory between 0° and 10° medially. **C,** The screws enter C-2 just above the C2-3 facet joint. An interspinous strut graft is wired to achieve a three-point fixation and to promote bone fusion (Sketches *modified from* Dickman *et al.* [11]; with permission.)

adjacent motion segments. The articular surfaces (*ie*, disk spaces or facets) of the segments to be fused should be obliterated, and bone grafts should be placed across them. Screw plates should fit flush against the bones that are intended to fixate. Anterior cervical plates are used to fixate adjacent vertebral bodies. Posterior plates are used to fixate adjacent cervical lateral masses. Hook plates [21], Y plates [8•], universal bone plates [23], and reconstruction plates [11] are available.

Screw plates act mechanically as a tension band and buttress plate to resist vertical and horizontal translation of the spine. Anterior screw plates provide a strong anterior tension band that resists extension; however, with a three-column spinal injury, anterior cervical plates weakly resist flexion and rotation. In comparison, posterior cervical plates or wires strongly resist flexion of the neck; however, these weakly resist extension. These biomechanical principles indicate that anterior or posterior cervical screw plate fixation should be supplemented by rigid external immobilization or additional fixation when three-column injuries of the cervical spine exist.

Although screw plates increase the internal stabilization of injured spinal segments, they do not always restore normal strength to the spine. The injured spine may remain weak. Surgeons should not exclusively or excessively depend on internal fixation devices. Instrumentation can fail if enough force, with the appropriate vectors, is applied to the spine. Instrumentation should be supplemented with an external orthosis. The type of orthosis depends on the type of injury and the type of internal fixation that is used. Only the development of an osseous union ensures spinal stability.

ANTERIOR CERVICAL SCREW PLATES

Anterior cervical plates fixate adjacent vertebral bodies and are useful when vertebrectomies or diskectomies are performed in the unstable spine. Screw plates improve the fusion rate associated with anterior cervical fusions, are useful for correction of spinal deformities, and prevent bone graft migration. Locking anterior cervical screw plates and trapezoidal screw plates have had extensive clinical use (Figure 13.9) [11,20,24,28,30].

Anterior plates fixed with bicortical screws

Technique

The Caspar anterior cervical plating system uses bicortical screws and has holes with variable positions. Other bicortical screw plates are also available. The Caspar plate can be contoured individually, and long plates are useful for long-segment fusions. Screws must be placed carefully to avoid intradural penetration with the screws. The cervical screw plates are fitted along the anterior portion of the vertebra and sized so they do not extend across the adjacent disk spaces. (Screws that extend into the adjacent disk spaces can loosen.) The depth and trajectory of the screws should be fluoroscopically visualized. The Caspar screw plates (Aesculap, San Francisco, CA) and Synthes H plates (SYNTHES, Paoli, PA) are fixated with bicortical screws and use similar principles. The drills and screws are directed through the anterior vertebral bodies at an angle of 10° to 15° toward the midline. A bicortical purchase is obtained. The posterior vertebral body cortex is penetrated with the drill,

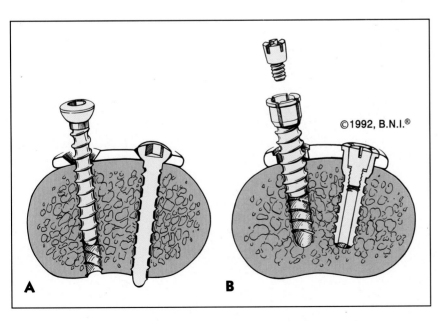

©1992, B.N.I.®

Figure 13.9

A, Bicortical screws for anterior cervical plate fixation. Pilot holes are drilled and tapped using fluoroscopic monitoring. The screws are angled 10° to 15° medially. **B,** Locking screw plates. The heads of the anchor screws are expanded by inserting a small locking screw into the anchor screw head. The anchor screw is compressed against the plate and the screws converge medially to avoid plate pullout. (*From* Dickman *et al.* [11]; with permission.)

tap, and screw. Fluoroscopic guidance and precise techniques are essential to avoid intradural penetration. Caspar plates have slots that permit a choice of screw sites. The screws can be repositioned if needed.

Analysis

The variability of the Caspar plates is better suited for long fusions, angular deformities, or the C2-3 interspace, where a superiorly angled trajectory of the screws may be needed [11,24]. Bicortical screw penetration, however, presents a potential risk of neurologic injury and can be difficult to achieve in the lower cervical spine, which cannot be seen adequately with fluoroscopy, especially in patients with short necks and large shoulders.

LOCKING SCREW PLATES

Technique

Anterior cervical locking screw plates were developed by Morscher. Anchor screws are positioned in a triangular configuration into the bone to resist pullout. The insertion of a second screw, the locking screw, into the head of the anchor screw expands the anchor screw head. The locking screw compresses the anchor screw against the plate hole and locks the screw to the plate. The screw heads have a flat profile. The predetermined screw trajectory must be used. Solid or hollow fenestrated 4-mm wide anchoring screws are used.

Analysis

The major advantage of the locking screw system is that the risk of neurologic injury from penetrating the posterior vertebral body with the screw is avoided. Fluoroscopy should still be employed to avoid placing the screws in the disk spaces and to size and position the plates correctly. The locking screw plates cannot be contoured excessively without altering the locking mechanisms. Locking screws cannot be removed easily once they are locked into position. The plates are simple and relatively safe.

POSTERIOR CERVICAL SCREW PLATES

Posterior cervical screw plates are more versatile than the anterior screw plates. Y plates have been used for occipitocervical fusion and hookplates, and lateral mass plates have been used for fixation of adjacent posterior cervical segments. Screws may be placed into the C1-2 facet, the C-2 pedicle, or the C-3 to C-7 lateral masses. Posterior cervical screw plates are excellent alternatives to wiring and are especially useful when the laminae or spinous processes are missing or incompetent. The plates may reduce some of the surface area available for bone fusion. These techniques may be supplemented by decorticating the facet joints to allow the facet surfaces to fuse and adding bone grafts to all available bone surfaces.

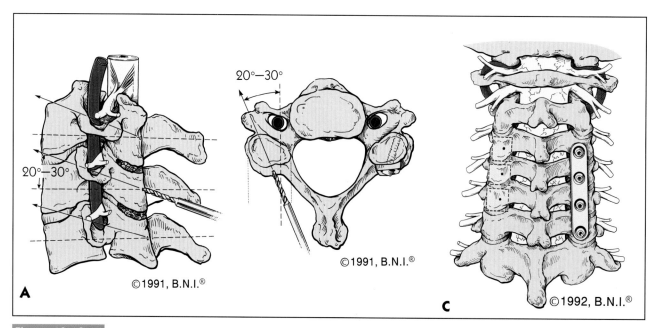

Figure 13.10

Lateral mass screw trajectories are angled 20° to 30° superiorly (**A**) and 20° to 30° laterally (**B**). Screw insertion is begun 1 mm medial to the center of the lateral mass (**C**). (*From* Cherny *et al.* [41]; with permission.)

Lateral mass screw placement

Technique

Correct screw placement is critical [11,16,17,22,23]. Lateral mass screws are placed into C-3 through C-7 with the following techniques. A posterior cervical exposure is performed, and the extreme edges of the lateral masses are exposed. The landmark for the center of the lateral mass is identified using the lateral and medial facet margins and the rostral and caudal aspects of the facets. Screw placement is begun 1 mm *medial* to the center of the lateral mass. A bone awl is used to pierce the cortical bone to mark the starting point to ensure a good drill purchase. For C3-7, the drill is angled 20° to 30° laterally and 20° to 30° rostrally. The trajectory must follow these guidelines to avoid the vertebral artery and nerve root (Figure 13.10). Spinal subluxations are reduced before plate application and screw placement. The spinous processes can be grasped with Allis clamps and pulled together to reduce subluxations. If a multiple-holed plate is placed, the distal holes should be drilled first. The plate is fitted and screwed into position. Next the middle holes are drilled, and the final screws are placed.

C-2 PEDICLE SCREW PLACEMENT

Technique

The posterior C-2 pedicle is fixated by a similar technique. The angling of the drill, however, is 20° to 30° rostrally and 20° to 30° *medially*. The screws are directed into the central axis of the C-2 pedicle (Figure 13.11) [11].

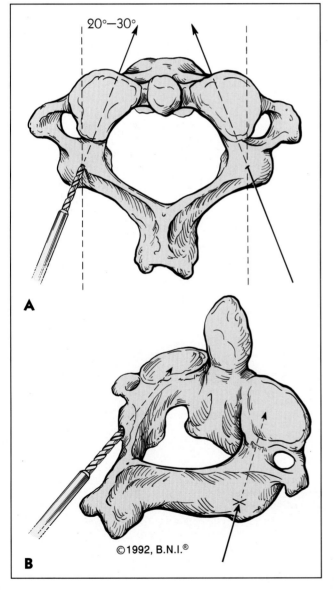

Figure 13.11

Screws are placed into the C-2 pedicle with a trajectory 20° to 30° medially (**A**) and 20° to 30° rostrally (**B**) through the center of the C-2 pedicle. (*Modified from* Dickman *et al.* [11]; with permission.)

20°—30°

A

©1992, B.N.I.®

B

LAMINAR HOOK-SCREW PLATE FIXATION

Technique

Screw plates or hookplates may be fixated with lateral mass or C-2 pedicle screws [11,21,29]. Hookplates fixate the lamina of the adjacent inferior cervical level and the lateral mass of the superior level. Hookplates should be used with an H graft, compressed between the spinous processes of the levels to be fused. The bone graft prevents overreduction, prevents hyperextension, and facilitates fusion (Figure 13.12).

Analysis

Anatomic studies for posterior screw plate fixation have demonstrated that the vertebral artery, spinal cord, and nerve root are relatively safe with the standard technique for lateral mass screw placement [16,17]. The C-7 vertebrae, however, is a transitional level and has a thin lateral mass. Screws in the C-7 lateral mass may potentially injure the nerve root [16].

CERVICAL INTERBODY FUSION WITH ALLOGRAFT

Technique

Awasthi and Voorhies [31] reported a modified technique for cervical vertebrectomy and interbody fusion using a banked fibular strut graft. The fibular strut graft is fashioned into a rectangular shape. The receptor site is a rectangular trench with a posterior ledge. The rectangular strut graft is countersunk into the rectangular receptor site. The posterior ledges prevent the graft from displacement toward the spinal cord. Figure 13.13 compares this technique with other methods of interbody fusion.

Variable results have been reported with fibular allograft for anterior cervical fusion. Fernyhough and colleagues [32] discovered a high nonunion rate for allograft and autograft bone among 126 consecutive cases. A nonunion rate of 27% occurred with autograft and 41% with allograft for one-level anterior fusions. The nonunion rate increased significantly with increasing numbers of motion segments fused. Zdeblick and Ducker [33] analyzed 87 patients undergoing Smith-Robinson anterior cervical fusions. They compared autograft and allograft tricortical iliac crest bone. At 1 year, nonunion occurred in 8% with autograft and in 22% with allograft. Delayed union occurred in 7% of the autografts and 21% of the allografts. Nonunion for one-level procedures was identical (5%) for both autograft and allograft. In two-level procedures, the nonunion rate was 17% for autograft

and 63% for allograft. Graft collapse was more commonly seen with freeze-dried allograft than with autograft (30% vs 5%). Clinically, relief of neck and arm pain was similar in both groups. Grossman and colleagues [34] found an 88% "good clinical result" in 83 anterior cervical levels fused after diskectomy among 42 patients with freeze-dried fibular allograft. Ninety-two percent of the grafts obtained complete or partial union by 6 months after surgery.

Analysis

Allograft bone provides immediate structural strength, but it undergoes remodeling and reabsorption. Allografts become progressively weaker after several months. Allograft bone should therefore be supplemented with other methods whenever possible to ensure solid fusion. Fibular strut grafts that are filled with cancellous autograft bone are useful. Allograft is

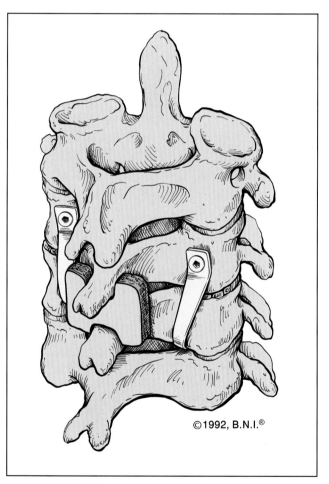

©1992, B.N.I.®

Figure 13.12

Laminar hook plates are positioned after performing a laminotomy to seat the hook correctly. The plates are screwed into the lateral masses at the superior level. An H graft provides additional stability since it prevents hyperextension. (*Modified from* Dickman *et al.* [11]; with permission.)

nonliving tissue that has infectious and immunologic risks. However, allograft avoids pain and other donor-site complications. Although several studies report successful results with anterior cervical reconstruction with allograft bone, when possible, autograft bone is still preferable. Autograft bone fuses more readily and contains active cells, morphogenic proteins, and structural elements of bone.

METHYL METHACRYLATE AND RESINS

Duff and colleagues [35] reported on 52 patients treated with methyl methacrylate internal fixation for fractures and dislocations without bone grafts. Two patients developed early failure, and 50 patients had stable constructs after a follow-up ranging from 6 months to 9 years. The average follow-up was not specified. Four technical factors were suggested as important for success for methyl methacrylate stabilization. The acrylic inlay must be provided with an anchor to the bone. The anchor must be of the type that does not usually erode through the bone. Wire must be included in a manner that allows each strand

to be completely encased in the acrylic. The cross-sectional area of the inlay is critical.

In this chapter, methyl methacrylate is used as an alternative to an external orthoses. Methyl methacrylate is a foreign body, can retain bacteria, and reduces the surface area available for formation of bony fusion. A pseudomembranous capsule, which forms around methyl methacrylate, may cause loosening and failure of the construct. Methyl methacrylate provides a temporary splint but does not promote bone fusion. It is not accepted for fractures or arthritis where bone fusion is the proven method of primary treatment. Methyl methacrylate tolerates tensile forces poorly; however, it is stronger under compression [36].

Segal and colleagues [37] used visible light-curing resin for vertebral body replacement in a rat corpectomy model. Vertebrectomies were compared with light-curing resin or conventional methyl methacrylate. Spinal cord function tests, spinal implant stability assessments, and histologic evaluations were performed. No animal developed neurologic deficits or radiographic instability. There were no adverse reactions by the surrounding tissue. Morphologic investigation of the resin-bone interface at 6 months

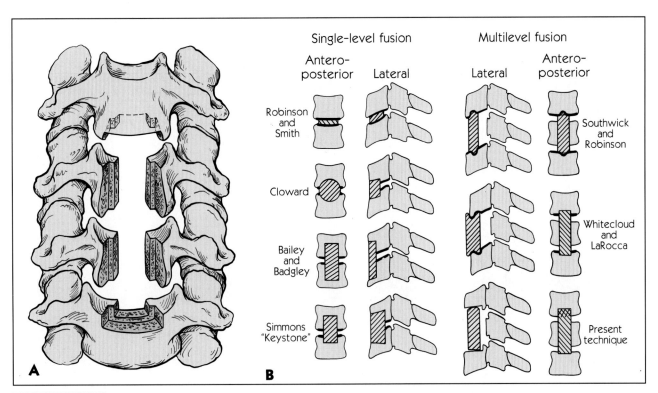

Figure 13.13

A, Rectangular receptor site with ledges to prevent posterior graft displacement. **B,** Comparison of different techniques of interbody fusion. (*From* Awasthi and Voorhies [31]; with permission.)

revealed very good implant anchorage. Visible light-curing resin was experimentally superior to methyl methacrylate for spinal reconstruction. Resin had a waxy consistency and was easy to handle. It remained pliable until ultraviolet light was applied. This allowed for adjustments in shape and for well-fitted implants without time constraints. The resin may be applied in layers, and adjustments can be made after polymerization of the previous layer. Further investigation with light-curing resin is warranted.

Shapiro [38] used tobramycin-impregnated methyl methacrylate for cranioplasty, vertebral body replacement, or spinal fusion among 65 patients. There was no tobramycin-related toxicity. One infection occurred among the 65 patients. It was suggested that tobramycin-impregnated methyl methacrylate was safe and that tobramycin may reduce the incidence of infection. If infections occur in these cases, superinfections or resistant strains of bacteria may develop.

CERVICAL SPINE FUSIONS IN RHEUMATOID ARTHRITIS

Chan and colleagues [39] evaluated 19 patients with rheumatoid arthritis who underwent upper posterior cervical fusion. There were 11 C1-2 fusions and eight occiput C-2 fusions. A fusion rate of 94% was achieved with an average follow-up of 5 years. A Gallie type fusion with autogenous iliac bone graft and monofilament wire was used. All patients were placed in a halo brace or cast for 3 months postoperatively. The authors emphasized that a high success rate of fusion may be achieved with upper cervical fusions in rheumatoid arthritis with supplemental external cervical immobilization, meticulous internal fixation, and supplemental autografts.

Papadopoulos and colleagues [40] examined 17 patients with rheumatoid arthritis treated with an atlantoaxial interspinous fusion. They recommend fusions for mobile atlantoaxial subluxations exceeding 6 mm. The risks of sudden death and spinal cord compression increased dramatically with more extensive subluxations. Thirteen patients developed stable osseous unions, two patients developed well-aligned fibrous unions, one patient developed a malaligned fibrous union, and one patient died before evaluation of fusion stability. Patients with rheumatoid arthritis are at risk for nonunion and fibrous union. Placing bone grafts under compression, thoroughly decorticating the bone surfaces, and obtaining contact of

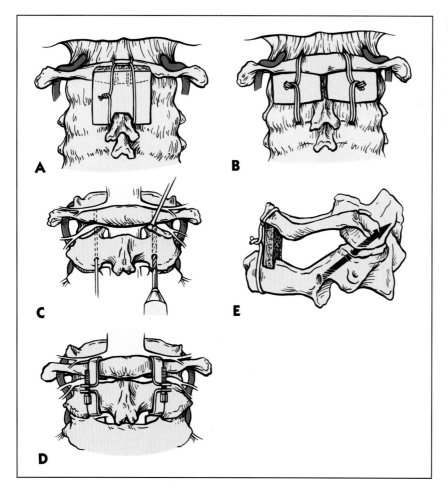

Figure 13.14

The four atlantoaxial fixation techniques compared biomechanically. Posterior views of the Gallie (**A**), the Brooks (**B**), the Magerl (**C**), and the Halifax (**D**) techniques. Lateral view of the Magerl technique (**E**). (*From* Grob *et al.* [3••]; with permission.)

cancellous bone of the adjacent surfaces to fuse are essential for success. Supplemental halo immobilization maximizes C1-2 fusion in rheumatoid arthritis.

BIOMECHANICAL STUDIES OF CERVICAL SPINE FIXATION DEVICES

Several recent outstanding reports provided *in vitro* laboratory biomechanical comparisons of different techniques for cervical spine fixation. Grob and colleagues [3••] compared four different techniques for posterior atlantoaxial fusion. The authors analyzed the Gallie wiring-graft method, the Brooks wiring-graft method, bilateral Halifax clamps, and bilateral transarticular atlantoaxial screws plus a Gallie wiring (Figure 13.14). Specimens were tested for stiffness in flexion, extension, axial rotation, and lateral bending to determine the physical response to loading. Pure moments were applied using techniques developed by Panjabi [3••,36].

Each of the internal fixation methods restricted C-1 motion considerably compared with the intact and injured spine. The Gallie method of wiring was the weakest method for atlantoaxial stabilization. The Gallie fusion allowed significantly more rotation in flexion, extension, axial rotation, and lateral bending than the other three techniques.

Posterior atlantoaxial facet screws combined with a Gallie wire graft provided the best rotational stability of any of the fixation techniques. There was no significant difference in the amount of flexion, extension, and lateral bending among the Brooks, Halifax clamps, and transarticular screw techniques.

Axial rotation and flexion-extension are the predominant movements of the atlantoaxial joint [36]. Three-point fixation with facet screws and a posterior bone graft offers the best immediate three-dimensional stability [36]. The optimum form of internal fixation of the atlantoaxial segment is three-point fixation. The effectiveness of a three-point internal fixation increases with increasing distance of the bone graft from the instantaneous axis of motion [36]. The instantaneous axis of rotation of C-1 is at the center of the dens [36]. The transarticular screw technique provides two points of fixation anteriorly in the C1-2 facet joints. One additional point of strong posterior fixation is achieved when using supplemental wire and bone grafts.

Hanson and colleagues [10] examined the biomechanical characteristics of posterior atlantoaxial transarticular screws supplemented with Gallie wiring. Screw fixation plus wires provided greater stiffness and stability than wired or control specimens (Figure 13.15). These data confirm the data presented by Grob *et al.* However, no data have been published

analyzing the strength of C1-2 screws without posterior wire and grafts. Eliminating atlantoaxial rotation and translation, which is difficult to achieve with wire alone, is the greatest advantage of C1-2 screw fixation. Rigid segmental internal fixation is desirable because it promotes spinal fusion.

Ulrich and colleagues [9] evaluated *in vitro* stiffness of a variety of instruments in human cadaver cervical spines. Posterior cervical hookplates, sublaminar wiring, anterior H plates, and combinations of anterior and posterior fixations were analyzed. The spinal segments were sequentially destabilized by sectioning

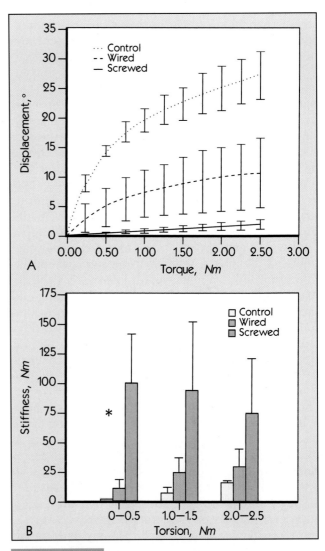

Figure 13.15

Stiffness data for C1-2 screws. **A,** Average torque versus displacement curves. *T-bars* represent 1 SD. All points except 0.75 Nm are significantly different (*P*<0.05) **B,** Stiffness values are taken from torque versus displacement (in radians) curves and calculated as the slope between the given intervals. *T-bars* represent 1 SD. Values at 0 to 0.5 Nm are significantly different (*P*<0.05). (*From* Hanson *et al.* [10]; with permission.)

the posterior ligaments, then removing the disk. Single subaxial motion segments were tested after each destabilizing procedure and after fixation. Flexion and torsion were evaluated; however, extension and lateral bending were not analyzed. Force-displacement data were derived using stiffness testing methods.

Anterior cervical plates alone were very weak when all three columns of the cervical spine were completely disrupted. Anterior cervical plates failed by bending open like a hinge under flexural loads. Anterior plates combined with posterior fixation (hookplates or posterior sublaminar wires) showed the highest stability. Only the posterior hookplate alone or its combination with the anterior cervical plate achieved a stability greater than that of the intact specimen. All other fixations were weaker than the normal spine.

This study demonstrates that after the disk and ligaments have been severed completely (*ie*, three-column instability), a single cervical fixation device is inadequate to restore normal strength to the spine. Combined anterior and posterior stabilizations or supplemental external fixation (*ie*, halo brace) should be strongly considered for individuals with three-column spinal injuries.

Cybulski and colleagues [30] clinically demonstrated that isolated posterior fixation can be inadequate for three-column cervical spine instability. Twenty-one patients had three-column cervical spine injuries that failed a single-stage posterior stabilization procedure. Patients were treated with a second fixation anteriorly or a combined, staged, anterior and posterior arthrodesis. Patients with flexion-distraction injuries with locked facets or teardrop compression-flexion injuries comprised high-risk groups. Posterior fixation alone failed universally in patients with three-column instability. Three-column spinal instability was manifested radiographically by 1) retrolisthesis and angulation, 2) distraction of the posterior interspinous ligaments, 3) subluxation or dislocation of the facets, 4) a shear dislocation of the vertebrae, and 5) disruption of the disk space and anterior and posterior longitudinal ligaments.

Combined posterior and anterior approaches for stabilization and fusion should be considered for such cases. If a single operative approach is performed (such as an anterior interbody fusion with plating or posterior fusion), it should be used with an external orthosis (*ie*, halo) to obtain adequate stability. These data emphasize that treatment of multicolumn injuries with multidirectional instability requires addressing all three columns of the cervical spine. One should not depend on internal fixation devices to restore normal strength to the incompetent spine.

Raynor and Carter [25] analyzed cervical facet injuries with subsequent posterior plate application.

Human cadaver cervical spines were destabilized with a facetectomy that removed the medial half of the facet joints. Posterior cervical screw plates were applied to the single destabilized motion segment. Flexion moments were applied until the plates failed. The screws all failed by fracturing the bone across the screw hole into the damaged joint. Additionally, when facet destruction was present, screw holes weakened the bone. Under stress, the remaining bone can fracture easily. Screws should not be placed in fractured facets.

If a facet is fractured, the fractured level should be spanned. Posterior screws can be used to fixate facets adjacent to the level of the fractured facet. Raynor and Carter's study demonstrates an important caveat for posterior lateral mass screw plates. Injured facets should not be fixated with a screw. Such fixation creates an inadequate purchase, and the internal fixation device fails.

Pelker and colleagues [29] evaluated posterior cervical spine stabilization using wiring, grafts, and methyl metha-crylate. A three-dimensional biomechanical evaluation of rotational stability, stiffness, and failure mechanisms was performed. Human cadaver cervical spines using two-motion segments were evaluated. Posterior spinous wiring, laminectomy with facet fusion, H grafting, and facetectomy with H grafting were evaluated. Each technique was tested before and after supplementation with methyl methacrylate.

Posterior spinous process wiring offered good stability in flexion but lacked sufficient stability with other motions. The repairs without methyl methacrylate were all relatively unstable in extension. Posterior cervical wiring appeared inadequate to prevent cervical extension. Supplementation with methyl methacrylate added considerable immediate stability to all of the constructs.

These data reinforce the concept that surgical stabilization of the posterior column is inadequate to prevent deformity with three-column spinal instability. Although methyl methacrylate can add stability internally, it is not preferred clinically except for tumor patients with reduced life expectancies.

CONCLUSIONS

With the advent of sophisticated cervical instrumentation, the techniques for cervical spine fusion have dramatically improved. All fusion techniques are guided by the biomechanics of the segments to be fused (in an attempt to correct what the disease process has destroyed). The hardware (wire, hooks, plates, screws, or clamps) are adjuncts to immobilize the bone rigidly while a solid fusion forms.

REFERENCES AND RECOMMENDED READING

Papers of particular interest, published within the annual period of review, have been highlighted as:
- •Of special interest
- ••Of outstanding interest

1. Aldrich EF, Crow WN, Weber PB, *et al.*: Use of MR imaging–compatible Halifax interlaminar clamps for posterior cervical fusion. *J Neurosurg* 1991, 74:185–189.

2. • Moskovich R, Crockard HA: Atlantoaxial arthrodesis using interlaminar clamps: an improved technique. *Spine* 1992, 17:261–267.

A technique is presented to improve the stabilizing effect of Halifax clamps. Bone struts are used between the posterior arches of C1-2 to prevent hyperextension, limit rotation, and avoid overreduction.

3. •• Grob D, Crisco III JJ, Panjabi MM, *et al.*: Biomechanical evaluation of four different posterior atlantoaxial fixation techniques. *Spine* 1992, 17:480–490.

This is a well-designed, carefully conducted biomechanical analysis of the *in-vitro* stiffness of several methods for C1-2 fixation. The authors compare wiring techniques, Halifax clamps, and transarticular facet screws.

4. • Dickman CA, Sonntag VKH, Papadopoulos SM, *et al.*: The interspinous method of posterior atlantoaxial arthrodesis. *J Neurosurg* 1991, 74:190–198.

A wiring technique for C1-2 is presented that differs from existing wiring methods. A bone strut is wired so that it is compressed between the posterior arches of C-1 and C-2. This technique can be used when C-1 is posteriorly dislocated, avoids sublaminar wire passage at C-2, and is mechanically effective for atlantoaxial stabilization.

5. Sonntag VKH, Dickman CA: Occipitocervical and high cervical stabilization. In *Neurosurgical Operative Atlas*, vol 1. Edited by Rengachary S, Wilkins R. Baltimore: American Association of Neurological Surgeons; 1991:327–337.

6. Dickman CA, Douglas RA, Sonntag VKH: Occipitocervical fusion: posterior stabilization of the craniovertebral junction and upper cervical spine. *BNI Quarterly* 1990, 6:2–15.

7. •• Magerl F, Seemann PS: Stable posterior fusion of the atlas and axis by transarticular screw fixation. In *Cervical Spine I*. Edited by Weidner PA. New York: Springer-Verlag; 1987: 322–327.

The operative technique for posterior atlantoaxial facet screw fixation is presented. This is a highly rigid, mechanically advantageous method to fixate C1-2. Precise techniques are required to avoid complications from screw malpositioning (*ie*, vertebral artery or dural injury).

8. • Grob D, Dvorak J, Panjabi M, *et al.*: Posterior occipitocervical fusion: a preliminary report of a new technique. *Spine* 1991, 16(suppl):S17–S24.

A rigid screw-plate fixation technique is presented for occipitocervical stabilization. This method, which has several merits, is an alternative to wiring techniques.

9. Ulrich C, Woersdoerfer O, Kalff R, *et al.*: Biomechanics of fixation systems to the cervical spine. *Spine* 1991, 16(suppl):S4–S9.

10. Hanson PB, Montesano PX, Sharkey NA, *et al.*: Anatomic and biomechanical assessment of transarticular screw fixation for atlantoaxial instability. *Spine* 1991, 16:1141–1145.

11. Dickman CA, Sonntag VKH, Marcotte PJ: Techniques of screw fixation of the cervical spine. *BNI Quarterly* 1992, 8:9–26.

12. • Songer MN, Spencer DL, Meyer Jr PR, *et al.*: The use of sublaminar cables to replace Luque wires. *Spine* 1991, 16(suppl):S418–S421.

This paper presents the biomechanical data pertaining to multistranded, braided, flexible cables. The operative techniques, mechanical characteristics, and fatigue and failure data are discussed.

13. Huhn SL, Wolf AL, Ecklund J: Posterior spinal osteosynthesis for cervical fracture/dislocation using a flexible multistrand cable system: technical note. *Neurosurgery* 1991, 29:943–946.

14. Nielsen CF, Annertz M, Persson L, *et al.*: Posterior wiring without bony fusion in traumatic distractive flexion injuries of the mid to lower cervical spine: long-term follow-up in 30 patients. *Spine* 1991, 16:467–472.

15. Esses SI, Bednar DA: Screw fixation of odontoid fractures and nonunions. *Spine* 1991, 16(suppl):S483–S485.16.

16. An HS, Gordin R, Renner K: Anatomic considerations for plate-screw fixation of the cervical spine. *Spine* 1991, 16(suppl):S548–S551.

17. Heller HG, Carlson GD, Abitbol J-J, *et al.*: Anatomic comparison of the Roy-Camille and Magerl techniques for screw placement in the lower cervical spine. *Spine* 1991, 16:S552–S557.

18. Etter C, Coscia M, Jaberg H, *et al.*: Direct anterior fixation of dens fractures with a cannulated screw system. *Spine* 1991, 16(suppl):S25–S32.

19. Montesano PX, Anderson PA, Schlehr F, *et al.*: Odontoid fractures treated by anterior odontoid screw fixation. *Spine* 1991, 16(suppl):S33–S37.

20. Aebi M, Zuber K, Marchesi D: Treatment of cervical spine injuries with anterior plating: indications, techniques, and results. *Spine* 1991, 16(suppl):S38–S45.

21. Jeanneret B, Magerl F, Ward EH, *et al.*: Posterior stabilization of the cervical spine with hook plates. *Spine* 1991, 16(suppl):S56–S63.

22. Nazarian SM, Louis RP: Posterior internal fixation with screw plates in traumatic lesions of the cervical spine. *Spine* 1991, 16(suppl):S64–S71.

23. Anderson PA, Henley MB, Grady MS, *et al.*: Posterior cervical arthrodesis with AO reconstruction plates and bone graft. *Spine* 1991, 16(suppl):S72–S79.

24. Tuite GF, Papadopoulos SM, Sonntag VKH: Caspar plate fixation for the treatment of complex hangmen's fractures. *Neurosurgery* 1992, 30:761–765.

25. Raynor RB, Carter FW: Cervical spine strength after facet injury and spine plate application. *Spine* 1991, 16(suppl):S558–S560.

26. Dickman CA, Mamourian A, Sonntag VKH, *et al.*: Magnetic resonance imaging of the transverse atlantal ligament for the evaluation of atlantoaxial instability. *J Neurosurg* 1991, 75:221–227.

27. Montesano PX, Juach EC, Anderson PA, *et al.*: Biomechanics of cervical spine internal fixation. *Spine* 1991, 16(suppl):S10–S16.

28. Segal J, Cahill D: Placement of anterior cervical instrumentation without intraoperative radiography. *J Spinal Disord* 1992, 5:162–169.

29. Pelker RR, Duranceau JS, Panjabi MM: Cervical spine stabilization: a three-dimensional, biomechanical evaluation of rotational stability, strength, and failure mechanisms. *Spine* 1991, 16:117–122.

30. Cybulski GR, Douglas RA, Meyer PR Jr, *et al.*: Complications in three-column cervical spine injuries requiring anterior-posterior stabilization. *Spine* 1992, 17:253–256.

31. Awasthi D, Voorhies RM: Anterior cervical vertebrectomy and interbody fusion: technical note. *J Neurosurg* 1992, 76:159–163.

32. Fernyhough JC, White JI, LaRocca H: Fusion rates in multilevel cervical spondylosis comparing allograft fibula with autograft fibula in 126 patients. *Spine* 1991, 10(suppl):S561–S564.

33. Zdeblick TA, Ducker TB: The use of freeze-dried allograft bone for anterior cervical fusions. *Spine* 1991, 16:726–729.

34. Grossman W, Peppelman WC, Baum JA, *et al.*: The use of freeze-dried fibular allograft in anterior cervical fusion. *Spine* 1992, 17:565–569.

35. Duff TA, Khan A, Corbett JE: Surgical stabilization of cervical spinal fractures using methyl methacrylate: technical considerations and long-term results in 52 patients. *J Neurosurg* 1992, 76:440–443.

36. White AA III, Panjabi MM: *Clinical Biomechanics of the Spine*. Philadelphia: JB Lippincott; 1978.

37. Segal R, Alsawaf M, Tabatabai A, *et al.*: The use of visible light-curing resin for vertebral body replacement. *J Neurosurg* 1991, 75:91–96.

38. Shapiro SA: Cranioplasty, vertebral body replacement, and spinal fusion with Tobramycin-impregnated methylmethacrylate. *Neurosurgery* 1991, 28:789–791.

39. Chan DPK, Ngian KS, Cohen L: Posterior upper cervical fusion in rheumatoid arthritis. *Spine* 1992, 17:268–272.

40. Papadopoulos SM, Dickman CA, Sonntag VKH: Atlantoaxial stabilization in rheumatoid arthritis. *J Neurosurg* 1991, 74:1–7.

41. Cherny WB, Sonntag VKH, Douglas RA: Lateral mass posterior plating and facet fusion for cervical spine instability. *BNI Quarterly* 1991, 7:2–11.

Chapter 14

Percutaneous Automated Lumbar Diskectomy

Joseph C. Maroon
Gary Onik
Danko Vidovich

Progressively less invasive techniques are becoming the standard for the treatment of many common disorders. Laparoscopic abdominal procedures, transluminal angioplasty, endovascular occlusions of aneurysm and arteriovenous malformations, and stereotactic endoscopic brain surgery are but a few examples. Percutaneous lumbar diskectomy is another scientific advancement in the evolution toward less invasive approaches to treat lumbar disk disease. Although the concept of chemonucleolysis and biochemical degradation of disks introduced the percutaneous intervention in the disk space, it was Hijikata [1•] who first devised instrumentation for the percutaneous removal of lumbar disks in 1975. Although he initially reported a 70% success rate, he encountered a major vascular injury in his series.

In 1983, Kambin and Gellman [2] and Kambin and Shaffer [3••] developed a separate set of instrumentation to be used percutaneously and subsequently reported an 87% success rate in their series of 100 patients. Additional modifications were introduced by Schreiber and colleagues [4••] in Switzerland, who used a contralateral percutaneous approach and inserted a fiberoptic *diskoscope* to visualize the material being removed. Although they had a 72% success rate over an 8-year period, they reported a 7% incidence of diskitis as well as an injury to the lumbar plexus in two patients and an iliac artery perforation in another [4••]. Friedman [5] evaluated the straight lateral percutaneous method introduced by Jacobson, which involved the insertion of a 40 F chest tube into the disk space. He concluded that this procedure was unsafe because of the potential of bowel and nerve root injury [5]. All these percutaneous techniques involved the manual removal of disk fragments with specially designed pituitary-like grasping forceps. The large size of the instrumentation resulted in a relatively high incidence of vascular and nerve root injury and also created more difficulty for entering the L5-S1 interspace.

After evaluating all available techniques, Onik and colleagues [6,7] in 1985 corroborated with engineers and designed an automated percutaneous diskectomy system that used a reciprocating suction-cutter for removing disk material. The instrument consisted of a 2-mm blunt-tipped device with a single side port

and a guillotine-like knife that morselized disk material as it was aspirated through the side port and amputated at approximately 180 times per minute by the cutter. This smaller sized instrumentation, which was automated, eliminated the major drawbacks of the other percutaneous techniques [8]. Maroon and Onik [9] published their initial series in 1987 and reported a 79% success rate.

Since then, approximately 80,000 patients have had the procedure of automated percutaneous diskectomy. Over 3000 surgeons have participated worldwide in instructional courses. In over 20 studies from separate institutions in the United States and Europe, the success rate remains between 66% and 80% [10••]. It also appears to be the safest procedure for the removal of selected lumbar disks.

This chapter reviews patient selection and also speculates on future developments for the percutaneous treatment of lumbar disk disease.

PATIENT SELECTION

As with any surgical procedure, success is extremely dependent on patient selection (Table 14.1). Automated percutaneous lumbar diskectomy is effective in treating those patients with small to moderate, well-contained disk herniations that show evidence clinically and radiographically of nerve root compression. Clinically, the most important symptoms are those in a

Table 14.1
Characteristics in patient selection for percutaneous diskectomy

Characteristics for candidacy

Leg pain (sciatica) with or without back pain; back pain only, except in unusual circumstances (centrally herniated nucleus pulposus), should not be indication for procedure

Physical findings that confirm nerve root irritation (positive straight leg raising test), weakness, sensory change, reflex alteration

CT or MR image showing a contained herniated nucleus pulposus with no evidence for extruded or free fragment; myelography is not adequate for this purpose

Absolute contraindications

Progressive clinically significant neurologic deficit, such as foot drop or cauda equina syndrome

Severe spinal stenosis

Large herniated disk with 50% or more of the thecal sac visible on MR imaging or CT

Skin infection in the area of the puncture site

CT—computed tomography; MR—magnetic resonance.

patient with more leg pain than back pain who has failed all conservative measures and remains significantly disabled by pain. A history of paresthetic discomfort in a specific dermatomal distribution is significant. Physical findings usually include a positive straight leg raising examination, slight weakness of the extensor hallucis longus or plantar flexors of the foot, mild sensory disturbances, and reflex alterations in a specific dermatome. Posterior leg pain that does not radiate below the knee is viewed with suspicion, particularly if it is not associated with other physical findings. The disruption of other soft tissues, such as facet joints, can cause referred leg pain of this nature, and careful palpation and evaluation of flexion, extension, and rotation of the lumbosacral spine are indicated. If there is marked weakness in any muscle group, bowel or bladder disturbances, or profound sensory loss, this procedure should not be considered. Also, a cross-positive straight leg raising sign is usually a strong indication of a sequestered fragment and contraindicates the use of percutaneous diskectomy. A demonstrated radiographic abnormality on computed tomography (CT), magnetic resonance (MR) imaging, or intrathecally enhanced CT and myelography must be present and correlate with the patient's physical findings. The ideal candidate is one who has a small to moderate sized focal herniation or bulge that makes an impression on the thecal sac consistent with the patient's symptoms (Figure 14.1). Patients with degenerative disk disease and diffuse annular bulging extending out from the entire circumference of the vertebral body are not candidates for this procedure. Also to be excluded are patients with lateral recess stenosis, calcified disk herniations, diffuse spinal stenosis, or evidence of instability such as anterior or posterior listhesis.

A major source of poor results is that of determining whether the disk is contained by the annulus or posterior longitudinal ligament or whether it has extruded through the posterior longitudinal ligament. The most definitive criterion for a sequestrated disk is the demonstration of a fragment superiorly or inferiorly from the disk space by the radiographic means. In the axial view, because of partial volume averaging, it is possible, in contained herniations, to see some disk material above or below the disk space. It is important to demonstrate, however, that the epicenter or the largest portion of the herniation is at the disk level, and sagittal MR imaging can be helpful in this determination. Also, there must be contiguous axial sections on MR imaging and CT scans from L-3 through S-1 with no associated gaps to exclude far lateral herniations as well as migrated fragments (Figure 14.2).

The size of the herniation is also used in determining whether it has extruded or not. It has been shown that herniations that compromise the thecal sac by 50% or more had a 90% correlation with sequestration. Therefore, any herniation of that size should not be considered for percutaneous diskectomy. A further radiographic point is the angle of the herniation. The angle of the herniation should be obtuse. Acute angulations indicate the extrusions and contraindicate percutaneous diskectomy.

Finally, diskography, although controversial, may be helpful in excluding those patients likely to have extruded disk fragments. The most important criterion of diskography is whether the herniation fills with contrast medium injected into the center of the disk. If the herniation is well outlined by contrast material and is contained by the posterior longitudinal ligament, good results may be anticipated (Figure 14.3).

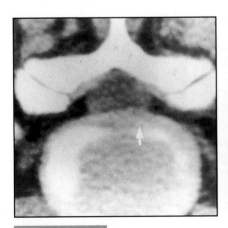

Figure 14.1

Computed tomographic scan of an "ideal" herniation for percutaneous diskectomy. The disk is contained and has smooth, obtuse margins (*arrow*).

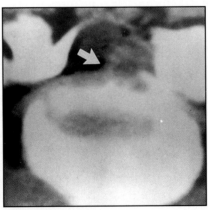

Figure 14.2

Computed tomographic scan of a very large disk that takes up 50% or more of the thecal sac (*arrow*). This scan indicates a contraindication for percutaneous diskectomy.

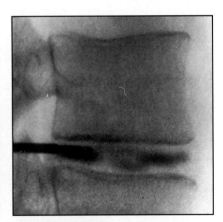

Figure 14.3

Lateral projection of a lumbar diskogram, showing contrast in the disk space with no flow of contrast medium beyond the longitudinal ligament. This is a well-contained herniation that responded well to percutaneous diskectomy.

If there is extravasation of contrast material up and down the spinal canal, invariably poor results may be anticipated. It is conceivable that a false-positive diagnosis for extrusion can occur if contrast medium flows behind the posterior longitudinal ligament, but generally, if this occurs, we do not do the procedure. At times, particularly at the L5-S1 level, results of the plain diskogram may be equivocal. In these instances, diskography followed by a CT scan shows subtle amounts of contrast extravasation into the epidural space.

TECHNIQUE

The safety of automated percutaneous lumbar diskectomy relies on guiding the Nucleotome (Surgical Dynamics, San Leandro, CA) into the disk space with precise radiographic control. Because a small but significant number of patients positioned prone have the colon posterior to the psoas muscle, a localizing CT scan is obtained to rule out this possibility. Using this localizing scan, it is also possible to select a tentative entry site using the cursor on the scanner on the same side as the patient's symptoms (Figure 14.4).

The procedure is performed with the patient in either the prone or lateral decubitus position. To open the disk space posteriorly and decrease the lumbar lordosis, the patient is flexed by inserting a roll under the abdomen or iliac crest using fluoroscopy. The patient must be perfectly straight and not rotated. When using the fluoroscope, one must count up from the sacrum viewing with continuous fluoroscopy so the inadvertent disk space is not punctured owing to the small fluoroscopic image on some C arms. Because all structures such as great vessels, bowel, and nerves that one must avoid lie anteriorly, the anteroposterior view is inadequate for monitoring. We

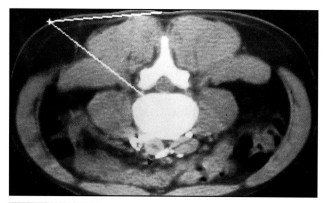

Figure 14.4

Nonmagnified computed tomographic scan of the abdomen showing the path that percutaneous diskectomy takes to the disk space. No bowel is traversed, and the path avoids the psoas muscle, which is traversed by branches of the lumbar plexus.

therefore use the lateral view initially and never insert the tip of the trocar anterior to a line that connects the posterior vertebral bodies unless the disk has already been encountered. Experience has shown that the trocar is at that line when the annulus is felt if the trajectory is correct. Any trocar placement that strikes the spine anterior to this line will have an anterior trajectory and will be an inadequate placement.

The procedure is performed with the patient under local anesthesia. A 22-gauge needle is used to anesthetize the skin and the deeper tissues. An 18-gauge introduction trocar is then placed into the correct position abutting the annulus. The insertion site is at a distance of 8 to 12 cm lateral from the midline. If a diskogram is to be performed, it is done through the 22-gauge needle placed within the annulus. Following this procedure, the 18-gauge trocar is placed in a tandem fashion next to this needle after correct positioning has been verified on both the anteroposterior and the lateral fluoroscopic modes. If there is radicular pain experienced with the insertion of the needle, redirection is indicated. The trocar, when lying against the annulus, should be lateral to a line that joins the medial border of the pedicles in the anteroposterior projection. When it is in this position, it can then be advanced into the center of the disk space. Because we want to be as close as possible to the disk herniation, any placement that has an anterior trajectory is not acceptable and needs to be corrected.

Once the trocar is in the correct position, the tissue dilator and then the cutting cannula are placed over the trocar down to the annulus. The dilator is then removed, and the cannula is pushed the extra few millimeters to rest on the annulus.

At this point, the fluoroscopic beam is brought perpendicular to the cannula (Figure 14.5). This view ensures that the cannula is absolutely down to the annulus. When this oblique view confirms that the cannula is against the annulus, the trephine is placed over the trocar and through the cannula, and the annulus is incised. Only after the incision is made with the trephine can the trocar be removed along with the trephine.

The Nucleotome is then placed into the disk through the cannula and confirmed to be within the disk space on both anteroposterior and lateral views. At this point, the disk is then aspirated by activating the foot pedal–controlled suction-cutting device. The procedure is monitored by watching the disk material in the aspiration line. Because the disk is avascular, the aspiration contents should be essentially bloodless. By rotating, elevating, and depressing the Nucleotome at different depths, access to the disk material is obtained (Figure 14.6). The procedure is terminated when disk material can no longer be aspirated. This usually takes from 20 to 40 minutes.

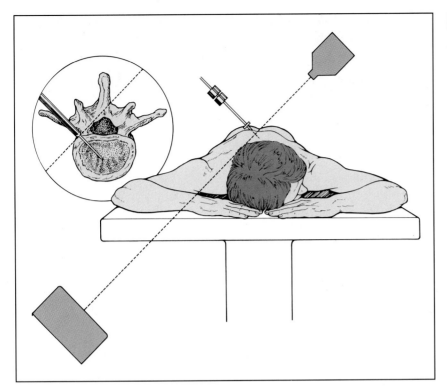

Figure 14.5

A fluoroscopic beam is brought perpendicular to the cannula. Thus the x-ray beam can visualize the interface between the cannula and the edge of the vertebral body.

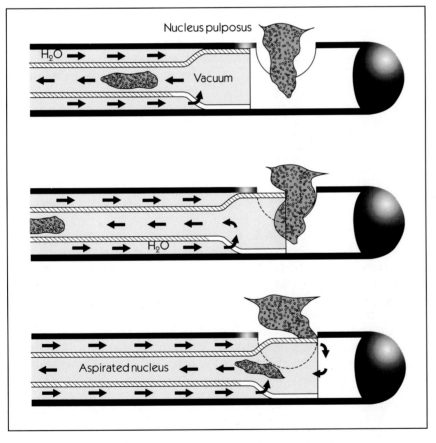

Figure 14.6

The action of the Nucleotome (Surgical Dynamics, San Leandro, CA).

PERCUTANEOUS DISKECTOMY AT THE L5-S1 LEVEL

Because of the iliac crest and the rather oblique projection that must be made to enter the L5-S1 disk space, a point must be selected that allows for enough medial entry into the disk while still being far enough laterally to allow a central to posterior placement. The starting entry point is determined by fluoroscopy. A line drawn tangential to the outside portion of the sacroiliac joint and extending superiorly until it intersects the iliac crest is a reasonable starting point from which to begin the procedure. A line is then drawn to the top of the iliac crest, and the top of the iliac crest is marked fluoroscopically along its length so when the instruments are placed they are as close to the iliac crest as possible. We begin the insertion where these two lines intersect.

Under fluoroscopy, the needle for anesthesia is placed in its trajectory toward the disk, and its angle with the disk is assessed. If the angle is steep, this is the entry point that is used; a curved cannula helps bring the Nucleotome more posterior in the disk if needed. If the anesthesia needle is in the plane of the disk, the entry point for the procedure is empirically moved laterally by approximately 2 cm, and the anesthesia needle to the disk is marked again. If the needle is in the plane of the disk or only slightly angled to the disk, the entry point is again moved empirically laterally to a maximum of approximately 10 cm to the midline. In this way, using a small-gauge spinal needle, the point can be found that is farthest lateral and still allows entry into the disk space. By moving laterally as far as possible, the difficulty of getting to the center or posterior margin of the disk is minimized. Besides the height of the iliac crest, the space between the transverse process of L-5 and the sacrum may be the most critical factor determining entry into the L5-S1 space. As this space decreases, the likelihood of being able to complete the procedure is also decreased. Also, if the disk space is quite narrow, the procedure becomes more difficult. Once the Nucleotome is positioned through the cannula and into the disk space, disk removal can be safely accomplished. If the Nucleotome slips out of the disk space, however, it may be impossible to reinsert it without repeating the entire process.

EXTREMELY FAR LATERAL HERNIATIONS

Extremely far lateral disk herniations present a diagnostic as well as a therapeutic challenge. Because by definition they lie outside the spinal canal and neural foramen, myelography is usually negative. It was not until cross-sectional imaging techniques became available that this entity was consistently diagnosed. Automated percutaneous diskectomy appears to be an excellent alternative to either of these methods. The path to the disk is excellently placed in relationship to the position of the herniation. The instruments pass extremely close in proximity to the herniation and may actually go through the herniation in many instances. Because the procedure is done with the patient under local anesthesia, the possibility of nerve root injury is greatly minimized. If a patient experiences radicular pain during the procedure, the position of the trocar can be changed. In addition, the procedure, because of its approach, does not violate the spinal canal, eliminating the problem of epidural fibrosis. Lastly, there is no bone removal with the later possibility of instability.

RESULTS

From 1984 to 1987, a prospective, multi-institutional study was carried out by 18 different investigators to evaluate the safety and efficacy of automated percutaneous lumbar diskectomy. Patients were prospectively assessed using the criteria outlined here. Patients for this study were excluded if they had any of the following: history of previous lumbar surgery; previous chymopapain injection; Worker's Compensation claim, or any cause of their pain as revealed by CT such as severe degenerative facet disease, lateral recess stenosis, spinal stenosis, or evidence of a free fragment disk. Although investigators were encouraged to stay within this study protocol, patients prospectively were operated on outside the protocol and recorded as such. Of 522 patients, 11 patients were lost to follow-up, whereas 316 patients met the prospective study criteria; 195 patients were knowingly operated on outside the protocol. The mean patient age was 41 years. There were 302 men and 220 women. The mean duration of preoperative conservative treatment was 11.6 months. Eighty percent of the procedures were performed at L4-L5 and approximately 20% at L5-S1.

Of the 316 patients within the protocol with a 1-year or longer follow-up, the success rate was 75.9%. Considered failures were 24.1%. In those patients operated on outside the protocol, 53.3% were successful, and 46.7% were unsuccessful. The success involved moderate to total relief of radicular pain, freedom from the use of narcotic analgesics, and a functional status enabling the patient to resume his or her usual activities. In addition, the patient had to be satisfied with the result of the procedure, noting the satisfaction by direct questioning or obtaining a completed questionnaire.

Of the 76 patients within the protocol considered to be failures, 41 underwent a laminectomy, a microdiskectomy, or subsequent fusion. Nineteen patients had a repeated percutaneous diskectomy, whereas 16 patients had not had any other procedure. Of the 41 patients undergoing a subsequent open procedure, 30 had free fragments of disks that were undetected by preoperative imaging, six had spinal stenosis, one had a vertebral fracture, and the remaining patients had bulging disks with no evident cause for failure.

Complications included one patient with diskitis successfully treated with antibiotics. Another patient had transient paresthesias in the thigh, and a third had a psoas hematoma that was not hemodynamically significant but manifested as groin pain on the side of the procedure. Three patients had transient severe paravertebral spasms, whereas most experienced only mild discomfort in the area of needle insertion. The mean hospital stay for the procedure was 0.3 days, with the majority of procedures performed as an outpatient procedure.

The safety and efficacy of the procedure have now been confirmed by other multiple studies. At least 22 studies have now been reported comprising over 3600 patients. Twenty-three studies reported results between 70% and 90%, with only one study (comprising 37 patients) reporting less than a 70% success rate [4••,11–21,22•,23–26,27••,28–30,31•,32,33]. Most important of all, however, is that the safety of the procedure was reproduced with no serious complications reported in these studies. A diskitis rate of 0.2%, three to five times lower than that for open diskectomy, was reported. Patients may obtain immediate complete relief from sciatica occasionally. The majority of patients note immediate moderate relief of pain, then gradual resolution over 6 weeks or longer. We have seen an occasional patient with minimal, if any, relief up to 4 weeks and then progressive improvement. We therefore wait at least 6 weeks before considering the procedure a failure. Thus far, patients who fail to get well have not been made worse by the procedure.

Postoperatively patients enter a rehabilitation program to correct postural and weight problems with trunk stabilization and strengthening of abdominal and back muscles. Patients with sedentary jobs usually return to work within the first week or two following the procedure. All patients who do heavy manual labor go through a work-hardening program before being allowed to return to work 6 to 12 weeks after the procedure. We consider this to be important because most patients have been off work engaging in some form of conservative therapy and have experienced subsequent loss of muscle tone and strength.

COMPLICATIONS

Before clinical introduction of automated percutaneous lumbar microdiskectomy, our most serious concern was for the potential misplacement of the probe, either into the spinal canal or into the retroperitoneal space, with the potential complications of serious neural and vascular trauma. Despite the extremely good safety record of this procedure relative to standard surgical and microsurgical techniques, there have recently been two catastrophic neural injuries of which we are aware. Epstein [34] as well as our group [35] have published papers describing patients from outside institutions with severe cauda equina injury from probe misplacement. It is absolutely imperative that the procedure be done with the patient under local anesthesia and that strict radiographic landmarks are adhered to for placement of instrumentation. Otherwise, just as a pituitary rongeur inadvertently used can grasp a root, the dura, or the cauda equina, this instrumentation inappropriately placed can cause similar trauma or damage.

FUTURE DEVELOPMENTS

A flexible Nucleotome was recently introduced. Once in position in the disk, the flexible part of the Nucleotome can be directed in desired positions within the disk and its position monitored under radiographic control. This allows further versatility of the Nucleotome, allowing more disk material to be evacuated (Figure 14.7).

Despite the generally good to excellent results achieved with automated percutaneous lumbar diskectomy, investigators have pursued even less invasive techniques by using laser fibers through 18- to 20-gauge needles for vaporization of lumbar disks. Currently there is considerable laboratory and clinical interest in assessing which laser system would be optimal and also the potential risks and complications of this use of laser energy. Available lasers that may be passed through fiberoptic cables and directed intradiskally include Neodymium:Yttrium-aluminum-garnet (Nd:YAG) (1.06 μ), Holmium:YAG (2.1 μ), and Erbium:YAG (2.9 μ). Experimental work conducted in our laboratories presently suggests that laser disk removal is characterized by an optimal and specific energy requirement, which, if exceeded, results only in unwanted disk space heating [36]. The Erbium:YAG laser is attractive in terms of its absorption characteristics, but there are serious problems in terms of the fiberoptics with this system. We and others have preliminarily found that the Holmium:YAG laser may be superior in practical use because of its absorption coefficient as well as its ability to be transmitted through optical fibers. Such a flexible cannula, including a malleable and directable Holmium:YAG laser fiber and irrigation and optical fiber, is currently under investigation in our laboratories as designed by Coherent Medical Group (Palo Alto, CA). Once the rigid cannula is placed into its proper position, the malleable multifiber is inserted under visual control. With visual control one can thus vaporize disk material through a 1.9-mm cannula, while the patient is under local anesthesia. Constant irrigation allows cooling of the disk space to avoid possible thermal injury. This new technology allows the neurosurgeon to visualize for the first time the intradiskal space while removing the intradiskal mass with low energy. It may be a definitive step forward in intradiskal therapy and in endoscopic neurosurgery (Figures 14.8 and 14.9).

CONCLUSIONS

Automated percutaneous lumbar diskectomy appears to be a low-risk procedure effective in 70% to 80% of appropriately selected patients. Advantages include the use of local anesthesia, minimal tissue disruption, performance on an outpatient basis, and an earlier return to former activities. Because the spinal canal is not violated, epidural fibrosis and scarring are absent, and, therefore, a patient in whom percutaneous diskectomy fails can undergo an open procedure. Subsequent evaluation reveals minimal disk space narrowing; therefore, there should be a negligible biomechanical effect. The problem of differential sequestered versus contained disk remains and is primarily an imaging problem at this point. CT diskography may be beneficial in helping evaluate patients with questionable sequestration or tears in the posterior longitudinal ligament. The risks of automated percutaneous lumbar diskectomy are significantly less than those of traditional surgery, and, therefore, in selected patients consideration should be given to this procedure.

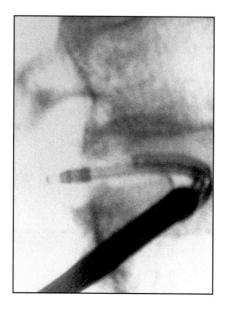

Figure 14.7

Lateral radiograph showing the Nucleotome II (Surgical Dynamics, San Leandro, CA) in situ. Note the malleability of the tip.

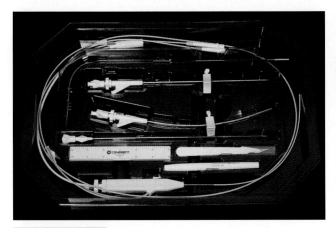

Figure 14.8

The coherent malleable LASE (laser-assisted spinal endoscopy; Coherent Medical, Palo Alto, CA) kit.

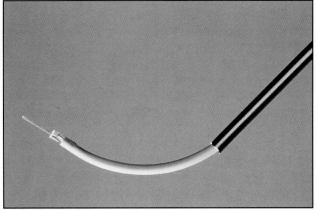

Figure 14.9

The tip of the LASE (laser-assisted spinal endoscopy; Coherent Medical, Palo Alto, CA) probe. Note the malleable part with the laser fiber at the tip. The probe's diameter is 1.8 mm.

REFERENCES AND RECOMMENDED READING

Papers of particular interest, published within the annual period of review, have been highlighted as:
• Of special interest
•• Of outstanding interest

1. • Hijikata S: Percutaneous nucleotomy: a new concept technique and 12 years' experience. *Clin Orthop* 1989, 238:9–23.
This article discusses the concept and theoretical considerations of percutaneous nucleotomy. There was a 72% success rate in 136 patients who were followed up.

2. Kambin P, Gellman H: Percutaneous lateral discectomy of the lumbar spine. *Clin Orthop* 1983, 174:127–132.

3. •• Kambin P, Shaffer JL: Percutaneous lumbar discectomy: review of 100 patients and current practice. *Clin Orthop* 1989, 238:23–34.
Prospective study in 100 patients with an 87% success rate based on meticulous selection of patients for the procedure.

4. •• Schreiber A, Suezawa MSD, Leu H: Does percutaneous nucleotomy with discography replace conventional discectomy? Eight years of experience and results in treatment of herniated lumbar discs. *Clin Orthop* 1989, 238:35–42.
Diskoscopy with an adapted arthroscopy kit for more effective percutaneous nucleotomy yielded a 72.5% success rate.

5. Friedman WA: Percutaneous discectomy: an alternative to chemonucleolysis? *Neurosurgery* 1983, 13:542–547.

6. Onik G, Helms CA, Ginsberg L, *et al.*: Percutaneous lumbar discectomy using a new aspiration probe: porcine and cadaver models. *Radiology* 1985, 155:251–252.

7. Onik G. Helms CA, Ginsberg L, *et al.*: Automated percutaneous discectomy: initial patient experience. *Radiology* 1987, 162:129–132.

8. Blankenstein A, Rubenstein E, Ezra E, *et al.*: Disc space infection and vertebral osteomyelitis as a complication of percutaneous lateral discectomy. *Clin Orthop* 1987, 225:234–237.

9. Maroon JC, Onik G: Percutaneous automated discectomy: a new method for lumbar disc removal. *J Neurosurgery* 1987, 66:143–146.

10. •• Onik G, Mooney V, Maroon JC, *et al.*: APD: a prospective multiinstitutional study. *Neurosurgery* 1990, 26:228–233.
Series of 327 patients who met selection criteria for automated percutaneous diskectomy. There was a 72.5% success rate.

11. Bocchi L, Ferrata P, Passarello F, *et al.*: La nucleoaspirazione secondo Onik nel trattzamento dell'ernia discale lombare: analisi multicentrica dei primi risultati su oltre 650 trattamenti. *Riv Neuroradiol* 1989, 2(suppl 1):119–122.

12. Bonaldi G, Belloni G, Prosetti D, *et al.*: Percutaneous discectomy using Onik's method: three years experience. *Neuroradiology* 1991, 33:516–519.

13. Bonneville JF, Runge M, Paris D *et al.*: Le discque intervertebral lombaire apres nucleotomie percutanee par aspiration: etude tomodensitometrique. Comparaison avec la chimionucleolyse. *Rachis* 1989, 1:113–121.

14. Cartolari R, Davidovits P, Gagliardelli M: Automated percutaneous lumbar diskectomy. In *Percutaneous Lumbar Diskectomy.* Edited by Mayer HM, Brock M. Berlin: Springer- Verlag; 1989:157–162.

15. Cooney FD: Comparison of chemonucleolysis with chymopapain to percutaneous automated discectomy: a

surgeon's first 50 cases of each. In *Percutaneous Lumbar Diskectomy*. Edited by Mayer HM, Brock M. Berlin: Springer-Verlag; 1989:163–168.

16. Corkhill G, Kimple J, Corkhill R: Automated percutaneous nucleotomy by pain scale. In *Percutaneous Lumbar Diskectomy*. Edited by Mayer HM, Brock M. Berlin: Springer-Verlag; 1989:169–172.

17. Davis GW, Onik G, Helms C: Automated percutaneous discectomy. *Spine* 1991, 16:359–363.

18. Gill K, Blumenthal SL: Clinical experience with automated percutaneous diskectomy: the Nucleotome system. *Orthopedics* 1991, 14:757–760.

19. Goldstein TB, Mink JH, Dawson EG: Early experience with automated percutaneous lumbar discectomy in the treatment of lumbar disk herniations. *Clin Orthop* 1989, 238:77–82.

20. Hammon W: Percutaneous lumbar nucleotomy. *Neurosurgery* 1989, 24:635.

21. Hoppenfeld S: Percutaneous removal of herniated lumbar discs: 50 cases with 10-year follow-up periods. *Clin Orthop* 1989, 238:92–97.

22. • Kahanovitz N, Viola K, Goldstein T, *et al.*: A multicenter analysis of percutaneous discectomy. *Spine* 1990, 15:7134–7135.

Study stating that percutaneous diskectomy does not appear to be as successful as surgical diskectomy.

23. Kaps H, Cotta H: Early results of automated percutaneous lumbar diskectomy. In *Percutaneous Lumbar Diskectomy*. Edited by Mayer HM, Brock M. Berlin: Springer-Verlag; 1989:153–156.

24. Lesoin F, Autricque A, Clarisse J, *et al.*: La nucleotomie precutanee automatisee en pathologie discal lombaire. *J Chir (Paris)* 1989, 126:185–188.

25. Luft C, Weber J, Horvath W, *et al.*: Automated percutaneous lumbar discectomy (APLD) method and one year follow-up. *Eur Radiol* 1991, 163(suppl 1):163.

26. Magalhaes AC, Pedrosa F: Percutaneous discectomy on an ambulatory basis. *Eur Radiol* 1991, 163(suppl 1):163.

27. •• Maroon JC, Allen RC: A retrospective study of 1,054 APLD cases: a twenty month clinical follow up at 35 US centers. *J Neurol Orthop Med Surg* 1989, 10:335–337.

Largest retrospective study of percutaneous diskectomies with emphasis on patient selection and meticulous technique.

28. Monteiro A, Lefevre R, Peters G, *et al.*: Lateral decompression of a pathological disc in the treatment of lumbar pain and sciatica. *Clin Orthop* 1989, 238:56–63.

29. Rezaian SM, Silver ML: Percutaneous diskectomy: personal observations of 27 cases. In *Percutaneous Lumbar Diskectomy*. Edited by Mayer HM, Brock M. Berlin: Springer-Verlag; 1989:173–176.

30. Schweigel J: Automated percutaneous discectomy: comparison with chymopapain. In *Automated Percutaneous Discectomy*. San Francisco: Radiology Research and Research Foundation; 1988:71–77.

31. • Swiecicki M: Results of percutaneous lumbar discectomy compared to laminectomy and chemonucleolysis. In *Percutaneous Lumbar Microdiscectomy*. Edited by Mayer HM, Brock M. Berlin: Springer-Verlag; 1989:133–137.

All three surgical techniques were compared.

32. Vanneroy F, Courtheoux F, Huet H, *et al.*: A new deal with far lateral lumbar disc herniations (FLDH), automated percutaneous discectomy. *Eur Radiol* 1991, 163(suppl 1):163.

33. Weigand H: Perkutane Neukleotomie: Eine nicht-operative Bahandlungsmethode des lumbalen Bandscheibenvorfalls. In *Jahrbuch der Radiologie*. Edited By Gunter RW, Gockel HPO. Zulpich, Germany: Bierman Verlag; 1991:169–176.

34. Epstein NE: Surgically confirmed cauda equina and nerve root following percutaneous discectomy at an outside institution: a case report. *J Spinal Disord* 1990, 3:380–383.

35. Onik G, Maroon JC, Jackson R: Cauda equina syndrome secondary to an improperly placed Nucleotome probe. *Neurosurgery* 1992, 30:412–415.

36. Quigley MR, Shih T, Elrifai A, *et al.*: Laser discectomy: comparison of Ho:YAG and Nd:YAG systems. *Surg Forum* 1991, 62:507–509.

Chapter 15

Peripheral Nerve Reconstruction

Hanno Millesi

THE PROBLEM

Peripheral nerve reconstruction is intended to create optimal conditions in a damaged peripheral nerve in order to promote nerve regeneration. To achieve this aim, a sequence of events must take place at different levels.

First, the neuron develops metabolic activities to produce axon sprouts. Neuron activity reaches a peak after about 3 weeks [1–5]. Second, axon sprouts originate from the ultimate intact segment of the axon. If this segment is close to the end of the stump, the axon sprouts reach the space between the stumps rapidly. If the ultimate segment of the proximal stump is damaged and develops fibrosis, however, the axon sprouts must proceed like a neuroma along this segment and are delayed in reaching the space between the stumps. Therefore, a resection is necessary. Third, axon sprouts need an ideal environment—Schwann cells—when traversing the space between two stumps.

Because the normal ratio of Schwann cells to fibroblasts is 9 to 1 in the endoneurium [6], a large number of Schwann cells are needed in the space between the two stumps. Unfortunately, epineurial fibroblasts invade this space earlier than endoneurial fibroblasts, perineurial fibroblasts, and Schwann cells, respectively [7]. Weiss and Taylor [8,9] rejected the idea of neurotropism. However, since the late 1970s, sufficient evidence has been collected to prove a certain degree of tissue and organ specificity [10–17]. Fourth, in the distal stump, a sufficient number of Schwann cells must survive [18] in order to be able to support arriving axon sprouts, and the axon sprouts must be able to mature further by enlargement and myelination by the Schwann cells. Of course, a sufficient number of axon sprouts must enter the distal stump at the correct level, find the correct pathway, and proceed toward the correct end-organ. Finally, the target organs (eg, end-plates of skeletal muscles, different sensory end-organs) must survive, and then be met by the proper axon sprouts.

RESEARCH

Several controversies exist regarding peripheral nerve regeneration, including whether the new evidence will influence surgical techniques. It is not possible to discuss all the papers published in the field of peripheral nerve reconstruction. I have restricted this review to neurotropism, neurotrophy, and the mechanical properties of peripheral nerves.

Neurotropy

Brushart and Seiler [19] demonstrated a selective reinnervation of distal motor pathways by proximal motor axons. They showed that this phenomenon was not detectable if the distance between the two stumps was only 2 mm but was clear if the distance was 5 mm. Brushart and Mesulam [20] performed a double-labeling study using horseradish peroxidase and fluoro gold. After 2 weeks motor and sensory fibers were randomly distributed, indicating that no selectivity took place. After the third week there were twice as many motor fibers in the correct motor pathways. This distribution did not change at 8 weeks. Apparently, some of the motor axon sprouts had entered a distal motor as well as a distal sensory pathway. The motor axons in the distal sensory pathway were not well supported by the Schwann cells of the distal stump and consequently degenerated. The axons in the other part, being in a correct distal pathway, survived, producing the significant rise of motor fibers in correct motor pathways starting at about the third week. This result is more an argument for the trial-and-error system of Weiss and Taylor [8,9] than a proof for neurotropism. Brushart (Brushart TM. Papers presented at the Annual Meeting of the American Society of Reconstructive Microsurgery; September, 1990; Toronto; and the Symposium of Peripheral Nerve Surgery Today; November, 1991; Vienna) repeated these experiments with peripheral nerve stumps that had been transected farther distally a second time, excluding any influence from the target organ. The result of these experiments did not differ from that of the aforementioned one, indicating that the decisive factor is located in the distal stump and not in the target organ. Carlstedt and colleagues (Carlstedt T, et al. Symposium of Peripheral Nerve Surgery Today; 1991) noted the absence of neurotropism in spite of functional restitution after implantation of avulsed ventral roots in primate brachial plexus injuries. Ochi and colleagues (Ochi M, et al. Symposium of Peripheral Nerve Surgery Today; 1991) reported on selective sensory and motor nerve regeneration in silicone Y-chambers. Machi (Machi Y. Symposium of Peripheral Nerve Surgery Today; 1991) found selectivity for regenerating motor axons only.

Neurotrophy

The discovery of nerve growth factor by Levi-Montalcini [21] opened a wide field for research. It became evident that particular nerve fibers need particular trophic factors. So far, only a limited number of trophic factors are known. In particular, the application of tubes or chambers between the two stumps permits the use of different substances (eg, different groups or factors such as nerve growth factor) expected to promote regeneration. Attempts have been made to use nerve growth factor for mixed nerves, although it is well known that nerve growth factor acts only on sensory and sympathetic nerve fibers. Brilliant surveys on this problem have been conducted by Lundborg (Lundborg G. Symposium of Peripheral Nerve Surgery Today; 1991) and Semiuk [22•]; the latter author concluded that initial attempts at manipulating the nerve conduit environment have met with limited success.

Mechanical properties of peripheral nerves

Little attention has been given to the problem of the passive motion of nerves against their surroundings. Any object at a certain distance from the plane of motion, whether on the flexor or the extensor side of an extremity, moves against the surrounding tissue when the extremity is flexed or extended. At the wrist level, for instance, the median nerve moves against the retinaculum flexorum with wrist flexion. A point in neutral position proximal to the carpal tunnel gets 9.6 mm inside the carpal tunnel because the retinaculum flexorum moves in the proximal direction. If the wrist is dorsiflexed, the nerve moves 3.5 mm in the proximal direction against the retinaculum flexorum or, in other words, the retinaculum flexorum moves in the distal direction against the median nerve. However, if the fingers are extended in this position, the nerve is drawn into the carpal tunnel, again by 9.6 mm [23••].

Zöch and colleagues [24••] developed a technique to establish a relationship between the length of the median nerve after excision and the length of the nerve bed in various positions of the upper extremity. The result of these cadaver studies was as follows. The median nerve had a mean length of 516.6 mm ± 10.4 mm. The length of the bed varied between 538.7 ± 10.6 mm in full extension and 438.2 ± 11.9 mm in full flexion. Therefore, the nerve had to slack down by 14.9% to adjust to full flexion, and had to be elongated by 4.3% to cope with full extension. Stress-strain studies have made it possible to calculate the tension of the median nerve in full extension (elongation by 4.3%) with 0.5 N/mm^2.

Millesi and colleagues [23••] and Zöch and colleagues [24••,25••] studied the stress-strain relationship of different nerve segments in situ and after excision (Figures 15.1 and 15.2). When the median nerve was studied after excision from the cadaver, 0.5 N/mm^2 was necessary to elongate the nerve by 4.3%. When the whole length of the median nerve (axilla and wrist) was studied in situ, the corresponding value was 2.5 N/mm^2. The necessary stress dropped to approximately 1.1 N/mm^2 if all the branches were transected. A similar value was measured in a segment without branches (the median nerve of the upper arm). The significant influence of the branches

on the stress-strain relationship becomes apparent. The difference between the stress-strain relationships in situ and after excision (1.1 vs 0.5 N/mm^2, respectively) represents the friction provided by the gliding tissue. Mechanical studies of excised nerves cannot be applied to a clinical situation. The relationship to the next set of branches must be considered.

If an elongation of 6% is attempted, 1 N/mm^2 is needed after excision. In situ, however, a more than threefold stress must be exerted because of the steep rise of the stress-strain curve. This view is supported by others. Wall and colleagues [26••] demonstrated that a 6% strain decreased the amplitude of the axon potential by 70% at 1 hour's duration but returned to normal during the recovery period. At 12% strain, conduction was completely blocked by 1 hour and recovery was minimal. Histologically, after 1 hour of elongation no changes could be seen, but we can assume that if the elongation had continued, fibrotic responses would have been inevitable. Clark and colleagues [27••] observed a 50% decrease of blood flow with an elongation of 8%. Blood flow returned to normal. After 15% elongation there was an 80% decrease in blood flow with minimal recovery. The authors concluded that elongation of a nerve by 8% may lead to a detrimental ischemia.

It was believed that stress relaxation may be exploited to decrease tension during elongation of a nerve [28•]. The relaxation phenomenon is well known in viscoelastic tissues. If such tissue is elongated with a certain force and by a certain percentage and the elongation is kept constant, the force necessary to maintain elongation decreases due to viscoelastic phenomena. The nerve also behaves as a viscoelastic tissue. Wall and colleagues [28•] showed that with 6% elongation, the force necessary to main-

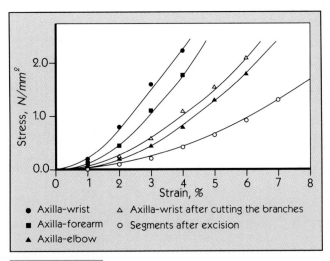

Figure 15.1

Stress-strain diagram of the median nerve.

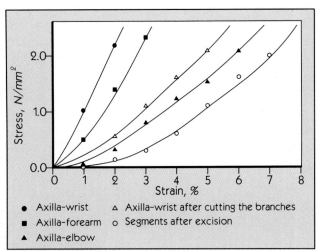

Figure 15.2

Stress-strain diagram of the ulnar nerve.

tain elongation dropped to 52.5% of the original force. If the elongation was 9% or 12%, relaxation decreased tension to about 69% of the original level. It is tempting to believe that such a phenomenon may keep elongation constant with reduced tension. In reality, however, this idea is in error. The decrease of tension is valid only while elongation is maintained. If a limb is immobilized in flexion, reducing elongation to zero for 10 minutes only, the tissue recovers and exactly the same amount of tension is necessary for a second elongation as for the first. The stress relaxation phenomenon, therefore, applies only if the suture site of the nerve is kept under tension (even reduced tension) and no protective flexion is used.

The mechanical properties induce another phenomenon. If a tissue is elongated in one direction, it becomes more narrow perpendicular to the elongation. This narrowing can be detected only by biaxial studies, as were performed by Zöch [25••]. These studies showed that Poisson's ratio was constant up to 6% elongation, but dropped at more than 6%, indicating structural damage to the tissue. The narrowing along an elongated tube, such as a perineurial tube, causes a decrease in volume. Measurement proved that 4% elongation decreases volume by 1%; 6% elongation decreases volume by 1.5%; and 8% elongation decreases volume by 2%. All this evidence shows how complicated the problem is and how carefully surgeons should avoid elongation.

CLASSIFICATION OF NERVE DAMAGE

Because of a particular trauma, a nerve may lose its ability to conduct. Complete paralysis and complete loss of sensation in the area of this nerve will be the result. If only a certain percentage of nerve fibers, *eg*, the more peripheral ones, are damaged, there will be a partial loss of function. The loss of conductivity can go along with different degrees of local damage.

Table 15.1
Classification of nerve injuries*

Degree of damage	Definition
I	Conduction block, morphologically normal, axons intact
II	Axonotmesis, axonolysis, other structures normal
III	Endoneurium disrupted, fascicular pattern intact
IV	Fascicles disrupted, epineurium in continuity
V	Loss of continuity

*From Sunderland [30]; with permission.

Table 15.2
Nerve injury classification as the basis for selection of surgical procedure

Combined classification	Classification according to the continuity of different tissue layers (Sunderland I–V)	Classification according to the tissue response (A, B, C, N, S)
I	Conduction block, continuity of all structures preserved	—
I A	Same as I	Fibrosis of the epifascicular epineurium: A
I B	Same as I	Fibrosis of the interfascicular epineurium: B
II	Axonolysis, endoneurium intact	—
II A	Same as II	Fibrosis of the epifascicular epineurium: A
II B	Same as II	Fibrosis of the interfascicular epineurium: B
III	Axonolysis, endoneurium destroyed, perineurium intact	—
III A	Same as III	Fibrosis of the epifascicular epineurium: A
III B	Same as III	Fibrosis of the interfascicular epineurium: B
III C	Same as III	Fibrosis of the endoneurium: C
IV N	Continuity preserved by connective tissue only	Connective tissue link invaded by a neuroma
IV S	Same as IV N	Neuroma did not reach the distal stump
V	Complete loss of continuity	—

Many attempts have been made to achieve accurate classifications.

Seddon [29] distinguished three different degrees of nerve damage: neurapraxia, axonotmesis, and neurotmesis. Sunderland [30] introduced five different degrees of damage (Table 15.1). Both classification systems are based on loss of continuity of different tissue layers within the peripheral nerves. However, they do not account for the connective tissue reaction that develops as a consequence of the traumatic influence. Millesi [31,32] tried to close this gap by distinguishing three different degrees of fibrosis according to localization. Type A fibrosis extends mainly in the epifascicular epineurium all around the nerve. The whole nerve trunk is compressed by shrinkage. This compression impedes the spontaneous regeneration that might otherwise occur due to the lesser degree of damage of the fascicular tissue itself. Type B fibrosis extends into the interfascicular tissue (interfascicular fibrosis). Type C fibrosis develops within the fascicles and replaces the original endoneurial structures. These fascicles become indurated and regenerative efforts cannot proceed (intrafascicular fibrosis).

This classification was selected because it provides a basis for selecting surgical procedures (Table 15.2). The stratification of fibrosis can be combined with Sunderland's five-degree system for classifying damage [30]. For patients who have suffered degree IV damage according to Sunderland, two typical situations are distinguished: formation of a neuroma, in which the neuroma invades the remaining connective tissue, and formation of scar tissue. The remaining connective tissue link consists only of connective tissue and is converted into scar tissue. The possible combinations are shown in Table 15.1.

CLASSIFICATION OF THE PROXIMAL AND THE DISTAL STUMP

Surgical reports usually read: "The two stumps were resected until normal nerve tissue was encountered. . ." It is evident that "normal" nerve tissue is required at the proximal and distal stumps to avoid a delay of the outgrowing axons from the proximal stump. Frequently, one of the consequences of severe trauma is a long transient zone between completely damaged nerve tissue and normal nerve tissue. Questions include how much to resect and how to define "normal" nerve tissue. For an exact description of the morphologic situation at the proximal and the distal stumps, a classification system was developed (Millesi H and Kovac W. Symposium of Peripheral Nerve Surgery Today; 1991). This system is based on the classification system of lesions in continuity and uses the morphologic criteria of degree I to degree IV damage according to Sunderland [30], complemented by the description of type A, B, and C fibrosis according to Millesi [31,32].

Prospect of spontaneous recovery	Diagnosis	Surgical therapy
Very good	Conductivity preserved in spite of muscle paralysis	None
Very good after decompression	Conductivity preserved in spite of muscle paralysis	Epineuriotomy
Very good after decompression	Conductivity preserved in spite of muscle paralysis	Partial epineuriotomy
Good	Spontaneous regeneration	None
Good after decompression	At surgery	Epineuriotomy
Good after decompression	At surgery	Partial epineuriotomy
Possible	At surgery	None
Possible after decompression	At surgery	Epineuriotomy
Possible after decompression	At surgery	Partial epineuriotomy
None	At surgery: induration	Resection and nerve grafting
Very poor	At surgery	Resection and nerve grafting
None	At surgery	Resection and nerve grafting
None	At surgery	Neurorrhaphy or nerve grafting

Proximal stump

A normal segment of the proximal stump shows degree I damage, according to Sunderland [30], which by definition does not present morphologic changes. In a ruptured nerve, all different degrees of damage can be assumed; degrees II through IV may be present in sequence. The amount of fibrosis seen in secondary repairs can be indicated by the A, B, C system. In this system, *N* defines the formation of a neuroma (seen in secondary repair only), which can develop within a fascicle along with degree III damage (IIIN) or ultimately degree IV damage (IVN) (Figure 15.3).

Distal stump

The distal stump can be classified in a similar way, with two main exceptions. First, a degree I situation is not possible because axons and wallerian degeneration always occur. Consequently, a normal-looking

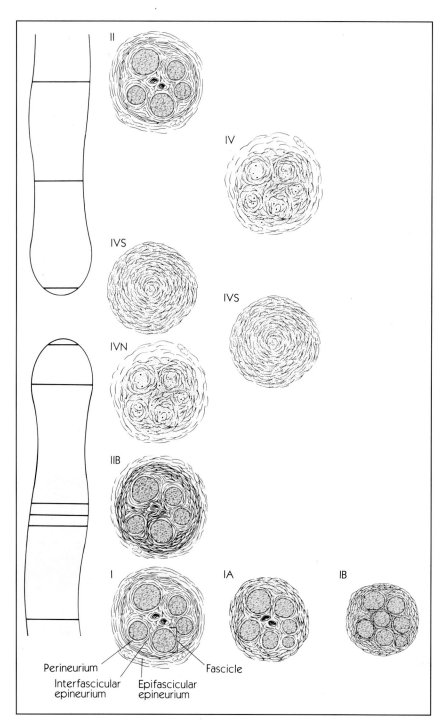

Perineurium
Interfascicular epineurium
Epifascicular epineurium
Fascicle

Figure 15.3

Example of a secondary nerve repair. **Bottom, Proximal stump**: IVS—Resection from the end shows scar tissue only. IVN—More proximal to this a neuroma can be seen. IIB—More proximal to this the fascicles look quite normal, but the endoneurium does not protrude. There is a lot of fibrous tissue around and between the fascicles. Histology shows the endoneurium intact. No axons or myelin sheath is found. IB—More proximal to this the fascicles look normal, with a lot of fibrous tissue around and between the fascicles. Histology shows the axons and myelin sheath intact. IA—More proximal to this the fascicles look normal. Fibrous tissue can be seen around the fascicles. Histology shows the axons and myelin sheath intact. **Top, Distal stump**: IVS— Resection from the end shows scar tissue only. IV—More distal to this there is nerve tissue but no fascicular structure. II—More distal to this the fascicles are rather small but not indurated. Connective tissue is normal. (*From* Millesi [32]; with permission.)

distal stump would present a degree II situation that might also have a type IIA or IIB fibrosis. Second, as might be expected, neuromalike structures cannot be seen in the distal stump after complete loss of continuity. Consequently, there can be no degree IIIN or IVN situation.

This system allows exact classification using simple histologic techniques, such as a frozen section colored with hematoxylin and eosin, which allows viewing of axons without special staining; and paraffin sections colored with hematoxylin and eosin, van Gieson's stain, and a myelin stain.

LESION IN CONTINUITY

A lesion in continuity can be the result of a traction injury, which may cause degrees of damage from I to IV in sequence according to the amount of traction. It may be the result of compression by an external force against a stiff background or of compression by a bony fragment, a foreign body, or scar tissue. A lesion in continuity with corresponding fibrosis also develops under ischemic conditions, *eg*, in compartment syndrome. Entrapment of a nerve in a narrow canal causes similar injury. In all situations, if a peripheral nerve is compressed, it is necessary to consider not only the compressing force as such, but also the fact that the nerve is prevented from moving, which causes traction damage in addition to the compression.

Characteristically, in all situations, the gliding tissue that links the nerve to the surrounding tissue becomes obliterated so that the nerve has no opportunity for passive motion and becomes adherent. This gliding tissue is termed *adventitia, paraneurium,* or *conjunctiva nervorum* [33].

External neurolysis

After exposure, the nerve is separated from the surrounding tissue by transection of the adhesions. New adhesions form if the nerve remains in a poor, scarry environment. However, if the nerve is in soft tissue well supplied with blood, the gliding tissue has a good regenerative capacity, or the nerve can be enveloped in a gliding tissue flap (Millesi H. Paper presented at the Annual Meeting of the Deutschprachige Arbeitsgemeinschaft für Handchirurgie; 1984; Strassburg; and Millesi H and Rath Th. Paper presented at the 8th Symposium of the International Society of Reconstructive Microsurgery; July, 1985; Paris) [34,35••].

Internal neurolysis

In internal neurolysis, the epineurium at least is fully transected. The first and most superficial step is the epifascicular epineuriotomy (Figure 15.4), which can be performed in a multiple way around the circumference of a nerve to achieve decompression in type A fibrosis. If type B fibrosis has partially invaded the

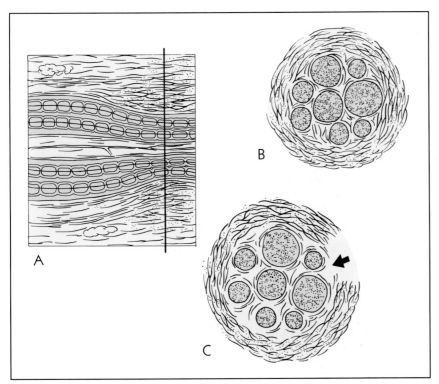

Figure 15.4

Fibrosis of the epifascicular epineurium (type A) with compression of the fascicles. Treatment is decompression by partial epifascicular epineuriotomy. **A,** Longitudinal section. Note two fascicles with two nerve fibers (*left side*), normal epifascicular epineurium (*top* and *bottom*), normal interfascicular epineurium (*center*), and compression of the fascicles due to fibrosis of the epifascicular epineurium (*right side*). **B,** Cross-sectional view according to the vertical line in *A.* **C,** Cross-sectional view of *A* after epifascicular epineuriotomy (*arrow*). (*From* Millesi [32]; with permission.)

interfascicular epineurium, the fibrotic epineurium can be resected all around the nerve (epifascicular epineuriectomy). If the interfascicular epineurium is highly fibrotic, compressing the fascicles of a polyfascicular nerve, the fibrotic parts are resected (interfascicular epineuriectomy; Figure 15.5). This procedure is always performed partially because it is never necessary to excise all the interfascicular tissue to isolate the fascicles completely and deprive them of blood supply. Such an extensive procedure also cuts the connections between the fascicles and may cause the formation of many small neuromas within the nerve. The aim of neurolysis in such cases is always decompression, which requires that fibrotic parts of the epifascicular epineurium be excised. If decompression is achieved, the procedure is immediately stopped. Few vessels or interconnecting fascicles are left in highly fibrotic tissue, and therefore the damage is minimal.

Internal neurolysis has become a controversial issue because in its early phases, many surgeons did not observe the rule that neurolysis must stop immediately if decompression is achieved (Table 15.2). If a nerve cannot move against the surrounding tissue, fascicle movement within the nerve increases to compensate for the necessary passive motion [23••]. This compensatory movement may lead to an internal entrapment, with fixation of the fibers in a meandering fashion [23••,36,37]. This deformity of the fascicles is corrected by partial interfascicular epineuriectomy.

LOSS OF CONTINUITY

Loss of continuity is equivalent to degree V damage, or neurotmesis [29,30]. Restoring continuity is the goal of all surgical efforts to provide favorable conditions for nerve regeneration. Clinicians must differentiate between two situations. First, in the case of *sharp transection*, the nerve tissue of the two stumps has not suffered damage. According to stump classification, this nerve tissue resembles a degree I lesion in the proximal stump and a degree II lesion in the distal stump. Surgical repair must merely realign the structures of the two stumps. Next, if a *blunt trauma* has destroyed or damaged the tissue of the proximal and distal stumps, this tissue will not survive as nerve tissue but will undergo fibrosis. In this case a certain amount of tissue must be resected. Realignment of the structures is impossible because of the structural differences along the course of the peripheral nerve (Figure 15.3). In either case a gap is left between the two stumps.

In a degree I lesion, the gap is caused by elastic retraction in the nerve stumps and does not represent a defect. In blunt trauma, the gap consists of the length of elastic retraction plus the real defect due to traumatic loss of nerve tissue. The distance to be overcome is further increased by the defect at the two stumps caused by the necessary resection of the damaged nerve tissue.

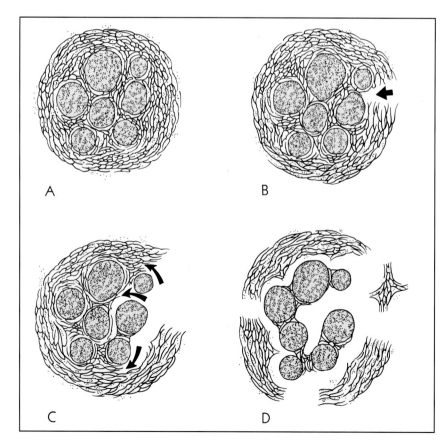

Figure 15.5

Fibrosis of the interfascicular epineurium (type B). Treatment is partial interfascicular epineuriectomy. **A,** Cross-section of a nerve with epi- and interfascicular fibrosis. **B,** An epineuriotomy (*arrow*) did not decompress the fascicles (in contrast to Figure 15.4). **C,** To achieve decompression it is necessary to dissect the interfascicular epineurium (*arrows*). **D,** Decompression was achieved by resection of the epifascicular epineurium and part of the interfascicular epineurium. The fascicles are still connected to each other by the remaining interfascicular epineurium, which contains preserved vessels and interfascicular connections. The fascicles are never completely isolated. Decompression is the goal. (*From* Millesi [32]; with permission.)

It is evident that damage of degrees IVS (*S* denotes scar tissue) and IVN in secondary repairs must be resected. It is also clear that damage of degrees IIIC and IIIN must be resected in secondary repairs. It is still an open question whether degree II damage must be resected. No study has yet been performed with this emphasis.

The technique of managing nerve defects is discussed below. In this connection there are only two questions of interest. Should a primary or a secondary nerve repair be performed? Should end-to-end neurorrhaphy or nerve graft, or alternative techniques to nerve grafting, be elected?

Primary versus secondary nerve repair

A great advantage of primary nerve repair is that no secondary intervention is necessary. The anatomic situation is clear. It is imperative to repair other structures, especially severed vessels, because nerve regeneration is positively influenced if the transected vessels are repaired simultaneously (Merle M. Paper presented at the 1st Congress of the European Federation of Societies of Microsurgery; September, 1992; Rome).

Arguments against primary nerve repair are studies showing that neuron activity is highest at the third week [1–5]. The main argument is that the amount of nerve tissue damage at the ends of the two stumps cannot be evaluated at the moment of injury, but becomes evident only when the damaged tissue has undergone fibrosis. If paralyzed structures such as flexor tendons are to be repaired, there is the danger of adhesions between nerves and tendons if the repairs are performed simultaneously. In some institutions, a surgeon experienced in peripheral nerve surgery may not always be available.

It is evident that the arguments against primary repair do not weigh as heavily in cases of sharp transection; therefore primary repair is without doubt the technique of choice in such cases. Conversely, in cases of blunt trauma, the difficulty in estimating the amount of damage is important. If there is a defect, a secondary repair is my treatment of choice. Between these two extremes there may be a transient zone where either technique might lead to equally good results.

End-to-end neurorrhaphy versus nerve graft or alternative techniques

In the past, many surgeons tried to avoid nerve grafting at any cost and accepted tension at the site of repair. Even Seddon [38,39], with his experience that a defect over 2.5 cm causes a sharp decrease of the percentage of useful recovery, stated in the second edition of his book, *Surgical Disorders of Peripheral Nerves* [39], that "an impressive development comes from Millesi. There is no doubt that the sutured nerve subjected to great tension may be so damaged that recovery will be prevented. Any degree of tension is harmful, and I believe that there is no use for stretching in moderation after suture. The normal elasticity of nerves, at the very least 6%, is ignored."

Many surgeons retain this opinion (Mackinnon SE: written communication, 1992). Applying current knowledge about the mechanical properties of nerve tissue in situ and after excision leads to the following conclusions: 1) in a normal nerve without adhesions, the tension necessary to overcome the elastic retraction can easily be accepted, and end-to-end nerve repair will not cause any problem; 2) if a secondary repair is necessary in a nerve that has lost its normal elasticity and has developed adhesions, the situation is completely different. Even overcoming the elastic retraction by accepting tension at the site of repair is in many cases doubtful; 3) normal nerve tissue in situ is constructed to be elongated by 4% to meet the requirement of full extension. If there is a nerve defect, tension must be applied not only to overcome the elastic retraction, but also to elongate the nerve by the amount lacking. Because the site of nerve repair is immobilized in the flexed position, elongation of the nerve is postponed until after mobilization is started again and elongation can be performed gradually. Conversely, in adhesions that develop during the period of immobilization, especially at the site of repair, the distribution of the necessary elongation is not equal along the length of the nerve. Shorter segments may be exposed to more elongation than others, passing the critical threshold. Mechanical studies have shown that the tension necessary to elongate a given nerve segment is very much influenced by the presence or absence of branches. Therefore, the site of the injury in relation to branches must be considered. To achieve the same elongation in a branched segment at least three times as much tension is needed than if the same study were performed with the nerve after excision.

In summary, the tension needed to overcome elastic retraction in primary repair can be easily accepted. Slight elongation of the nerve may be possible to overcome a small defect, especially if it is done as a primary repair and if there is no fibrosis or adhesions. The above statements regarding primary end-to-end neurorrhaphy do not apply to nerve grafts. Free nerve grafts are extremely sensitive to tension, which must be absolutely avoided in this situation. As a recent study stated, ". . .any degree of tension at the graft repair site has a deleterious effect on functional nerve regeneration" (Kim D. Symposium of Peripheral Nerve Surgery Today; 1991) [40,41•].

NEURORRHAPHY

The purpose of neurorrhaphy is to allow axons to cross a free space between the proximal and distal stumps in order to reach the latter. This section discusses two aspects of neurorrhaphy.

Steps to nerve repair

The fascicular tissue must be coapted to make the space between the two stumps as narrow as possible. A nerve repair is performed in four steps.

The first step is *preparation of stumps*. Damaged and fibrotic tissue must be resected. Either resection of the whole stump or interfascicular dissection can be performed, transecting individual fascicles or fascicle groups at different levels (Figure 15.5). Second, the two stumps must be *approximated*. It is here that all the questions of tension discussed in the previous section become significant.

Third, the surgeon attempts to *coapt* the fascicular tissue as closely as possible. How well this can be done depends on the fascicular pattern of the two stumps. With a monofascicular pattern (only one fascicle), coaptation is easy. If the nerve trunk consists of two to four fascicles, fascicular coaptation is not a problem if there is no defect and if the pattern of the two stumps corresponds. However, if there is an oligofascicular pattern involving, for example, five to 12 large fascicles, trunk-to-trunk coaptation is not automatically satisfactory. In this case a better coaptation is achieved if these five to 12 large fascicles are isolated and a fascicular repair is performed. From Hentz and colleagues [42] we learn that perineurial (*ie*, fascicular) repair yielded electrophysiologically better results than did epineurial sutures. Other studies did not show much difference between the two techniques in animal experiments, but it must be remembered that at present, techniques for evaluating results are far too crude to allow proper differentiation.

In the case of a polyfascicular pattern, in which many fascicles are consequently smaller and less manageable, coaptation cannot be performed as for an oligofascicular pattern. The surgical damage in trying to manipulate these small fascicles individually outweighs an eventual advantage of a fascicular repair. In this case, trunk-to-trunk repair, eventually using guide sutures, is the proper solution. If, in a polyfascicular pattern, the fascicles are arranged in groups, an alternative is group-to-group coaptation.

Many studies investigating the relative merits of epineurial (trunk-to-trunk) repair versus perineurial (fascicular) coaptation are irrelevant because they do not consider the fascicular pattern. Fascicular repair is an overtreatment if there are one to four or five fasci-

cles but cannot be applied if there are too many small fascicles. However, in certain cases the fascicular pattern contains a limited number of manageable fascicles. Only these cases are eligible for fascicular repair.

Finally, *coaptation* can be maintained by stitches that may be anchored in the epifascicular epineurium, the interfascicular epineurium, the perineurium, or the paraneurium. Because axon sprouts do not proceed irregularly if they have the chance to meet nerve tissue, watertight repair to prevent aberration of axon sprouts is obsolete. A few stitches are sufficient to keep the two nerve stumps together. If there is no tension or very limited tension, only a few stitches and consequently very little surgical manipulation are necessary. More tension requires more stitches and more surgical manipulation. These facts constitute an argument against the use of tension.

Coaptation can also be maintained by fibrin glue. We know now that fibrin glue, as it is provided today, is not an obstacle to axon sprouts (Palazzi S. Symposium of Peripheral Nerve Surgery Today; 1991). One of the dangers of gluing—that glue may penetrate between the fascicles and form an obstacle—is no longer relevant. The use of glue rather than many stitches shortens the time of surgery. (If the number of stitches is reduced to a minimum in cases without tension, this advantage is of little importance.) Fibrin glue can glue together several nerve grafts to concentrate the grafts to a smaller area (Narakas A. Paper presented at the Symposium Update and Future Trends in Fibrin Sealing in Surgical and Nonsurgical Fields; November, 1992; Vienna).

Ideal coaptation creates an ideal transient zone between the two stumps, with parallel arrangement of the nerve fibers and of the vessels (Greulick M, *et al.* Symposium of Peripheral Nerve Surgery Today; 1991). Without ideal coaptation, there is an irregular transient zone that consists of collagen and contains an irregular vascular pattern coming from epineurial vessels. From our own studies we know that these irregular transient zones are regularly present if the repair has been performed under tension [31,32].

A special technique of coaptation was developed by de Medinaceli and colleagues (de Medinaceli L, *et al.* Symposium of Peripheral Nerve Surgery Today; 1991) [43]. By using a special device, the terminal segment of the two stumps is frozen before trimming and during coaptation. By this maneuver, the cellular environment, as far as electrolyte concentration and other factors are concerned, is kept constant. A ribbon relieves the tension in end-to-end repair. Preliminary clinical results of this technique were presented by Merle (Merle M. Symposium Update and Future Trends in Fibrin Sealing in Surgical and Nonsurgical Fields; 1992). Other authors have developed special devices to relieve tension at the site of coaptation by ribbons to achieve approximation (Kafritas D, *et al.* Symposium of Peripheral Nerve Surgery Today; 1991).

Coaptation with the stumps separated

Lundborg and Hansson [10,11] showed how axons with accompanying structures proceed along a gap within a tissue chamber. The tissue chamber protects the nerve from invasion by cells from the surrounding tissue. The tissue chamber technique has been used not only for studying neurotropism and neurotrophism but also to enhance nerve regeneration by local application of substances (Haas G; Kafritas D, *et al.*; and Danielson N. Symposium of Peripheral Nerve Surgery Today; 1991) [44] and Schwann cells. The chamber technique was used successfully in an ulnar nerve repair, keeping the two stumps separated by 3 to 4 mm (Lundborg G. Symposium of Peripheral Nerve Surgery Today; 1991) [45].

Hentz and colleagues [42] suggested applying tubulization at the fascicular level. Prospective studies must be performed before we can evaluate this approach.

NERVE GRAFTING AND ALTERNATIVES

Management of nerve defects

There are three basic ways to manage a nerve defect. One way is to shorten the distance between the two stumps, which can be achieved by resection of a bony segment or transposition of a nerve into a shorter bed. In both cases, the distance that can be overcome is limited. The classic example of nerve transposition into a shorter bed is the transposition of the ulnar nerve to the palmar side of the elbow joint. This maneuver offers two possibilities: 1) the nerve is situated in a shorter bed and is now too long (the gain in length with an extended elbow joint is about 2 cm); or 2) the elbow joint is flexed, which allows an additional defect to be overcome but is followed by an elongation of the nerve, as discussed later.

Another method of managing nerve defects is to elongate the nerve tissue. The problem of the stress-strain relationship of peripheral nerves is discussed above. To cope with the mechanical requirements of free motion of the upper extremity, the median nerve must be able to be elongated by about 4%. If a nerve defect is managed by elongation and free motion of the extremity must still be provided, the elongation must extend beyond 4%. Acute elongation is tolerated only in a limited way, and stress relaxation does not help. Constant elongation beyond a certain limit consequently leads to fibrosis of the nerve stumps mainly at the site of repair [45–48]. The consequences of overelongation can be reduced if the necessary elongation is distributed over a longer nerve segment. This distribution is possible only if the nerve has preserved its elasticity, if the gliding tissue has remained intact, and if there are no branches. It is consequently not effective in secondary repairs.

The second technique for diminishing the consequences of elongation is gradual elongation distributed over a longer time interval. This can be achieved by presurgical elongation, using an expanderlike device, as described by Van Beek and colleagues (personal communication, June 1980). The literature has reported only a few such cases, with limited success. There is significant danger of damaging the nerve (Brunelli G. Symposium of Peripheral Nerve Surgery Today; 1991). A final method of managing a nerve defect is by providing additional nerve tissue. This procedure is done by nerve grafting or one of the alternative methods.

Nerve grafting

If the distance between the two stumps is bridged by an autologous nerve graft, the axon sprouts must cross from the proximal stump into the graft. If the graft has survived the grafting procedure in good condition, the fibrosis cells meet all the necessary requirements by the Schwann cells of the graft and are able to proceed along the structures of the graft to the distal stump. There they must cross again into the distal stump. The axon sprouts must cross two lines of coaptation, but both coaptations must have been performed under the ideal conditions without tension.

The literature frequently reports on the mutual advantages and disadvantages of grafting and neurorrhaphy. These reports are without value if the technique of the grafting procedure has not been well described. Nerve grafts can be performed in many different ways and can be classified according to four parameters.

The origin of nerve grafts is important; autologous nerve grafts are the technique of choice. Allografts or xenografts cause an immunologic response that attacks mainly the connective tissue and the cellular part of the nerve graft. Axon sprouts and basal membrane have the chance to survive if they have been established. The problems of the immunologic reaction and immune suppression have been studied carefully [49–53]. One clinical case was treated with limited success. The symposium "Peripheral Nerve Surgery Today: Turning Point or Continuous Development?" in Vienna in November 1991 resulted in the conclusion that clinical application of allografts should not yet be advocated (Mackinnon SE and Berger A. Symposium of Peripheral Nerve Surgery Today; 1991).

The donor nerves are also important. Free transplantation of a nerve is possible only if the spontaneous revascularization is fast enough to establish circulation before the central part of the nerve has suffered ischemic damage. A free grafted nerve is only then revascularized fast enough if a relatively large surface is in contact with a recipient site well supplied with blood, and if the diameter of the nerve does not pass a certain limit. Cutaneous nerves, for example, usually survive free grafting very well, but only if these grafts are transplanted individually and if each graft has sufficient contact with the surrounding tissue. This contact is not secured for cable grafts. Seddon [39] described his technique: "Grafts are cut to the correct length (15% greater than the gap). The grafts are assembled to form a cross-sectional area equal to that of the proximal stump." In this way each graft loses part of its surface for contact with the recipient site and revascularization is retarded. In fact, these cable grafts have not proven successful, but similar techniques are still advocated.

If a trunk graft should be used, a problem of excessively large caliber must be solved. Two techniques are possible: maintaining or immediately restoring the circulation of the graft, and splitting the nerve graft into minor units by microsurgical dissection. Because the group pattern of nerves having a polyfascicular structure with group arrangement remains constant over a reasonably long distance, sufficiently long nerve grafts of an acceptable caliber can be dissected. This split nerve grafting has been used successfully in cases of brachial plexus lesions, when the ulnar nerve was available as a donor but could not be used as a vascularized nerve graft [32].

The mechanical aspects are another important factor. The final distance between the two nerve stumps is determined by elastic retraction, which may be fixed by fibrosis; the real nerve defect; and the amount of resection from the proximal and the distal stumps. This distance is influenced and can be manipulated by the position of the adjacent joints. Flexion of the adjacent joints minimizes the defect and with extension of the same joints maximizes it. This point is extremely important. Seddon [39] approximated the two ends of the defective nerve as far as possible and closed the "remaining" defect—after minimizing it—with a nerve graft (Figure 15.6A). Thus the disadvantage of a suture under tension was combined with the disadvantage of a nerve graft (two sites of coaptation). These results had to be worse than an end-to-end nerve repair. It is better to maximize the nerve gap by bringing the joints into at least neutral position, selecting the length of the graft in this position (Figure 15.6B). Then the two coaptations

can be performed without any problems and the healing is not adversely influenced by local tension. In all my papers I have underlined this fact as a condition for successful nerve grafting. This necessity was confirmed by Terzis and colleagues in 1975 [54] and by Kim and colleagues [40, 41•] in 1990 and 1991.

As a consequence, a longer graft segment must be used. The literature states that the quality of the result decreases with the length of the graft. This is not true. The quality of nerve grafting decreases with the length of the defect—which consequently needs longer grafts—but not with the length of the graft itself. This statement was recently confirmed by Frey and colleagues [55••], who showed that in sheep, saphenous nerve grafts 28 cm long without connection to a target organ were well neurotized if they remained on the same side of the body. They were less well neurotized if they crossed over to the contralateral side.

Why are free nerve grafts so sensitive to longitudinal traction? Nerve grafts survive by forming adhesions with the recipient site to allow rapid revascularization. They are therefore not moveable and cannot adapt, as a normal nerve does, to longitudinal traction during the motion of a limb. This fact is another common cause for failure of a nerve grafting procedure. If the length of the graft is selected correctly, according to the maximal distance between the two stumps in extended position, but the extremity is immobilized in flexed position, the graft forms adhesions in a relaxed state in flexed position. When mobilization is started, the graft cannot adapt to extension because of these adhesions, even if it was originally long enough (Figure 15.6C).

Finally, the circulatory aspects are important. A free nerve graft survives the grafting procedure by spontaneous revascularization from invading vessels of the recipient site. From Penkert and Samii (Penkert G and Samii M. Symposium of Peripheral Nerve Surgery Today; 1991) we know that revascularization of the autologous graft begins on the third postoperative day. Through regenerative sprouting, hyperemia develops on the fourth postoperative day. The longitudinal revascularization is of no great importance. Schwann cells are known to survive the free grafting procedure well [56–58]. To avoid this short period of ischemia, the techniques of the pedicled [59,60] and vascularized nerve grafts were developed [61,62]. This technique was further developed by Breidenbach and Terzis [63,64]. A vascularized nerve trunk can also be transferred as an island flap if the transfer is within the range of the vascular pedicle. Vascularized nerve grafts have the advantage of being independent of the quality of the recipient site. The gliding apparatus of the transplant remains intact. Consequently, these grafts are less sensitive to longitudinal traction than are free nerve grafts. Many attempts have been made to prove the theoretic superiority of these nerve grafts over "conventional" nerve grafts. These attempts were not very successful. Most authors concluded that regeneration occurs earlier in vascularized nerve grafts, but in the final outcome does not differ much if grafting has been performed under comparable conditions. Kanaya and colleagues [65•] reported on experiments with rats, showing that the vascularized nerve grafts looked morphologically and physiologi-

cally better 12 weeks after surgery. However, there was no difference as far as muscle weight and axon count were concerned. Mani and colleagues [66•] reported on similar experiments with rabbits but saw no significant difference in the rate of regeneration between vascularized and nonvascularized nerve grafts. Doi and colleagues [67••] reported on 27 vascularized and 22 conventional sural nerve grafts in patients with comparable upper extremity injuries. They found that vascularized nerve grafts did better if the defect was longer than 6 cm and associated with a

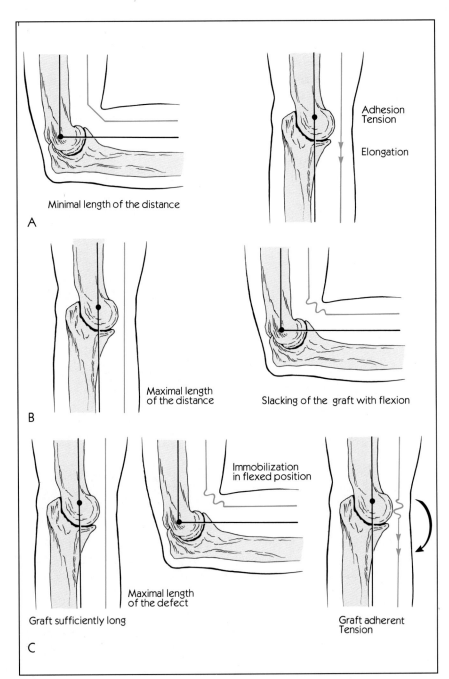

Figure 15.6

Maximal and minimal length of the graft. **A,** The length of the graft was selected according to the minimal distance between the two stumps in flexion of the adjacent joint. The graft is too short when the joint is mobilized. **B,** The length of the graft was selected according to the maximal distance between the two stumps with the joint in extension. When mobilization starts, the graft is slacked down but not extended. **C,** The length of the graft was selected correctly according to the maximal distance between the two stumps. Immobilization in flexed position. The necessary adhesions form in flexed position. When mobil-izations starts, the graft cannot be adapted and is exposed to traction.

Minimal length of the distance

A

Adhesion Tension

Elongation

Maximal length of the distance

Slacking of the graft with flexion

B

Immobilization in flexed position

Graft sufficiently long

Maximal length of the defect

Graft adherent Tension

C

massive skin defect, or if the graft was performed after reimplantation. Otherwise results achieved with "conventional" grafts were equally good. Therefore, the conclusion has been drawn that vascularized nerve grafts are indicated in certain situations but are not by definition better than free nerve grafts.

To achieve optimal results with free nerve grafting, the stumps must be prepared carefully by interfascicular dissection, separating the individual fascicle groups if these are present. These fascicle groups are transected at different levels. The length of the graft is estimated with extended joints and joints in neutral position, respectively. The grafts are placed into the defect individually to provide maximal contact with the recipient site. Coaptation to corresponding fascicle groups of the proximal and distal stumps is performed by one stitch to avoid damage by touching the

graft with forceps or other instruments. If the stitch is placed correctly, an optimal coaptation usually can be achieved. In a few instances, when the graft end tends to rotate, a second stitch may be necessary (Figure 15.7). The coaptation is maintained by normal fibrin formation, which secures adherence of the graft on the cross-section to the corresponding fascicle group, and also to the site of neighboring fascicles. Because the stump has been prepared in fascicle groups of different lengths, an interdentation between fascicles and fascicle groups can be achieved (Figure 15.8). Many authors advocate additional use of fibrin glue. In my opinion, fibrin glue is not necessary if tension is really zero and the length of the graft is sufficient.

Special care must be taken to close the skin without dislocating the grafts. After skin closure, the extremity is immobilized by a plaster cast for 8 days in

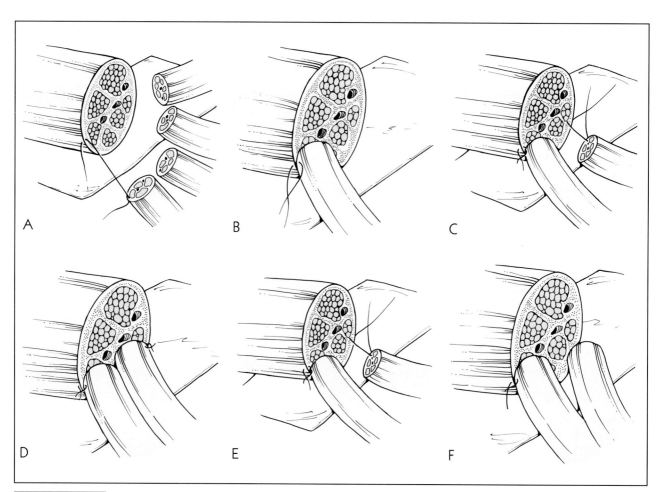

Figure 15.7

Management of a nerve defect by cutaneous free nerve grafts with a monofascicular nerve. Four segments of the sural nerves are used (**A**). The first graft is coapted to the lower portion of the fascicular area by one stitch (**B**). The second nerve graft is approximated (**C**).

If the stitch is placed properly, the coaptation is satisfactory (**D**). If the stitch is not placed properly, (*eg*, too low [**E**]), the graft rotates in the wrong direction (**F**).

(Continued.)

exactly the position it held during the operation. After 8 days, mobilization can begin without danger of dislocation and rupture because the graft is not exposed to longitudinal traction.

Alternatives to nerve grafting

A transected peripheral nerve forms a regenerative neuroma. Axon sprouts originate terminally or laterally from the most distal segment of any intact proximal axon. These axon sprouts are accompanied by Schwann cells, capillaries, and epi- and perineurial fibroblasts. The fibroblasts tend to form sheathlike structures to envelop several axon sprouts, producing minifascicles. If no distal stump is available, the outgrowth is irregular and a tumorlike structure develops. In many instances such neuromas may cause

pain syndromes. If there is a minimal gap, there might be a chance for such a neuroma to reach a distal stump and produce a spontaneous recovery. It is known that in animals, even relatively long distances between two nerve stumps can be bridged by such neuromas. Usually, however, if no distal stump is encountered, the neuroma stops growing, apparently because the impetus to proceed is exhausted.

If there is a structure available, a neuroma may proceed for a certain distance. This phenomenon was studied by Schröder and Seiffert [68] using lyophilized nerve segments and was termed *neuromatous neurotization*. It immediately became clear that bridging a defect by mesothelial chambers [10,11] may be an alternative to nerve grafting. The advantages over nerve grafting would be that in the free space, the neurotropic influences can be fully effective. Lacking

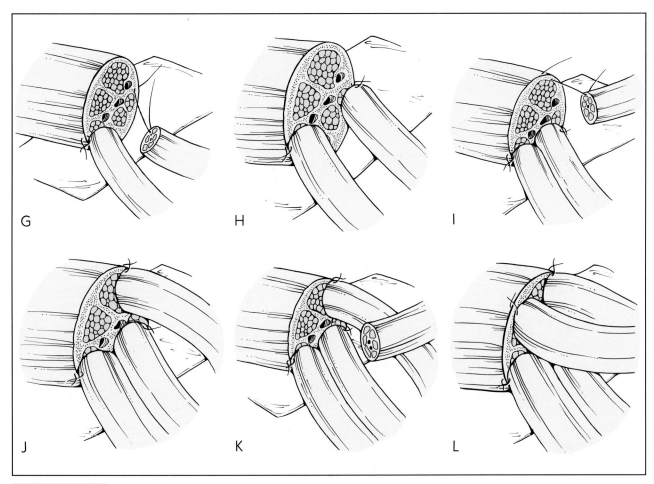

Figure 15.7   (continued)

If the stitch is located too high (**G**), the graft rotates in the other direction. Exact positioning of the stitch is, therefore, extremely important (**H**). The second graft is well placed and the third graft

is an approximation (**I**). The third graft is coapted (**J**). The fourth graft is an approximation (**K**). The whole fascicular area is covered by four grafts (**L**). (*From* Millesi [32]; with permission.)

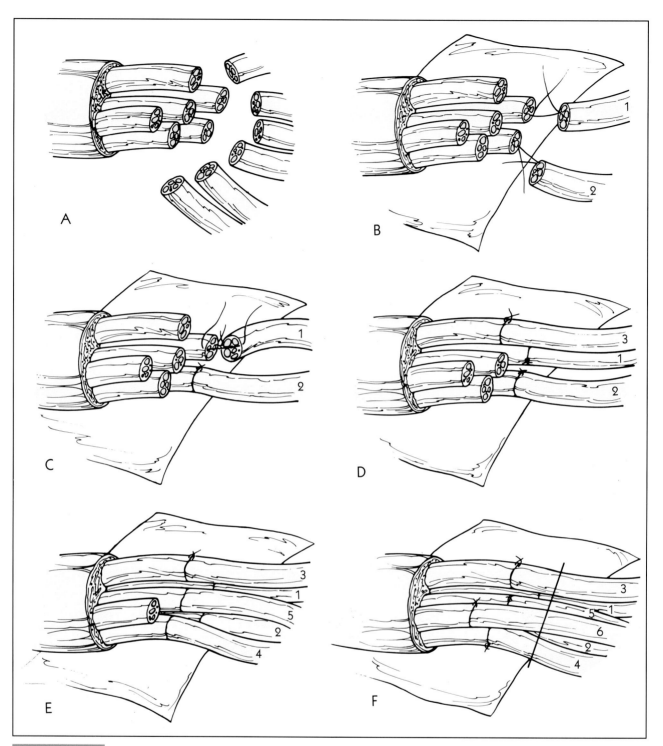

Figure 15.8

Management of a nerve defect by free cutaneous nerve grafting. The proximal stump consists of five fascicle groups and one large fascicle. Six segments of the sural nerve are prepared for nerve grafting. The stump has been prepared by interfascicular dissection (resection of the epi- and interfascicular epineurium). The fascicle groups are resected at different levels (**A**). Two segments of the cutaneous nerve segments are approximated by one stitch each (**B**). Graft number one is approximated by one stitch. A second stitch is necessary to achieve good coaptation. Graft number two is perfectly coapted by one stitch (**C**). Three grafts are coapted (**D**). Five grafts are coapted (**E**). All six grafts are coapted (**F**). Stability is provided by side-to-side contact between grafts and protruding fascicle groups. (*From* Millesi [32]; with permission.)

a given structure, the axons might be able to find their way according to neurotropic influences. Neurotrophy can affect regenerating nerve tissue through the insertion of different substances enhancing nerve regeneration into the tube.

The disadvantage is that the proceeding of the axons depends on the Schwann cells from the proximal stump. In contrast, in a surviving nerve graft, the axons meet Schwann cells within the graft. With nerve grafts, axons from a certain point of the proximal stump could be directed to a selected point of the distal stump. The decisive question is for how long a distance the Schwann cells from a proximal stump can proceed.

The following alternatives are available: classic mesothelial chamber, silicone tubes, bioresorbable polyglycolic acid tubes, veins, and frozen and thawed muscle.

Animal experiments to compare the results after autogenous and allogeneic nerve grafting with tubes yielded different results. Müller and colleagues [69,70] and Gibson and Daniloff [71] presented results in favor of nerve grafting over tubes. Archibald and colleagues [72] stated that the results after nerve grafting and tubes are equal up to a defect of 4 mm in length. Lundborg and colleagues [73], Molander and colleagues [74], Bora and colleagues [75], Dellon and Mackinnon [76], and Mackinnon and Dellon [77] could not detect statistical differences between nerve repair by grafts or by tubes. Zhao [78] compared silicone tubes, interfascicular nerve grafts, nerve trunk grafts, muscle bridge, and peri- and epineurial sutures. He demonstrated that repair with silicone tubes, perineurial sutures, and interfascicular nerve grafts was superior to repair with nerve trunk grafts, muscle bridge, and epineurial sutures with respect to the specificity of muscle reinnervation. However, recovery of muscle tetanic force was best after repair with epineurial sutures. Müller [44] reported many favorable aspects of the repair by silicone tubes. The results were, however, inconsistent. With autologous nerve grafts after 12 weeks, defects of 13 to 16 mm were bridged in 10 of 11 cases. With silicone tubes such a distance could be bridged in only five of 34 cases. Danielson (Danielson N. Symposium of Peripheral Nerve Surgery Today; 1991) concluded that promising results have also been achieved with intubation. This technique cannot yet be recommended as a clinical routine alternative to nerve grafting.

Lundborg and colleagues [79] had already shown successful clinical cases using the mesothelial chamber. However, they reported that in animal experiments a distance of over 10 mm could not be bridged. Mackinnon and Dellon [80] and Dellon (Dellon AL. Symposium of Peripheral Nerve Surgery Today; 1991) reported on the successful bridging of digital nerve

defects with polyglycolic acid tubes up to 3 cm but admitted that the results were inferior to autologous nerve grafting and recommended this technique only in less important nerves.

Vein grafts have also proven successful [81–84]. Clinical application to cover digital nerve defects has been reported [85]. Brunelli and colleagues [86] stated that in animal experiments only defects of 5 mm could be successfully overcome. Rigoni and colleagues [83] had comparable results between vein grafts and autologous nerve grafts only when the defect was smaller than 10 mm. The distance to be overcome could be increased to 40 mm if a piece of nerve tissue containing living Schwann cells was introduced into the middle of the vein graft. Zöch and Lassmann (Zöch G and Lassmann G. Symposium of Peripheral Nerve Surgery Today; 1991) reported a significant superiority of autologous nerve grafts over vein grafts.

Glasby and colleagues [87] demonstrated that the remaining structure of a muscle with parallel fiber pattern, after this muscle was frozen and thawed, could serve as a rail for axon sprouts. Successful animal experiments even in brachial plexus repairs [88•] have been reported in clinical cases (Calwer JS and Norris RW. Symposium of Peripheral Nerve Surgery Today; 1991). However, a recent paper [89] stated that no reliable repair with muscle was achieved in defects over 5 cm. In the experiments of Zöch and colleagues [24••], the outcome was significantly in favor of autologous nerve grafts as compared with frozen and thawed muscle. At present the question of alternatives to autologous nerve grafting may be summarized as follows.

Some alternatives provide surprisingly good results for short distances. The results remain inferior to autologous nerve grafts. In clinical use these techniques can be recommended for less important nerves, for which the sacrifice of an autologous nerve graft might not be justified, or as an adjunct to increase the available grafting material. There are indications that the lack of Schwann cells plays a role in limiting outgrowth. This possibility justifies experiments using cultivated Schwann cells, such as the studies by Ikeda and colleagues and Kim (Ikeda E, *et al.*; and Kim D. Symposium of Peripheral Nerve Surgery Today; 1991).

HOW PRECISE SHOULD COAPTATION BE?

Two views have thus far been discussed. These are whether coaptation should be as precise as possible, as was accepted without controversy a few years ago, or whether to leave a space protected by a tubular structure between the two stumps. This method is based on Lundborg's [10,11] and Brushart's [19,20] concept of the mesothelial chamber and was used by Lundborg in clinical cases and in Brushart and Seiler's study on neurotropism [19]. The answers to these questions depend on the range of neurotropic activity, which can take place within a fascicle, within a fascicle group, or between fascicle groups over the whole cross-section of a nerve trunk.

As has already been stated, exact coaptation can never be achieved—especially if a nerve defect must be overcome and if nerve grafts are used—because of the different fascicular patterns of a fascicle group and a nerve graft. But in spite of this inexactness, excellent results can be achieved [90]. With our present techniques, if we want to achieve fascicular or fascicle group coaptation, we are to a certain degree dependent on neurotropic activities. Only if it could be proven that neurotropic activity can act between fascicle groups over the whole cross-section of the nerve trunk will we have to change our technical approach.

Therefore, I believe that coaptation as precise as possible should be attempted. This point brings up the question of identification of corresponding fascicle groups. Identification should not be a problem in cases of clean transections, but becomes increasingly difficult with longer defects because the fascicular pattern changes. In more distal levels, identification of the fascicular pattern, with its characteristic fibrous qualities in the distal stump, is easy by retrograde tracing. The nerve is exposed to its division, and the fascicular groups forming the branches are traced along the distal stump to the site of the lesion. Then the location of the proximal stump is estimated after the orientation in space is defined by exploring the proximal stump to the next branch in the proximal direction. Hakstian [91], Gaul [92], and Jabaley (Jabaley ME. Paper presented at the Meeting of the Suner-

land Society in Bishop's Lodge; May, 1983) advocated electric stimulation in awake patients. Local anesthesia is used in these procedures.

Riley and Lang [93] recommended coloring sensory fibers with carboanhydrase. Because motor axons contain more acetylcholinesterase than sensory fibers do, they can be specifically colored by histochemical techniques. This technique was applied for motorsensory differentiation by Gruber and Zenker [95] and clinically used by Freilinger and colleagues [96]. In the 1970s this method took 48 hours to give a result and was therefore not practical for clinical use. In the meantime it has been improved so that a result can be ready within 2 hours at the latest [97]. Clinical results of this technique have been presented (Deutinger M, et al. Symposium of Peripheral Nerve Surgery Today; 1991). Similar attempts were made by Sumita and Tajima [98], He and Zhong [99], and Kanaya and colleagues [100].

CONCLUSIONS

I have attempted to survey present trends in peripheral nerve surgery, on the basis of a literature survey and a symposium on peripheral nerve surgery held in Vienna in November 1991. My opinion after analyzing all the data is that all the new developments, as far as neurotrophism and neurotropism are concerned, must be followed carefully but are not ready for wider clinical application. More arguments now exist for the use of minimal tension if an end-to-end neurorrhaphy is performed, and for no tension at all if a free nerve grafting procedure is done. There are several alternative techniques for nerve grafting available, all of which provide some results in short defects. However, all these techniques are inferior to autologous nerve grafting.

REFERENCES AND RECOMMENDED READING

Papers of particular interest, published within the annual period of review, have been highlighted as:
• Of special interest
•• Of outstanding interest

1. Ducker TB, Kempe LG, Hayes GJ: The metabolic background for peripheral nerve surgery. *J Neurosurg* 1969, 30:270–280.

2. Ducker TB: Pathophysiology of peripheral nerve trauma. In *Management of Peripheral Nerve Problems.* Edited by Omer G, Spinner M. Philadelphia: WB Saunders; 1980:475–486.

3. Ducker TB: The central cell body and axonal degeneration. In *Posttraumatic Peripheral Nerve Regeneration: Experimental Basis and Clinical Implications.* Edited by Gorio A, Millesi H, Mingrino S. New York: Raven Press; 1981:7–11.

4. Grafstein B: The nerve cell body response to axotomy. *Exp Neurol* 1975, 48:32–51.

5. McQuarrie IG, Grafstein B: Axon outgrowth enhanced by previous nerve injury. *Arch Neurol* 1973, 29:53–55.

6. Ochoa AJ, Mair WGP: The normal sural nerve in man. *Acta Neuropathol (Berl)* 1969, 13:197.

7. Jurecka W, Ammerer HP, Lassmann H: Regeneration of a transected peripheral nerve: an autoradiographic and electronmicroscopic study. *Acta Neuropathol* 1975, 32:299–312.

8. Weiss P, Taylor AC: Repair of peripheral nerves by grafts of frozen dried nerves. *Proc Soc Exp Biol Med* 1943, 52:326–328.

9. Weiss P, Taylor AC: Further experimental evidence against "neurotropism" in nerve regeneration. *J Exp Zool* 1944, 95:233–236.

10. Lundborg G, Hansson HA: Regeneration of a peripheral nerve through a preformed tissue space. *Brain Res* 1979, 178:573–576.

11. Lundborg G, Hansson HA: Nerve lesions with interruption of continuity: studies on the growth pattern of regeneration axons in the gap between the proximal and distal nerve ends. In *Posttraumatic Peripheral Nerve Regeneration: Experimental Basis and Clinical Implications.* Edited by Gorio A, Millesi H, Mingrino S. New York: Raven Press; 1981:229–239.

12. Politis MJ, Ederle K, Spencer PS: Tropism in nerve regeneration in vivo: attraction of regenerating axons by diffusable factors derived from cells in distal nerve stumps of transected peripheral nerves. *Brain Res* 1982, 253:1–12.

13. Politis M, Spencer P: An in vivo assay of neurotrophic activity. *Brain Res* 1983, 278:229–231.

14. Williams LR, Longo F, Powell HC, *et al.*: Spatial-temporal progress of peripheral nerve regeneration within a silicone chamber: parameters for bioassay. *J Comp Neurol* 1983, 218:460–470.

15. Williams LR, Powell HC, Lundborg G, *et al.*: Competence of nerve tissue as distal inserts promoting nerve regeneration in silicone chamber. *Brain Res* 1984, 293:202–211.

16. Seckel BR, Ryan SE, Gagne RG, *et al.*: Target-specific nerve regeneration through a nerve guide in the rat. *Plast Reconstr Surg* 1986, 78:793–798.

17. Mackinnon SE, Dellon AL, Lundborg G, *et al.*: A study of neurotropism in a primate model. *J Hand Surg [Am]* 1986, 11:888–894.

18. Keynes RJ: Schwann cells during neural development and regeneration: leaders or followers? *Trends Neurosci* 1987, 10:137–139.

19. Brushart TM, Seiler WA: Selective reinnervation of distal motor stumps by peripheral motor axons. *Exp Neurol* 1987, 97:290–300.

20. Brushart ThME, Mesulam MM: Alteration in connections between muscle and anterior horn motor neurons after peripheral nerve repair. *Science* 1980, 208:603–605.

21. Levi-Montalcini R: The nerve growth factor: its mode of action on sensory and sympathetic nerve cells. *Harvey Lect* 1966, 60:217–259.

22. • Semiuk NA: Neurotrophic factors: role in peripheral neuron survival and axonal repair. *J Reconstr Microsurg* 1992, 8:399–404.
The role of neurotrophic factors in peripheral neuron survival and axon repair is described. So far the influence is still limited.

23. •• Millesi H, Zöch G, Rath Th: The gliding apparatus of peripheral nerve and its clinical significance. *Ann Hand Upper Limb Surg* 1990, 9:87–97.
The gliding apparatus of peripheral nerves is described.

24. •• Zöch G, Reihsner R, Beer R, *et al.*: Stress and strain in peripheral nerves. *Neuroorthopaedics* 1991, 10:371–382.
Stress and strain phenomena in peripheral nerves are outlined. Stress-strain curves are provided for different segments of cadaver nerves.

25. •• Zöch G: Über die Anpassung der peripheren Nerven an die Bewegungen der Extremitäten durch Gleiten und Dehnung: Untersuchungen am Nervus medianus. *Acta Chir Austriaca* 1992, 96(suppl):1–16.
In this paper stress-strain curves deriving from median nerves of cadavers in situ and after excision are studied. Stress-strain curves of nerve segments without branches and with branches are compared. The segments with branches are much stiffer but after transection of the branches the stress-strain curve comes closer to the curve in segments without branches.

26. •• Wall EJ, Massie AJ, Kwan MK, *et al.*: Experimental stretch neuropathy: changes in nerve conduction under tension. *J Bone Joint Surg [Br]* 1992, 74:126–129.
With experimental stretch the nerve conduction goes down significantly.

27. •• Clark WL, Trumble ThE, Swiontkowski MF, *et al.*: Nerve tension and blood flow in a rat model of immediate and delayed repairs. *J Hand Surg [Am]* 1992, 17:677–687.
With increasing tension the blood flow in a rat model is significantly decreased.

28. • Wall EJ, Kwan MK, Rydevik BL, *et al.*: Stress relaxation of a peripheral nerve. *J Hand Surg [Am]* 1991, 16:859–863.
The tension necessary to keep a nerve segment elongated to a certain percentage of elongation decreases significantly due to stress relaxation.

29. Seddon HJ: Three types of nerve injury. *Brain* 1943, 66:237.

30. Sunderland S: A classification of peripheral nerve injuries producing loss of function. *Brain* 1951, 74:491.

31. Millesi H: Eingriffe am peripheren Nerven. In *Chirurgische Operationslehre.* Edited by Gschnitzer F, Kern E, Schweiberer L. München-Wein: Urban & Schwarzenberg; 1986:1–88.

32. Millesi H: *Chirurgie der peripheren Nerven.* München-Wein: Urban & Schwarzenberg; 1992.

33. Lang J: Über das Bindegewebe und die Gefäße der Nerven. *Anat Embryol* 1962, 123:61–79.

34. Millesi W, Achhammer E: Gleitgewebslappen zur Deckung des Trigonum colli laterale. *Acta Chir Austr* 1988, 80(suppl):12–15.

35. •• Millesi W, Schober G, Bochdansky Th: Subpectoral gliding tissue flaps. *Plast Reconstr Surg* 1992, in press.
The clinical application of the subpectoral gliding tissue flap is presented. The gliding tissue of the median nerve in the carpal tunnel is described.

36. Millesi W, Leitner E: Subpektoraler Gleitgewebslappen zur Deckung des seitlichen Halsdreiecks. *Handchir Mikrochir Plast Chir* 1989, 21:26–28.

37. Rath Th, Millesi H: Das Gleitgewebe des Nervus medianus im Karpalkanal. *Handchir Mikrochir Plast Chir* 1990, 23:203–205.

38. Nicholson OR, Seddon HL: Nerve practice: results of treatment of median and ulnar nerve lesions. *BMJ* 1957, 2:1065–1071.

39. Seddon HJ: *Surgical Disorders of the Peripheral Nerves,* 2nd ed. Edinburgh: Churchill Livingstone; 1975.

40. Kim DH, Conolly SE, Voorhies RM, *et al.*: Initial evaluation of variable graft length and lesion length in the repair of nerve gaps. *J Reconstr Microsurg* 1990, 6:311–316.

41. • Kim DH, Conolly SE, Gillespie JT, *et al.*: Electrophysiological studies of various graft lengths and lesion lengths in repair of nerve gaps in primates. *J Neurosurg* 1991, 75:440–446.

In order to achieve a useful result, the graft has to be sufficiently long to avoid tension at the two sites of repair.

42. Hentz VR, Rosen JM, Xiao S-J, *et al.*: A comparison of suture and tubulization nerve repair techniques in a primate. *J Hand Surg [Am]* 1991, 16:251–261.

43. De Medinaceli L, Wyatt R, Freed WJ: Peripheral nerve reconnection: mechanical, thermal, and ionic conditions that promote the return of function. *Exp Neurol* 1983, 81:469–487.

44. Müller H: *Nervenregeneration: experimentelle Befunde.* Stuttgart: Georg Thieme Verlag; 1992.

45. Highet WB, Sanders FK: The effect of stretching nerves after suture. *Br J Surg* 1943, 30:355.

46. Highet WB, Holmes W: Traction injuries to the lateral popliteal nerve and traction injuries to peripheral nerves after suture. *Br J Surg* 1943, 30:212.

47. Lundborg G, Rydevik B: Effect of stretching the tibial nerve of the rabbit. *J Bone Joint Surg [Br]* 1973, 55:390–401.

48. Miyamoto Y, Watari S, Tsuge K: Experimental studies on the effects of tension on intraneural microcirculation in sutured peripheral nerves. *Plast Reconstr Surg* 1979, 63:398–403.

49. Zalewski AA, Gulati AK: Survival of nerve and Schwann cells in allografts after cyclosporin A treatment. *Exp Neurol* 1980, 70:219–255.

50. Zaleweski AA, Gulati AK: Survival of nerve allografts in sensitized rats treated with cyclosporin A. *J Neurosurg* 1984, 60:828–834.

51. Zaleweski AA, Silvers WK, Gulati AK: Failure of host axons in regenerate through a once successful but later rejected long allograft. *J Comp Neurol* 1982, 209:347–351.

52. Mackinnon SE, Hudson AR, Falk RE, *et al.*: The nerve allograft response: an experimental model in the rat. *Ann Plast Surg* 1985, 14:334–339.

53. Schaller E, Mailänder P, Becker M, *et al.*: Nervenregeneration im autologen und allogenen Transplantat des N.ischiadicus der Ratte mit und ohne Immunsuppression durch Cyclosporin A. *Handchir Mikrochir Plast Chir* 1988, 20:7–10.

54. Terzis JK, Faibisoff B, Williams HB: The nerve gap suture under tension versus graft. *Plast Reconstr Surg* 1975, 56:166–170.

55. •• Frey M, Koller R, Gruber I, *et al.*: Time course of histomorphometric alterations in nerve grafts without connection to a muscle target organ: an experimental study in sheep. *J Reconstr Microsurg* 1992, 8:345–357.

In this paper it is demonstrated that even a long graft that is attached to a motor nerve but not to a distal target is neurotisized.

56. Aguayo AJ: Construction of the graft. In *Posttraumatic Peripheral Nerve Regeneration: Experimental Basis and Clinical Implications.* Edited by Gorio A, Millesi H, Mingrino S. New York: Raven Press; 1981:365.

57. Aguayo AJ, Attiwell M, Trecarten J, *et al.*: Abnormal myelination in transplanted Trembler mouse Schwann cells. *Nature* 1977, 265:73–75.

58. Aguayo AJ, Kasarjian J, Skamene E, *et al.*: Myelination of mouse axons by Schwann cells transplanted from normal and abnormal human nerves. *Nature* 1977, 268:753–755.

59. Strange FGStC: An operation for nerve pedicled grafting: preliminary communication. *Br J Surg* 1947, 34:423–425.

60. Sheldon C, Pudenz H, McCarty CS: Two stage autografts for repair of extensive median and ulnar nerve defects. *J Neurosurg* 1947, 4:492–496.

61. Taylor GI, Ham FJ: The free vascularized nerve graft. *Plast Reconstr Surg* 1976, 57:413–426.

62. Taylor GI: Nerve grafting with simultaneous microvascular reconstruction. *Clin Orthop* 1978, 133:56–70.

63. Breidenbach W, Terzis JK: Vascularized nerve grafts (Scholarship Context). American Society for Plastic and Reconstructive Surgery Educational Foundation 1983.

64. Breidenbach W, Terzis JK: The anatomy of free vascularized nerve grafts. *Clin Plast Surg* 1984, 11:65–71.

65. • Kanaya F, Firrell J, Tsai T-S, *et al.*: Functional results of vascularized versus nonvascularized nerve grafting. *Plast Reconstr Surg* 1992, 89:924–930.

There is a very slight superiority of vascularized nerve grafts compared with free nerve grafts.

66. • Mani GV, Shurey C, Green CJ: Is early vascularization of nerve grafts necessary? *J Hand Surg [Br]* 1992, 17:536–543.

Early vascularization in the form of a vascularized nerve graft is not necessary.

67. •• Doi K, Tamaru K, Sakai K, *et al.*: A comparison of vascularized and conventional sural nerve grafts. *J Hand Surg [Am]* 1992, 17:670–676.

A comparison of vascularized versus free graft shows no significant difference. Vascularized nerve grafts are indicated if there is a very poor recipient site and in long defects.

68. Schröder JM, Seiffert KE: Die Feinstruktur der neuromatösen Neurotisation von Nerventransplantaten. *Virchows Arch [B]* 1970, 5:219–235.

69. Müller H, Shibib K, Friedrich H, *et al.*: Evoked muscle action potentials from regenerated rat tibial and peroneal nerves: synthetic versus autologous interfascicular grafts. *Exp Neurol* 1987, 95:21–23.

70. Müller H, Shibib K, Modrack M, *et al.*: Nerve regeneration in synthetic and autologous interfascicular grafts: II. Morphometric analysis. *Exp Neurol* 1987, 98:161–164.

71. Gibson KL, Daniloff JK: Comparison of sciatic nerve regeneration through silicone tubes and nerve allografts. *Microsurgery* 1989, 10:126–129.

72. Archibald SJ, Krarup C, Shefner J, *et al.*: A collagen based nerve guide conduit for peripheral nerve repair: an electrophysiological study of nerve regeneration in rodents and non-human primates. *J Comp Neurol* 1991, 306:685.

73. Lundborg G, Dahlin LB, Danielsen N, *et al.*: Nerve regeneration across an extended gap: a neurobiological view of nerve repair and the possible involvement of neurotrophic factors. *J Hand Surg [Am]* 1982, 7:580–587.

74. Molander H, Engkvist O, Hägglund J, *et al.*: Nerve repair using a polyglactin tube and nerve graft: an experimental study in the rabbit. *Biomaterials* 1983, 4:276–282.

75. Bora FM, Bednar JM, Osterman AL, *et al.*: Prosthetic nerve grafts: a resorbable tube as an alternative to autogenous nerve grafting. *J Hand Surg [Am]* 1987, 12:685–692.

76. Dellon AL, Mackinnon SE: An alternative to the classical nerve grafts for the management of the short nerve gap. *Plast Reconstr Surg* 1988, 82:849–856.

77. Mackinnon SE, Dellon AL: A comparison of nerve regeneration across a sural nerve graft and a vascularized pseudo sheath. *J Hand Surg [Am]* 1988, 13:935–942.

78. Zhao Q: *Nerve Regeneration in Silicone Tubes. A Study of Fibrin Matrix Formation and Specificity of Muscle Reinnervation.* Skurup, Sweden: Lidbergs Blankett; 1992.

79. Lundborg G, Dahlin LB, Danielsen N, *et al.*: Nerve regeneration in silicone chambers: influence of gap length and of distal stump components. *Exp Neurol* 1982, 76:361–375.

80. Mackinnon SE, Dellon AL: Clinical nerve reconstruction with a bioabsorbable polyglycolic acid tube. *Plast Reconstr Surg* 1990, 85:419–424.

81. Chiu DTW: Autogenous vein graft as a conduit for nerve regeneration. *Surg Forum* 1980, 31:550.

82. Chiu DTW, Janecka I, Krizek TJ, *et al.*: Autogenous vein graft as a conduit for nerve regeneration. *Surgery* 1982, 91:226–233.

83. Rigoni G, Smahel J, Chiu DTW, *et al.*: Veneninterponat als Leitbahn für die Regeneration peripherer Nerven. *Hand Chir* 1983, 15:227–231.

84. Suematsu N, Atsuta Y, Hirayama T: Vein graft for repair of peripheral nerve gap. *J Reconstr Microsurg* 1988, 4:313–318.

85. Chiu DTW, Lovelace RE, Yu LT, *et al.*: Comparative electrophysiologic evaluation of nerve grafts and autogenous vein grafts as nerve conduits: an experimental study. *J Reconstr Microsurg* 1988, 4:303–309.

86. Brunelli G, Fontana G, Jaeger C, *et al.*: Chemotactic arrangements of axons inside and distal to the venous graft. *J Reconstr Microsurg* 1987, 3:87–89.

87. Glasby MA, Gschmeissner SE, Hitchcock RJI, *et al.*: A comparison of nerve regeneration through nerve and muscle grafts in rat. *Neuroorthopaedics* 1986, 2:21–28.

88. • Glasby MA, Carrick MJ, Hems TEJ: Freeze-thawed skeletal muscle autografts used for brachial plexus repair in the non-human primate. *J Hand Surg [Br]* 1992, 17:526–535.

The results using freeze-thawed skeletal muscle autografts to manage nerve defects in brachial plexus repair with nonhuman primates are presented.

89. Hems TEJ, Glasby MA: Comparison of different methods of repair of long peripheral nerve defects: an experimental study. *Br J Plast Surg* 1992, 45:497–502.

90. Millesi H: How exact should coaptation be? In *Posttraumatic Peripheral Nerve Regeneration: Experimental Basis and Clinical Implications.* Edited by Gorio A, Millesi H, Mingrino S. New York: Raven Press; 1981:301–304.

91. Hakstian RW: Funicular orientation by direct stimulation: an aid to peripheral nerve repair. *J Bone Joint Surg [Am]* 1968, 50:1178–1186.

92. Gaul JS: Electrical fascicle identification as an adjunct to nerve repair. *J Hand Surg [Am]* 1983, 8:289–296.

93. Riley DA, Lang DH: Carbonic anhydrase activity of human peripheral nerves: possible histochemical aid to nerve repair. *J Hand Surg [Am]* 1984, 9:112–120.

94. Karnovsky MJ, Roots LA: A "direct-coloring" thiocholine method for cholinesterase. *J Histochem Cytochem* 1964, 12:219–221.

95. Gruber H, Zenker W: Acetylcholinesterase: histochemical differentiation between motor and sensory nerve fibres. *Brain Res* 1973, 51:207–214.

96. Freilinger G, Gruber H, Holle J, *et al.*: Zur Methodik der sensomotorisch differenzierten Faszikelnaht peripherer Nerven. *Hand Chir* 1975, 7:133–138.

97. Szabolcs MJ, Huber H, Schaden GE, *et al.*: Selective fascicular nerve repair: a rapid method for intraoperative motorsensory differentiation by acetylcholinesterase histochemistry. *Eur J Plast Surg* 1991, 14:21–25.

98. Sumita J, Tajima T: Distribution of motor fiber of human median nerve by Karnovsky stain. *Seikagaku* 1979, 30:1427–1429.

99. He Y, Zhong S: Acetylcholinesterase: a histochemical identification of motor and sensory fascicles in human peripheral nerve and its use during operation. *Plast Reconstr Surg* 1988, 82:125–130.

100. Kanaya F, Odgen L, Breidenbach WC, *et al.*: Sensory and motor fiber differentiation with Karnovsky staining. *J Hand Surg [Am]* 1991, 16:851–858.

Chapter 16

Positron Emission Tomography in the Evaluation of Patients for Epilepsy Surgery

Allen R. Wyler

RATIONALE FOR USE

The identification of an epileptogenic focus is more difficult than the identification of structural lesions excised by neurosurgeons. Unlike routine structural lesions such as vascular malformations or tumors, the focus is not easily identified on magnetic resonance (MR) or computed tomographic (CT) imaging. Furthermore, even when a particular lesion, such as a benign astrocytoma, is associated with the epileptogenic focus, there is no guaranteed correlation between the margins of the tumor and the margins of the focus. This is most likely because epilepsy is due to chronic subtle damage to neuronal cell bodies and dendrites, and this damage may extend beyond the present resolution of imaging techniques. The ambiguity in identifying the location and extent of an epileptogenic focus is part of the reason that even in the most carefully selected patient series only 90% of patients are helped by epilepsy surgery, and another 10% continue to have seizures after surgery. This is also the reason that new and innovative methods for identifying the location and extent of an epileptogenic focus are being researched.

Because it is assumed that focal epilepsy results from chronic damage to cortical gray matter (not white matter), localization of a focus has always been directed at identifying a cortical lesion. Because the lesion is often below our limits of resolution with present measuring techniques, most epileptologists agree that localization is maximal when a concordance exists among several methods of localization. These tests have included tests of anatomic, neurophysiologic, and functional integrity.

Historically, anatomic integrity has been investigated using skull radiology, then pneumoencephalography, then angiography. With the advent of digital computer use in radiology, CT and then MR imaging have improved our ability to image more subtle anatomic cortical abnormalities.

Neurophysiologic advances have included primarily the addition of ictal recordings. Prior to the introduction of long-term video electroencephalographic (EEG) monitoring, all EEG data were interictal, except for the serendipitous recording. During the past decade, the trend of including long-term intracranial ictal recordings as an integral part of the presurgical evaluation has developed.

In the past, functional studies were performed by neuropsychologists, based on the supposition that cortical damage would be mirrored by functional deficits on neuropsychologic tests. Although this is an attractive hypothesis, it has not been borne out in rigorous testing. With the introduction of positron emitters capable of crossing the blood-brain barrier and reflecting brain activity, there has been a resurgence of interest in using functional brain testing for two purposes: 1) localizing the epileptogenic focus and 2) investigating potential biochemical abnormalities of the focus, which may lead to greater understanding of the basic mechanisms of focal epilepsy.

HISTORY OF USE

Some of the first studies relating positron emission tomographic (PET) scans and epileptogenic foci were done at the University of California at Los Angeles (UCLA) [1,2]. These studies are of particular significance because many of the patients studied also had depth electrodes implanted, providing additional confirmation of the correlation between PET abnormalities and ictal onset. Initially these studies were interictal using ^{18}F-fluorodeoxyglucose (FDG). Of the first 50 patients studied, 35 (70%) had one or more zones of abnormal hypometabolism, and 15 (30%) had normal metabolic patterns.

One surprising finding from the UCLA studies was that the interictal PET focus was hypo- rather than hypermetabolic. This was surprising because laboratory models of focal epilepsy are characterized by neurons that fire in bursts of action potentials, which are assumed to require increased glucose utilization. A second interesting and unexplained finding was that the region of hypometabolism corresponding to the epileptic focus was much larger than the abnormality found at surgery [2]. In histopathologic studies on 25 patients who underwent anterior temporal lobectomies, 22 had hypometabolic lesions corresponding to pathologic abnormalities in 19 patients (mesial temporal sclerosis in 15). One patient had focal hypometabolism but normal findings on pathologic analysis. Three patients with normal PET scans had no pathologic abnormalities in the resected tissue. They reported that the area of hypometabolism was significantly greater than the amount of pathologic tissue. They suggest that this discrepancy was not an artifact of the technique but must represent either structural abnormalities below the resolution of routine histopathologic studies or functional inactivation of neuronal elements associated with the epileptogenic lesion.

The pioneering studies done at UCLA have been replicated at other major epilepsy centers with PET scan research capabilities [3–6] and show little variation from the original reported finding that approximately 70% of patients with partial epilepsy have a hypometabolic interictal PET lesion. These findings have also been corroborated with oxygen metabolism using ^{15}O, and blood flow using ^{13}N-ammonia and ^{15}O-water (reviewed by Engel [7••]). It has also been shown that if the positron emitter is given immediately before or at the onset of a seizure, the focus will appear hyper- rather than hypometabolic.

PROBLEMS

The use of PET scans as a routine tool for the evaluation of patients for epilepsy surgery involves several problems. First, the technique is not universally available; it requires an on-site medical cyclotron, highly trained personnel, and expensive equipment. However, newer PET systems are presently being developed with self-contained cyclotrons, and these are more compatible with the routine clinical setting with respect to facility and personnel requirements. Thus some of these problems may be moot years from now. Nonetheless, this imaging modality is still considered only a research tool, and the expense of a PET scan is not covered by most third-party carriers.

For several reasons, most studies correlating PET scan findings with other clinical data have used patients with temporal lobe epilepsy. First, these patients are the most likely to present for consideration of epilepsy surgery. Second, they have the highest likelihood of responding favorably to epilepsy surgery. Third, temporal lobe epilepsy is the most well-studied clinical model of focal epilepsy available. However, these are also the group with the best outcome from epilepsy surgery. Therefore, it is difficult to see what advantage PET scans provide in the evaluation of routine-surgery patients; its utility in routine cases is questionable.

In the 70% of seizure patients with positive FDG–PET studies, the hypometabolism is most commonly found in those with mesial temporal lesions, usually hippocampal sclerosis, but it is also found in those with other structural lesions such as tumors or hamartomas. These lesions are precisely those that MR imaging is good at identifying. In the past hippocampal sclerosis has not been easily recognized, but recently volumetric MR studies [8,9] have improved this capability, making the need for PET studies even less likely for this group of patients.

Positron emission tomographic abnormalities do not always correlate with the suspected site of seizure onset and therefore may be misleading if not interpreted with additional data. Patients with complex partial seizures from the frontal or occipital lobe may also have interictal temporal hypometabolism, presumably due to recurrent projection of ictal discharge into mesial temporal structures.

Although the presence of hypometabolism on FDG–PET scans may be extremely useful for identifying the site of an epileptogenic lesion for surgical purposes, the presence or absence of such a zone has no prognostic value with regard to surgical outcome [7••]. An example is found in our own series. The first patient (Figure 16.1) was found to have a hypometabolic focus in the left temporal lobe, which was removed. Postoperatively the patient still has auras, but no complex partial seizures 2 years later. The second patient (Figure 16.2) also had a left temporal lobe focus, but no abnormality on PET scan. He has been completely seizure-free since surgery. (PET scans were done at the University of Tennessee, Knoxville.)

The strongest argument in support of PET scanning in the selection of surgical patients is that it is a noninvasive procedure. If PET scanning can be developed to have greater selectivity and sensitivity than techniques presently available for the identification and

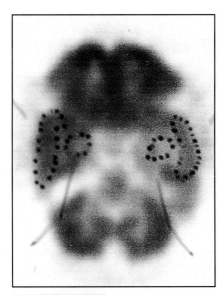

Figure 16.1

Interictal fluorodeoxyglucose scan from a 23-year-old woman with left temporal lobe epileptogenic focus. *Dotted regions* are areas of analysis on this slice. Left temporal lobe (*right*) shows a 33% decrease in glucose metabolism. Positron emission tomographic scan focus corresponds to electroencephalographic data and hippocampal sclerosis on pathologic examination of surgical specimen. Patient has had only auras since surgery.

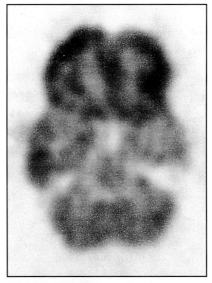

Figure 16.2

Interictal fluorodeoxyglucose scan from a 38-year-old man with left temporal lobe epileptogenic focus. This scan did not show an abnormality. Patient has been seizure-free since surgery and did in fact have hippocampal sclerosis on pathologic specimen.

selection of good surgical candidates, then it will likely replace many of the long-term invasive studies now being done. In the past year two excellent review articles have been published on FDG–PET scans in the evaluation of epilepsy surgery candidates [7••,10••].

RECENT ADVANCES

The pediatric neurosurgical unit at UCLA has recently developed an innovative application of FDG–PET in the localization of epileptogenic foci in a group of especially difficult cases. In their first investigation [11••], they studied eight children (aged 18 days to 5 years) with severe seizures. Three of the children had hemispherectomies and are subsequently seizure-free. Another child had a frontal lobe that was hypometabolic. Its subsequent removal has rendered this child also seizure-free. In their recent report, Chugani and colleagues [12••] described 13 children with infantile spasms of undetermined cause. Five of these female infants also showed FDG–PET hypometabolism in the parietooccipitotemporal regions. MR scans were also normal in four of these five infants, but in one, there was suggestion of cortical dysgenesis. Four of these infants underwent resection of the hypometabolic regions and were subsequently seizure-free. What is so impressive about these cases is that these children would ordinarily become progressively retarded and develop intractable seizures. Early follow-up suggests that these children are beginning to regain cognitive capabilities, and there is hope they may be spared retardation. If this is the case, these pioneering studies provide new hope to some patients with infantile spasms who may actually have a focal seizure disorder. In the past, it was thought that children with infantile spasms suffer from a generalized seizure disorder and that medication was the only treatment.

Although most research on the utility of PET scanning in epilepsy has been with FDG–PET scans, these scans have limitations. One problem is that glucose metabolism is not necessarily constant from moment to moment and is highly influenced by the metabolic activity at the time the positron emitter is taken up by the brain. This is why there is so much discrepancy between ictal and interictal FDG–PET scans. Because of this, newer tracers are being developed that may be more specific to the epileptogenic focus than is FDG. One such study looked at cortical benzodiazepine receptor binding in patients with focal and generalized epilepsy [13••]. The rationale for this study was that it is assumed in focal epilepsy that there is an imbalance between excitatory and inhibitory neurotransmitters. Because the γ-aminobutyric acid–ben-zodiazepine receptor complex is the main mediator of cortical inhibition in mammalian brain, this receptor seemed reasonable to assay. The ^{11}C-labeled benzodiazepine receptor antagonist Ro 15-1788 was used as ligand. For patients with partial epilepsy, the region suspected to be the focus always showed a significant reduction of benzodiazepine receptor density compared with homotopic cortex. These changes were not found in 10 patients with generalized epilepsy who were studied in a similar manner.

Another study based its hypothesis on evidence that central nervous system opioid peptides may be involved in the termination of seizures and that opiate receptors and endogenous opioid peptides may play a role in seizure mechanisms. Thus, the PET group at Johns Hopkins used PET scans to quantify μ and non-μ opiate receptors in patients with unilateral temporal lobe epilepsy [14••]. They used two opiate receptor ligands: the μ-selective opiate agonist ^{11}C-carfentanil and the opiate partial agonist ^{C}C-diprenorphine, which has similar affinity for μ, Δ, and κ opiate receptors. Carfentanil binding was found to be increased in the temporal neocortex and decreased in the amygdala on the side of the epileptic focus. Diprenorphine binding was not significantly different among regions in the focus and nonfocus temporal regions.

CONCLUSIONS

During the past few years, studies using PET scanning for improving localization of the epileptogenic focus have not been numerous. This is because the personnel and equipment requirements for mounting such a research effort are spectacularly horrendous, leaving only a few centers capable of maintaining viable research efforts. In addition, in the centers that have the capabilities, the research program is usually divided among several specialties, such as neurology, psychiatry, radiology, and cardiology. This makes for many logistical problems in using such research protocols. Finally, the clinical variables that must be strictly controlled, coupled with the constraints of active clinical practice, make it very difficult to conduct this type of research. Nonetheless, steady progress is being made.

With respect to FDG–PET, it is safe to say that this test remains confirmatory, because demonstration of epileptogenicity using electrophysiologic techniques is always a necessary component of the presurgical evaluation protocol. This is especially true when considering temporal lobe epilepsy, for which standard electrophysiology and newer MR imaging techniques provide excellent selection criteria. The most exciting role for this form of PET is probably the identification of pediatric patients who may be candidates for early corrective surgery.

What FDG–PET scans lack in specificity and selectivity for localizing epileptogenic foci may be improved on by ligands that can bind specific neurotransmitter receptors. Because abnormalities in the distribution or function of these receptors may be more specific to the pathology of focal epilepsy than is glucose metabolism, it is appealing to pursue this avenue. Early studies with benzodiazepine receptors and μ-agonists are encouraging because they suggest that such studies permit detection of biologic abnormalities specific to the epileptogenic focus that have previously been unrecognized. This may improve patient selection by permitting identification of patients with unilateral foci. In addition, with a further understanding of the biology as it exists in humans, as opposed to laboratory models, we should be able to understand the basic mechanisms of focal epilepsy better.

REFERENCES AND RECOMMENDED READING

Papers of particular interest, published within the annual period of review, have been highlighted as:
• Of special interest
•• Of outstanding interest

1. Engel Jr J, Brown WJ, Kuhl DE, *et al.*: Pathological findings underlying focal temporal lobe hypometabolism in partial epilepsy. *Ann Neurol* 1982, 12:518–528.

2. Engel J Jr, Kuhl DE, Phelps ME, *et al.*: Interictal cerebral glucose metabolism in partial epilepsy and its relation to EEG changes. *Ann Neurol* 1982, 12:510–517.

3. Abou Khalil BW, Siegel GJ, Sackellares JC, *et al.*: Positron emission tomography studies of cerebral glucose metabolism in chronic partial epilepsy. *Ann Neurol* 1987, 22:480–486.

4. Latack JT, Abou Khalil BW, Siegel GJ, *et al.*: Patients with partial seizures: evaluation by MR, CT, and PET imaging. *Radiology* 1986, 159:159–163.

5. Sperling MR, Wilson G, Engel Jr J, *et al.*: Magnetic resonance imaging in intractable partial epilepsy: correlative studies. *Ann Neurol* 1986, 20:57–62.

6. Theodore WH, Newmark ME, Sato S, *et al.*: [18F]Fluorodeoxyglucose positron emission tomography in refractory complex partial seizures. *Ann Neurol* 1983, 14:429–437.

7. •• Engel Jr J: PET scanning in partial epilepsy. *Can J Neurol Sci* 1991, 18:588–592.
This is one of the best state-of-the-art review articles on the role of PET scanning for defining the epileptogenic focus. It is concise and very inclusive although it focuses on glucose PET scanning.

8. Cascino GD, Jack CR, Parisi JE, *et al.*: Magnetic resonance imaging-based volume studies in temporal lobe epilepsy: pathological correlations. *Ann Neurol* 1991, 30:31–36.

9. Clifford Jr RJ, Sharbrough FW, Cascino GD, *et al.*: Magnetic resonance image-based hippocampal volumetry: correlation with outcome after temporal lobectomy. *Ann Neurol* 1992, 31:138–146.

10. •• Fisher RS, Frost JJ: Epilepsy. *J Nucl Med* 1991, 32:651–659.
An excellent review article on PET scanning that includes positron emitters other than glucose. Should be read by anyone interested in the relationship between PET scanning and localization of epileptogenic foci.

11. •• Chugani HT, Shewmon DA, Peacock WJ, *et al.*: Surgical treatment of intractable neonatal-onset seizures: the role of positron emission tomography. *Neurology* 1988, 38:1178–1188.
A landmark article reviewing the UCLA pediatric epilepsy surgery experience in treating children with infantile spasms. The implications of this work are far-reaching and worth monitoring.

12. •• Chugani HT, Shields WD, Shewmon DA, *et al.*: Infantile spasms: I. PET identifies focal cortical dysgenesis in cryptogenic cases for surgical treatment. *Ann Neurol* 1990, 27:406–413.
The second major article by this group describing results from their series of patients. This is potentially a major contribution to the treatment of infantile spasms if their long-term studies support the findings so far, because these children not only cease having seizures, but seem to reverse mental retardation.

13. •• Savic I, Widen L, Thorell JO, *et al.*: Cortical benzodiazepine receptor binding in patients with generalized and partial epilepsy. *Epilepsia* 1990, 31:724–730.
One of the few articles discussing benzodiazepine-receptor-binding PET scanning. Recommended reading for those interested in the general role of PET in epileptogenic focus localization.

14. • Ryvlin P, Philippon R, Cinotti L, *et al.*: Functional neuroimaging strategy in temporal lobe epilepsy: a comparative study of ^{18}FDG-PET and ^{99m}Tc-HMPAO-SPECT. *Ann Neurol* 1992, 31:650–656.
Compares the accuracy of PET and single-photon emission CT scans in MR-defined nonlesional and lesional temporal lobes. In nonlesional temporal lobes, the accuracy of PET scanning was 80%.

Index

idazoxan in, 7.8
intracellular calcium and, 7.8
opiate receptor antagonists in, 7.7
pharmacologic advances in, 7.1–7.8
rationales for, 7.2–7.4
steroids in, 7.7
volatile anesthetics in, 7.7
Cerebrovascular disease *see also specific type; specific treatment*
acquired, magnetic resonance angiography in, 8.9–8.14
Cervical spine fusion, 13.1–13.18
biomechanical studies of fixation devices for, 13.17–13.18
Halifax interlaminar clamps in, 13.2
interbody, with allograft, 13.14–13.15
methyl methacrylate in, 13.15–13.16
occipitocervical, 13.4–13.5
posterior, wire fixation for, 13.6–13.7
posterior atlantoaxial, wiring and bone grafting for, 13.2– 13.4
resins in, 13.15–13.16
in rheumatoid arthritis, 13.16–13.17
screw fixation techniques for, 13.7–13.10
screw plate fixation for, 13.10–13.14
Chondrosarcoma, stereotactic radiosurgery for, 5.9
Chordoma, stereotactic radiosurgery for, 5.9
Chromosomal abnormalities, brain tumors and, 1.3–1.4
Clamps, interlaminar, Halifax, 13.2
Coils, in endovascular occlusion of cerebral aneurysms, 9.6– 9.10, 9.11
Coma, Traumatic Coma Data Bank and, 6.1–6.7
Corticosteroids, in cerebral protection, 7.7
Cranial base meningiomas, 2.1–2.11 *see also* Meningiomas
Cranial nerves
optic nerve, cavernous sinus surgery and, 3.9
preservation of, stereotactic radiosurgery for acoustic tumors and, 5.4
reconstruction of, meningiomas and, 2.10
Cranioorbital zygomatic flap, 3.5–3.6
Craniopharyngiomas, cavernous sinus surgery and, 3.3 *see also* Cavernous sinus surgery
c-*sis* gene, 1.4
C-2 pedicle screw placement, cervical fixation and, 13.13
Cytogenetics of meningiomas, 2.3
Cytokinetics, meningiomas and, 2.3–2.4

Dilantin, in cerebral protection, 7.7
Diskectomy, lumbar *see* Percutaneous automated lumbar diskectomy
Distal stump, peripheral nerve reconstruction and, 15.5, 15.6– 15.7
Dopamine D_1 and D_2 receptors, meningiomas and, 2.2–2.3
Doppler scanning, transcranial, in preoperative carotid stenosis assessment, 12.6
Drugs *see* Pharmacologic agents
Duplex scanning, carotid, in preoperative stenosis assessment, 12.5
Dural opening, in cavernous sinus surgery, 3.8
Dural tail sign, meningioma and, 2.7

Edema
cerebral, meningiomas and, 2.2
radiation, after arteriovenous malformation radiosurgery, 11.7– 11.8, 11.10–11.11
Elderly, meningioma surgery in, 2.6
Electrolytes, in poor-grade aneurysm patient, 10.5
Embolization, meningioma, magnetic resonance imaging of, 2.7
Endarterectomy, carotid, 12.1–12.13
Endovascular occlusion of cerebral aneurysms, 9.1–9.13
balloons in, 9.2–9.6
coils in, 9.6–9.10
patient selection for, 9.10, 9.12
perioperative management in, 9.12–9.13
End-to-end neurorrhaphy *see* Neurorrhaphy
Epidemiology, of meningiomas, 2.4–2.5

Epilepsy surgery
positron emission tomography in evaluation for, 16.1–16.5
positron emission tomography in patient evaluation for
history of, 16.2
problems with, 16.2–16.4
rationale for use of, 16.1–16.2
recent advances in, 16.4
erb-B gene, 1.4
European Carotid Surgery Trial, 12.3
Evoked potential monitoring, in preoperative carotid stenosis assessment, 12.6–12.7
Extended frontal approach, to meningiomas, 2.8–2.9
Extracranial cerebrovascular disease, magnetic resonance angiography in, 8.9–8.12

Fixation, cervical spine *see* Cervical spine fusion
Flap, zygomatic, cranioorbital, 3.5–3.6
Focused beam irradiation *see* Radiosurgery
Fractures, cervical, wire without bone grafts for, 13.7
Free radical scavengers, in cerebral protection, 7.5–7.6
Frontal approach, extended, to meningiomas, 2.8–2.9
Fusion, cervical spine *see* Cervical spine fusion

Gangliosides, in cerebral protection, 7.6–7.7
Genetics
of astrocytoma, 1.1–1.6
of meningiomas, 2.3
Glial tumors, stereotactic radiosurgery for, 5.8–5.9
Glutamate antagonists, in cerebral protection, 7.5
Guglielmi detachable coils, 9.8–9.9
placement of, 9.9–9.10, 9.11

Halifax interlaminar clamps, in cervical spinal fusion, 13.2
Head injury
cerebral protection in, pharmacologic advances in, 7.1–7.8
classification of, 6.3
neuropsychologic and behavioral outcome after, 6.6
recovery from, alcohol abuse and, 6.6–6.7
Hemangiomas, cavernous sinus surgery and, 3.3 *see also* Cavernous sinus surgery
Hemorrhage *see* Intracerebral hemorrhage; Intraventricular hemorrhage; Subarachnoid hemorrhage
Herniations, lumbar disk *see* Percutaneous automated lumbar diskectomy
Hydrocephalus, intraventricular hemorrhage and, poor-grade aneurysm patient and, 10.13–10.14
5-Hydroxytryptamine-1A receptor agonists, in cerebral protection, 7.8
Hypertension, intracranial, critical levels of, 6.4–6.6

Idazoxan, in cerebral protection, 7.8
Intensive care management, endovascular occlusion and, 9.13
Interbody fusion, cervical, with allograft, 13.14–13.15
Interlaminar clamps, Halifax, in cervical spine fusion, 13.2
Internal carotid artery, subclinoid segment of, cavernous sinus surgery and, 3.8
Interstitial brachytherapy, 4.1–4.12
complications of, 4.5
experimental studies of, 4.2–4.3
failure of, 4.5
future strategies for, 4.10–4.12
for metastatic brain tumors, 4.5
in primary treatment of brain tumors, 4.4–4.5
for recurrent tumors, 4.3–4.4
technique for, 4.5–4.10
Intracavernous surgery *see* Cavernous sinus surgery
Intracellular calcium, cerebral protection and, 7.8
Intracerebral hemorrhage *see also* Subarachnoid hemorrhage

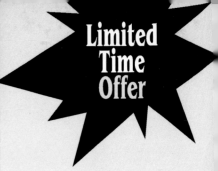
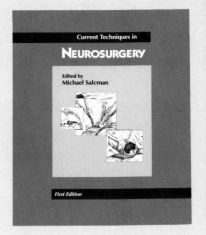